Acta Neurochirurgica Supplement 129

Series Editor
H.-J. Steiger

For further volumes:
http://www.springer.com/series/4

Giuseppe Esposito • Luca Regli
Yasuhiko Kaku • Tetsuya Tsukahara
Editors

Trends in the Management of Cerebrovascular Diseases

Springer

Editors
Giuseppe Esposito
Department of Neurosurgery
University Hospital Zurich
University of Zurich
Zurich, Switzerland

Luca Regli
Department of Neurosurgery
University Hospital Zurich
University of Zurich
Zurich, Switzerland

Yasuhiko Kaku
Department of Neurosurgery
Asahi Uni Murakami Memorial Hospital
Gifu, Japan

Tetsuya Tsukahara
Department of Neurosurgery
National Hospital Organization
Kyoto Medical Center
Kyoto, Japan

ISSN 0065-1419 ISSN 2197-8395 (electronic)
Acta Neurochirurgica Supplement
ISBN 978-3-030-08848-4 ISBN 978-3-319-73739-3 (eBook)
https://doi.org/10.1007/978-3-319-73739-3

Printed on acid-free paper

This Springer imprint is published by the registered company Springer Nature Switzerland AG
The registered company address is: Gewerbestrasse 11, 6330 Cham, Switzerland

Preface

The European–Japanese Cerebrovascular Congress (EJCVC) was initiated in Zurich, Switzerland, in 2001 by Prof. Y. Sakurai and Prof. Y. Yonekawa, under the name "Swiss–Japanese Joint Conference."

The second meeting was also organized in Zurich 2 years later.

The third meeting, under the name "European–Japanese Joint Conference for Stroke Surgery," was held in 2006 in conjunction with the 70th Anniversary of the Department of Neurosurgery, University Hospital Zurich.

The fourth meeting was organized in Helsinki, Finland, in 2008.

The fifth meeting was organized in Düsseldorf, Germany, in 2010.

The sixth meeting, under the name "European–Japanese Stroke Surgery Conference," was organized in 2012 in Utrecht, the Netherlands.

The seventh meeting was held in Verona, Italy, from June 25 to 28, 2014.

The eighth EJCVC meeting was held at University Hospital Zurich from June 22 to 25, 2016. This meeting represented a unique opportunity to gather the latest updates on neurovascular surgery and intervention for cerebrovascular diseases. The main topics of the meeting consisted of management of intracranial aneurysm, cerebrovascular neuroanatomy, management of arteriovenous malformations, cavernomas and dural arteriovenous fistulas, hemorrhagic and ischemic stroke, current trends in cerebral revascularization, and new concepts in cerebrovascular imaging.

The EJCVC has been able to facilitate networking among cerebrovascular specialists, maintaining the long-standing tradition of international exchanges in clinical neurosciences at University Hospital Zurich.

This volume presents the original papers resulting from the meeting.

Zurich, Switzerland	Giuseppe Esposito
Zurich, Switzerland	Luca Regli
Gifu, Japan	Yasuhiko Kaku
Kyoto, Japan	Tetsuya Tsukahara

Contents

Part IV Miscellaneous

Part I

Intracranial Aneurysms

Computational Fluid Dynamics Analysis and Correlation with Intraoperative Aneurysm Features

Alberto Feletti, Xiangdong Wang, Sandeep Talari, Tushit Mewada, Dilshod Mamadaliev, Riki Tanaka, Yasuhiro Yamada, Yamashiro Kei, Daisuke Suyama, Tukasa Kawase, and Yoko Kato

Abstract *Introduction.* There are many controversies about computational fluid dynamics (CFD) findings and aneurysm initiation, growth, and ultimate rupture. The aim of our work was to analyze CFD data in a consecutive series of patients and to correlate them with intraoperative visual aneurysm findings.

Methods. Hemoscope software (Amin, Ziosoft Corporation, Minato ward, Tokyo, Japan) was used to process images from 17 patients who underwent clipping of 18 aneurysms. Pressure (*P*), wall shear stress (WSS) gradient and vectors, normalized WSS, and streamlines (SL) direction and velocity were assessed. CFD data were compared to intraoperative visual findings. A total of 39 aneurysm wall areas were assessed.

Results. Red, thin aneurysm wall areas were more often associated with low WSS. However, the association of low WSS with high *P*, diverging WSS vectors, direct impact of SL, and high SL velocity more frequently matched with yellow, atherosclerotic aneurysm walls.

Conclusions. Low WSS alone is not sufficient to determine the thickness of an aneurysm wall. Its association with other parameters might enable one to distinguish preoperatively atherosclerotic, thick areas (high *P*, diverging WSS vectors, high flow velocity) from thin areas with higher rupture risk (parallel WSS vectors, lower flow velocity). The changing balance between these parameters can modify the features and the risk of rupture of aneurysm wall over time.

Keywords Computational fluid dynamics (CFD) · Aneurysm · Wall shear stress (WSS) · Pressure · Streamlines · Intraoperative

Introduction

The possibility to predict the natural history of unruptured intracranial aneurysms (UIAs) would be of the utmost importance for both patient and surgeon. Surgeons could more precisely assess the risk of rupture, therefore advising surgery only for those patients whose rupture risk is higher than the risks of the treatment. Moreover, surgeons could have a clearer preoperative knowledge of not only the shape and the position of the aneurysm, but also the features of its wall. Knowing in advance whether an area of the wall is thinner or thicker could help in the surgical planning, and potentially reduce the risks of intraoperative rupture. This would be even more important before starting coiling an aneurysm. Computational fluid dynamics (CFD) analysis is considered a promising tool in order to understand better aneurysm initiation, growth, and eventual rupture [1, 2]. The majority of studies have so far been focused on prediction of rupture [3–7]. However, the analysis of several CFD hemodynamic factors has led to controversial results [4, 8]. Moreover, only a few published papers have analyzed the correspondence between CFD parameters and the features of the aneurysm wall [1, 9].

With the aim of finding potential correlation between CFD hemodynamic factors and the characteristics of the aneurysm wall, we prospectively applied CFD analysis to a series of 18 UIAs, and compared the results with intraoperative anatomical findings.

A. Feletti, M.D., Ph.D. (✉)
Department of Neurosciences, Neurosurgery Unit, NOCSAE Modena Hospital, Modena, Italy

Department of Neurosurgery, Fujita Health University Hospital, Nagoya, Japan

X. Wang, M.D., Ph.D. · S. Talari, M.D. · T. Mewada, M.D.
D. Mamadaliev, M.D. · R. Tanaka, M.D.
Y. Yamada, M.D., Ph.D. · Y. Kei, M.D. · D. Suyama, M.D.
T. Kawase, M.D., Ph.D. · Y. Kato, M.D., Ph.D.
Department of Neurosurgery, Fujita Health University Hospital, Nagoya, Japan

G. Esposito et al. (eds.), *Trends in the Management of Cerebrovascular Diseases*, Acta Neurochirurgica Supplement, Vol. 129,
https://doi.org/10.1007/978-3-319-73739-3_1, © Springer International Publishing AG, part of Springer Nature 2018

Materials and Methods

Case Series

Eighteen UIAs clipped in 17 patients during 17 procedures between February and May 2016 have been included in the study. The population included 4 males and 13 females with a mean age of 64 years (range 41–77 years). Aneurysm locations, sizes, and patients' demographics are summarized in Table 1.

The study protocol was approved by the local ethics committee of our institution.

Computational Fluid Dynamics Modeling

Head digital subtraction angiography images were processed via manual cropping and thresholding, and converted into a triangulated surface through Ziosoft (Amin Corp, Minato ward, Tokyo, Japan), obtaining the geometry of blood vessels and aneurysms. An unstructured computational volumetric mesh was built from the triangulated surface. The mesh was composed of tetrahedrons and prism element layers to improve the analytic precision of the boundary layer. Hemoscope software (Amin Corp, Minato ward, Tokyo, Japan) used the Navier–Stokes equations to simulate blood flow on the computational mesh, assuming pulsatile laminar flow, zero pressure at the blood vessel outlet, Newtonian fluid, and rigid blood vessel walls with non-slip conditions. For each aneurysm we investigated instantaneous maximum pressure (*P*), instantaneous wall shear stress magnitude (WSSm), cycle variation WSS (cvWSS), wall shear stress vectors (WSSv), and streamlines velocity and direction (SL). WSS and velocity were also normalized by parent vessel values generated from the same CFD simulation to minimize the dependence on inlet conditions.

Table 1 Aneurysm data and patients' demographics

Patient	Sex, age	Aneurysm location	Aneurysm size (mm)
1	F, 57	Lt ICA bif	4
2	F, 65	Lt MCA M1	6
3	F, 77	Rt MCA M2	9
4	M, 41	Lt VA	10
5	F, 60	Lt ICA	6
6	F, 64	Acom	12
7	F, 73	Rt MCA	3
8	M, 76	Lt MCA	4
9	F, 71	Lt ICPC	6
10	F, 73	A2-A3	6
11	M, 57	Acom	8
12	F, 67	Lt MCA prox	4
		Lt MCA dist	3
13	F, 52	Rt ICA C2	8
14	F, 63	Lt MCA bif	5
15	F, 65	Acom	4
16	F, 70	Rt MCA	5
17	M, 62	Lt ICPC	8

Operative Procedure

All patients have been operated on using a ZeissFlow 800 OPMI Pentero surgical microscope (Zeiss, Oberkochen, Germany) with motor evoked potential (MEP) monitoring in selected cases. Pre-clipping and post-clipping ICG-VA were performed in all cases. A rigid endoscope (Machida, Japan) was always used to inspect eventual perforators and to have a better vision of the walls of the aneurysm that were not visible by the microscope. All operations have been video-recorded. For every aneurysm, we checked for the presence of eventual areas characterized by either red, translucent walls or white-yellow, atherosclerotic walls during surgery. As in previous studies, the surfaces with red color and translucence were defined as thin-walled (TW), compared with healthy areas of parent vessels. The surfaces with yellow-white color and opaqueness were defined as thick-walled and atherosclerotic (AW). A total of 39 areas have been identified, directly visually inspected, and compared with CFD data.

Statistical Analysis

Continuous data are shown as mean ± SD. We used the *t* test for the comparison of mean values. An overall significance level of $p < 0.05$ was adopted.

Results

Among 39 microsurgically-visualized areas, we identified 12 TW areas and 19 AW areas in 18 aneurysms (Table 2). We found that the association of high *P*, low WSS, divergent WSS vectors, and streamlines hitting the wall with high velocity is more often associated with AW areas (78.6% of cases; Fig. 1). In these cases, the mean normalized WSS was

Table 2 CFD data and intraoperative findings

Patient	Aneurysm	Area	nP	nWSS	nVel	hP, lWSS, dWSSv, hitSL	WSS	Intraop
1		1	99.7	5	38.1		Low	TW
		2	99.8	1	90.48	Yes	Low	AW
	Lt ICA bif	3	99.7	5	19.05		Low	AW
2	LtMCA	4	100	0.32	100	Yes	Low	AW
		5	99.9	0.32	40	Yes	Low	AW
		6	99.8	0.32	16.67		Low	AW
		7	99.8	96.77	83.33		High	Normal
3	Rt MCA	8	99.8	0.54	8		Low	TW
		9	99.8	0.54	8		Low	AW
4	Lt VA	10	99.8	74.2	87.23		Normal	AW
		11	99.7	0.64	6.38		Low	AW
5	Lt ICA	12	99.9	0.48	98	Yes	Low	AW
		13	99.7	70.97	50		High	TW
6	Acom	14	99.9	64.51	87.5		Normal	Normal
		15	99.8	29.03	70.83		Low	TW
7	Rt MCA	16	100	0.95	80	Yes	Low	AW
		17	99.9	2.38	10		Low	Normal
8	Lt MCA	18	99.9	1.42	80	Yes	Low	AW
		19	99.9	1.42	10		Low	TW
9	Lt ICPC	20	100	2.85	92.59	Yes	Low	AW
		21	99.8	85.71	59.26		Normal	Normal
10	A2-A3	22	100	100	91.67		High	Normal
		23	99.9	25	12.5		Low	AW
11	Acom	24	100	0.41	91.67	Yes	Low	AW
		25	99.9	0.4	41.67		Low	AW
	Lt MCA	26	100	0.2	66.67	Yes	Low	TW
		27	99.9	52	30		Normal	Normal
12	Lt MCA	28	99.7	0.2	66.67	Yes	Low	TW
		29	99.6	52	33.33		Normal	Normal
13	Rt IC A2	30	99.8	0.28	75	Yes	Low	AW
		31	99.4	0.28	33.33		Low	AW
14	Lt MCA	32	100	0.38	90.48	Yes	Low	TW
		33	99.9	0.38	47.62		Low	normal
15	Acom	34	99.8	342	75		High	TW
		35	100	0.71	85	Yes	Low	AW
16	Rt MCA	36	100	0.33	96.67	Yes	Low	AW
		37	99.9	100	90		High	TW
		38	99.9	0.33	33.33		Low	TW
17	Lt ICPC	39	99.9	1	33.33		Low	TW

nP: normalized pressure, *nWSS*: normalized wall shear stress, *nVel*: normalized velocity, *hP*: high pressure, *lWSS*: low wall shear stress, *dWSSv*: divergent wall shear stress vectors, *hitSL*: hitting streamlines, *WSS*: wall shear stress, *Intraop*: intraoperative, *TW*: thin wall, *AW*: atherosclerotic wall

0.8 ± 0.8% (range 0.3–2.9%), and the mean P was 99.9% compared to the parent vessel P (range 99.8–100%). The mean SL velocity was 84.5% compared to the parent vessel. Compared to aneurysm dome areas with normal appearance, normalized P, SL velocity and normalized SL velocity were significantly higher (p values 0.04, 0.02, and 0.004, respectively), whereas WSS, and normalized WSS were significantly lower (p values 0.0007 and 0.0002, respectively). In the other cases (20%) this association of parameters matched with TW areas (Fig. 2).

In TW areas, we identified low WSS (normalized WSS 4.6 ± 9.9%, range 0.2–29%) in the majority of cases (75%), along with high P (mean 99.9 ± 0.1% compared to parent vessel P, range 99.7–100%), and low streamline velocity (mean 48 ± 30% compared to parent vessel SL velocity, range 8–90.5%) (Fig. 3). WSS and normalized WSS were significantly lower than aneurysm dome areas with normal appearance (p = 0.006 and 0.003, respectively). We also found that, in the majority of cases, TW areas are characterized by parallel WSS vectors (75%) and curved streamlines (75%).

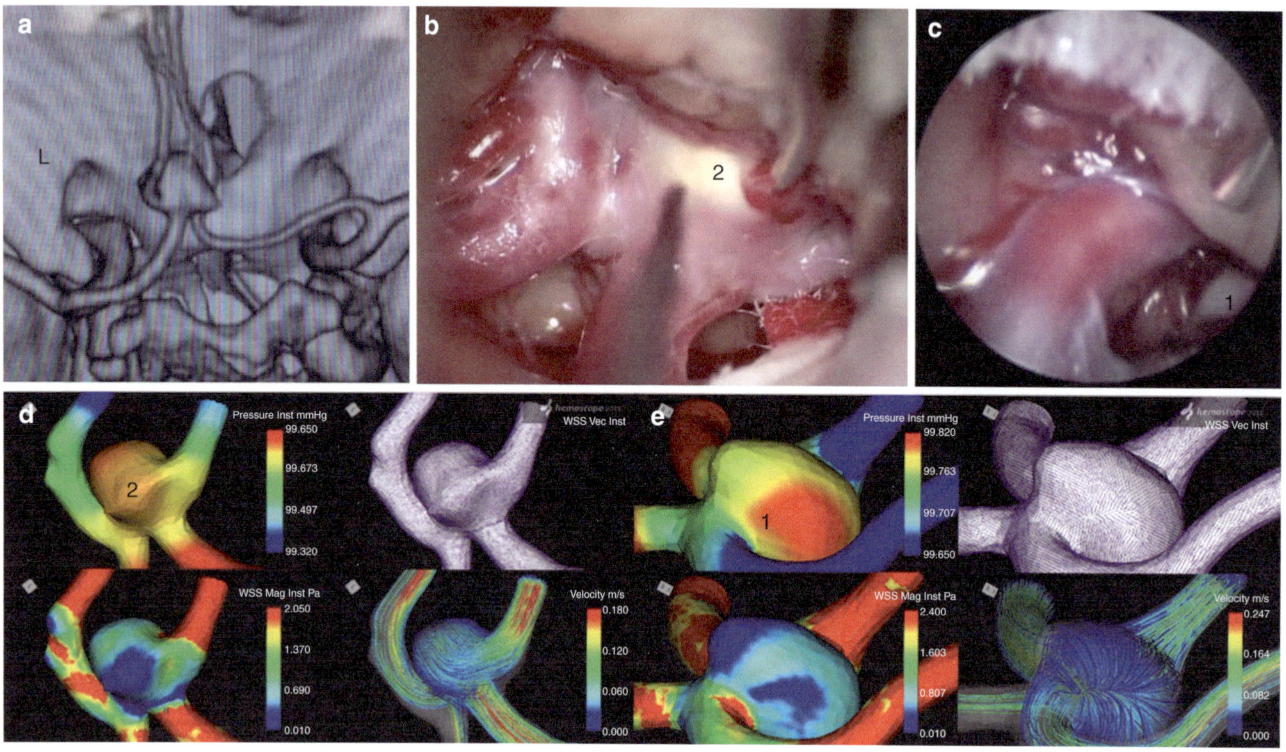

Fig. 1 Patient n.11. (**a**) 3D CT-scan reconstruction of the Acom aneurysm. (**b**) Intraoperative inspection demonstrating a yellowish and thick area (*2*). (**c**) Intraoperative endoscopic inspection revealing a second yellowish and thick area (*1*). (**d**, **e**) CFD analysis showing different characteristics of the areas *1* and *2*. In particular, area *1* reveals high *P*, low WSS, divergent WSS vectors, *streamlines* hitting the wall of the aneurysm with high velocity

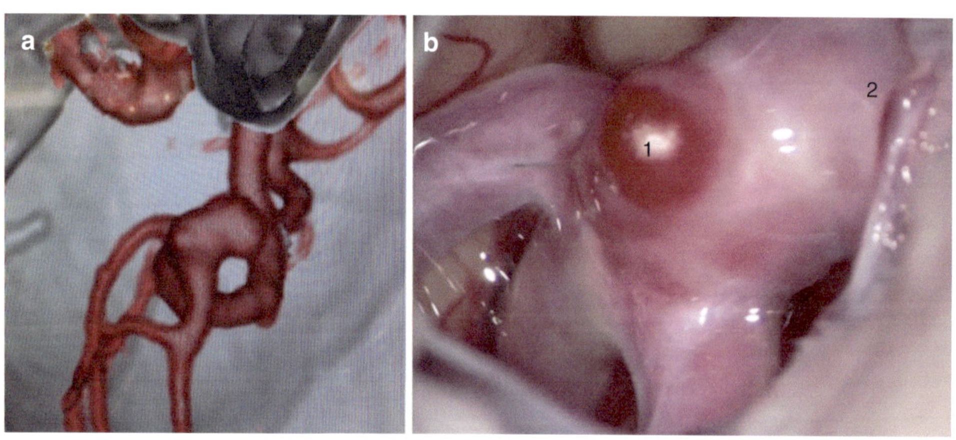

Fig. 2 Patient n.14. (**a**) 3D CT-scan reconstruction of the left MCA aneurysm. (**b**) Intraoperative direct visualization revealed a TW bleb (*1*), in contrast with a normal wall dome (*2*). (**c**) CFD analysis showed the TW bleb to have high *P*, low WSS, divergent WSS vectors, and SL hitting the bleb wall with high velocity

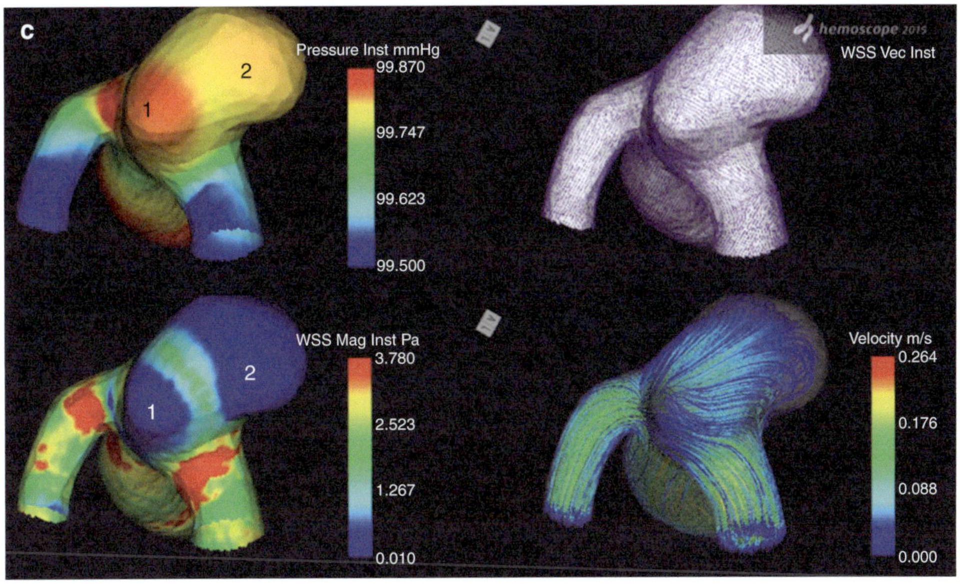

Fig. 2 (continued)

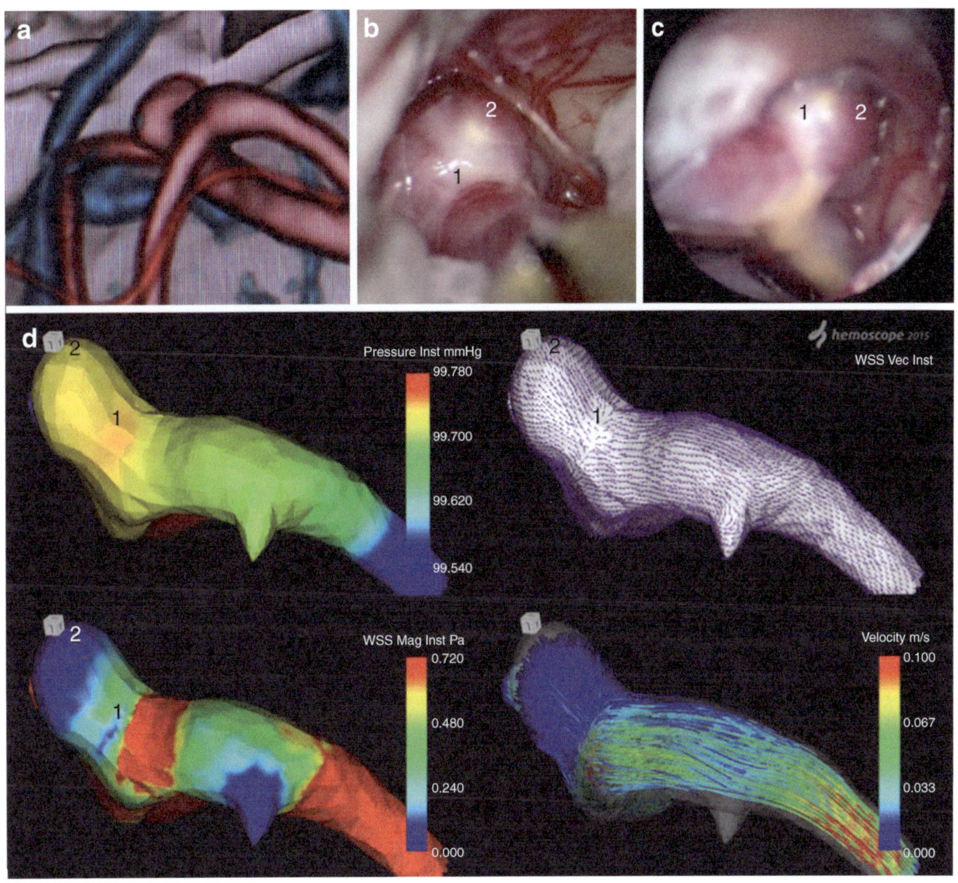

Fig. 3 Patient n.8. (**a**) 3D CT-reconstruction of left MCA aneurysm. (**b, c**) Intraoperative microscopic and endoscopic inspection revealing an AW area close to the neck of the aneurysm and a TW area at the tip of the dome. (**d**) CFD analysis showing the AW area with high *P*, low WSS, divergent vectors, and SL hitting with high velocity. The TW area has low WSS

Discussion

Computational fluid dynamics is a tool that allows the analysis of fluids through pipes and tube dilations. It has been applied to the study of intracranial vessels and aneurysms for more than 15 years, and is regarded as a promising instrument to predict the natural history of aneurysms. However, conflicting results have been published about the interpretation of CFD parameters. Two theories explaining the mechanisms of cerebral aneurysm rupture have been proposed. Some authors reported that ruptured aneurysms have higher

WSS compared with unruptured aneurysms, although others stated that ruptured aneurysms have a lower WSS and higher OSI [4, 8]. More recently, Takao et al. showed that a low WSS may be associated with aneurysm rupture, but statistical significance was noted only in ICA cases and not in MCA cases [10]. The same study also investigated pressure loss coefficient (PLc), which represents the pressure loss associated with the shape of pipes and obstacles to flow. Interestingly, they showed that high PLc is associated with a higher risk of aneurysm rupture. This might be consistent with our findings of high *P* in the areas of thicker walls. Miura published similar results showing that low WSS is associated with rupture of MCA aneurysms [6]. Fukazawa et al. applied CFD to 12 ruptured MCA aneurysms, showing an association between the rupture point seen during operation and low WSS, lower-velocity areas, and complex flow patterns [11]. Similarly, Omodaka et al. found that the time-averaged WSS at the rupture point of six ruptured MCA aneurysms was significantly lower than that at the aneurysm wall without the rupture point [7]. Also Lu et al. associated low WSS with higher risk of rupture [5]. Bleb formation seems, however, to be associated with high WSS, which later falls after the formation of the bleb [2, 3]. More recently, a unifying theory has been proposed, hypothesizing that both high and low WSS could drive intracranial aneurysms growth and rupture. Mural cell-mediated (high WSS) and inflammatory cell-mediated (low WSS) destructive remodeling pathways have been involved in this process [12, 13].

The possible correlation between CFD results and the risk of aneurysm rupture is very intriguing, as it could be of great importance to stratify rupture risk and tailor treatment accordingly. However, CFD parameters related to blood flow and wall stress can be of great importance, even irrespective of aneurysm eventual rupture. Actually, the potential ability of CFD to provide information about the structural characteristics of the aneurysm wall can be a valuable tool during surgical dissection or coiling. All the available current imaging techniques can show the morphology and the anatomical relationships of the vessels and the aneurysm with adjacent structures, but nothing can be used to detect the thickness of the aneurysm wall. Although the majority of studies on CFD focused on the risk of rupture, fewer publications are available about the correlation between CFD parameters and the characteristics of the aneurysm wall. Kadasi et al. first reported the colocalization of TWRs with areas of low WSS and focal pressure elevation [1]. Suzuki et al. recently published a paper where they assessed 50 aneurysm wall surfaces and investigated the correlation between pressure elevation and TWRs [9]. They found that most P_{max} areas (82%) corresponded with TWRs.

Our study also found a co-localization of low WSS and TWRs. However, low WSS can also be found in areas of the aneurysm dome that are not thin and red. Moreover, in some cases, red, thin walls do not show a low WSS (30% of cases in our series). We also noticed that when low WSS is associated with high pressure, divergent WSS vectors, and streamlines hitting the wall with high velocity, the surface is more likely thick, yellow, and atherosclerotic (78.6% of cases in our series).

We hypothesize that continuous high velocity blood flow hitting an area of the aneurysm could trigger a remodeling of the wall, ultimately leading to a reactive thickening. In this perspective, areas with low WSS but stagnating blood flow can be more prone to thinning remodeling as a consequence of an inflammatory process, as already described in other studies. We also think that, at this stage, CFD analysis can provide only a general but intriguing picture of the association between fluid dynamics parameters and intraoperative findings. This can be caused by many reasons. First, aneurysm initiation, growth, and eventual rupture are long and complex processes. By definition, aneurysm architecture often changes over time, and fluid dynamics in the aneurysm are likely to change accordingly. CFD analysis is a representation of the aneurysm fluid dynamics at a specific time point, and it is therefore very difficult to foresee the natural evolution of the aneurysm from a single static picture. CFD data from a very large population of patients could maybe provide a wider representation of different aneurysm stages at different locations, and finally help clinicians to refine the ability to predict the natural history of the disease. Another reason for the difficulty in providing a unique and comprehensive interpretation of CFD results is the fact that other factors different from fluid dynamics can influence aneurysm evolution, for example, genetics, and the environment around the aneurysm itself. Moreover, the currently available software, although advanced, might still be limited to provide a fully detailed analysis of the multiple variables playing a role in the fluid dynamics in vivo.

Our study is therefore affected by limitations that are common to previously published papers about CFD analysis. These limitations depend on the pre-processing assumptions of Newtonian fluid models with fixed density and viscosity, vessel rigidity. Moreover, we did not consider aneurysm histology, peri-aneurysm anatomy, or humoral and physiological parameters. The AW and TW areas evaluation method was subjective and based only on visual intraoperative findings. The boundary conditions were uniform across all cases, although patient-specific analysis requires boundary conditions established with magnetic resonance imaging and echocardiographic imaging.

Despite the current limitations of CFD analysis applied to clinical settings, and the limited number of patients, our results show that red, thin areas on aneurysm walls often have a low WSS, consistent with previously published papers. Therefore, attention must be taken when approaching areas with a low WSS. Moreover, we noticed that the association of high pressure, low WSS, divergent WSS vectors, and SL hitting the wall with high velocity is most often associated with thickening of the aneurysm wall.

Conflict of Interest The authors declare that they have no conflict of interest.

References

1. Kadasi LM, Dent WC, Malek AM. Colocalization of thin-walled dome regions with low hemodynamic wall shear stress in unruptured cerebral aneurysms. J Neurosurg. 2013;119:172–9.
2. Russell JH, Kelson N, Barry M, Pearcy M, Fletcher DF, Winter CD. Computational fluid dynamic analysis of intracranial aneurysmal bleb formation. Neurosurgery. 2013;73:1061–8.
3. Cebral JR, Castro MA, Burgess JE, Pergolizzi RS, Sheridan MJ, Putman CM. Characterization of cerebral aneurysms for assessing risk of rupture by using patient-specific computational hemodynamics models. AJNR Am J Neuroradiol. 2005;26:2550–9.
4. Cebral JR, Mut F, Weir J, Putman C. Quantitative characterization of the hemodynamic environment in ruptured and unruptured brain aneurysms. AJNR Am J Neuroradiol. 2011;32:145–51.
5. Lu G, Huang L, Zhang XL, Wang SZ, Hong Y, Hu Z, Geng DY. Influence of hemodynamic factors on rupture of intracranial aneurysms: patient-specific 3D mirror aneurysms model computational fluid dynamics simulation. AJNR Am J Neuroradiol. 2011;32:1255–61.
6. Miura Y, Ishida F, Umeda Y, Tanemura H, Suzuki H, Matsushima S, Shimosaka S, Taki W. Low wall shear stress is independently associated with the rupture status of middle cerebral artery aneurysms. Stroke. 2013;44:519–21.
7. Omodaka S, Sugiyama S, Inoue T, Funamoto K, Fujimura M, Shimizu H, Hayase T, Takahashi A, Tominaga T. Local hemodynamics at the rupture point of cerebral aneurysms determined by computational fluid dynamics analysis. Cerebrovasc Dis. 2012;34:121–9.
8. Xiang J, Natarajan SK, Tremmel M, Ma D, Mocco J, Hopkins LN, Siddiqui AH, Levy EI, Meng H. Hemodynamic-morphologic discriminants for intracranial aneurysm rupture. Stroke. 2011;42:144–52.
9. Suzuki T, Takao H, Suzuki T, Kambayashi Y, Watanabe M, Sakamoto H, Kan I, Nishimura K, Kaku S, Ishibashi T, Ikeuchi S, Yamamoto M, Fujii Y, Murayama Y. Determining the presence of thin-walled regions at high-pressure areas in unruptured cerebral aneurysms by using computational fluid dynamics. Neurosurgery. 2016;79:589–95.
10. Takao H, Murayama Y, Otsuka S, Qian Y, Mohamed A, Masuda S, Yamamoto M, Abe T. Hemodynamic differences between unruptured and ruptured intracranial aneurysms during observation. Stroke. 2012;43:1436–9.
11. Fukazawa K, Ishida F, Umeda Y, Miura Y, Shimosaka S, Matsushima S, Taki W, Suzuki H. Using computational fluid dynamics analysis to characterize local hemodynamic features of middle cerebral artery aneurysm rupture points. World Neurosurg. 2015;83:80–6.
12. Meng H, Tutino VM, Xiang J, Siddiqui A. High WSS or low WSS? Complex interactions of hemodynamics with intracranial aneurysm initiation, growth, and rupture: toward a unifying hypothesis. AJNR Am J Neuroradiol. 2014;35:1254–62.
13. Xiang J, Tutino VM, Snyder KV, Meng H. CFD: computational fluid dynamics or confounding factor dissemination? The role of hemodynamics in intracranial aneurysm rupture risk assessment. AJNR Am J Neuroradiol. 2014;35:1849–57.

Adenosine-Assisted Clipping of Intracranial Aneurysms

Torstein R. Meling

Abstract *Background.* Temporary parent vessel clip occlusion in aneurysm surgery is not always practical or feasible. Adenosine-induced transient cardiac arrest may serve as an alternative.

Methods. All patients who underwent microsurgical clipping of intracranial aneurysms under adenosine-induced asystole performed by the author between September 2011 and July 2014 were retrospectively reviewed.

Results. A total of 16 craniotomies were performed and 16 aneurysms were clipped under adenosine-induced asystole (in 8 basilar arteries, 7 internal carotid arteries, and 1 middle cerebral artery) in 14 patients (8 females, 6 males). Seven cases were elective and 7 were performed after subarachnoid hemorrhage. The patients' mean age was 54 years (range, 39–70 years). The indications for adenosine use were proximal control in narrow surgical corridors in 11 cases, aneurysm softening in 4 cases, and aneurysm rupture in 1 case. A single dose was used in 12 patients; 2 patients had multiple boluses. The median (range) total dose was 30 (18–60) mg. Adenosine induced bradycardia with concomitant arterial hypotension in all patients and the majority also had asystole for 5–15 s. Transient cardiac arrhythmias were noted in 1 patient (atrial fibrillation in need of electroconversion after two boluses).

Conclusion. Nine clinical scenarios were identified in which adenosine-induced temporary cardiac arrest and deep hypotension was an effective adjunct to temporary clipping during the microsurgical clipping of intracranial aneurysms.

Keywords Adenosine · Aneurysm · Cardiac arrest · Carotid artery · Basilar artery

T. R. Meling, M.D., Ph.D.
Department of Neurosurgery, Oslo University Hospital-Rikshospitalet, Oslo, Norway

Institute of Clinical Medicine, Faculty of Medicine, University of Oslo, Oslo, Norway

Introduction

Aneurysm surgery remains a neurosurgical challenge. Although the basic principles were established in the last century and modern microscopes and training have dramatically reduced the risks of aneurysm surgery, we are now, relatively speaking, confronted with more and more complex cases [1–3]. Furthermore, endovascular therapy has so far not turned out to be the panacea once thought for many aneurysms, including basilar tip aneurysms, leaving us with recurrent or partially coiled aneurysms in quite difficult locations.

The basic principles of safe aneurysm surgery include subarachnoid dissection, proximal and distal control, dissection of branches and perforators, dissection of the aneurysm neck, and complete circumferential exposure of the aneurysm (Fig. 1) [4]. Temporary clipping is an important technique, allowing aneurysm softening in the final stages of aneurysm neck and perforator dissection (Fig. 2, Table 1). Furthermore, softening of an aneurysm prior to permanent clip application can change seemingly unclippable aneurysms into clippable ones. In more challenging cases, temporary clipping has to be applied to both the afferent and efferent arteries (trapping) to facilitate both dissection and permanent clipping. Aneurysm trapping can be followed by deflation (suction-decompression), which can be used to facilitate clip reconstruction (Fig. 2) [5]. Lastly, temporary clipping is also an important technique for dealing with intraoperative aneurysm rupture [6].

However, the use of temporary clip occlusion can potentially injure the branches, perforators, and even the parent vessel, resulting in dissection, stroke, or vessel rupture. Furthermore, there is often a limited anatomical space for temporary clips to be applied, necessitating the use of brain retractors or the extensive removal of bone at the skull base.

Conceptually, another way of obtaining a low intra-aneurysmal pressure during aneurysm dissection and permanent clipping is to lower the systemic blood pressure (Fig. 3). Several techniques for transient cardiac standstill have been developed to allow for aneurysm softening. In 1966, Small et al.

G. Esposito et al. (eds.), *Trends in the Management of Cerebrovascular Diseases*, Acta Neurochirurgica Supplement, Vol. 129,
https://doi.org/10.1007/978-3-319-73739-3_2,

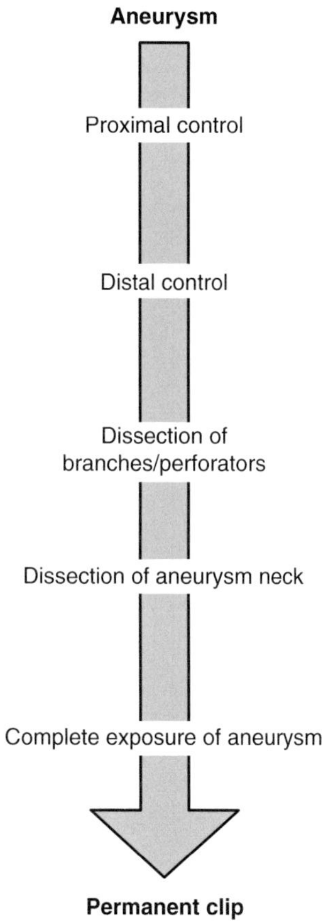

Fig. 1 The basic steps of safe aneurysm clipping

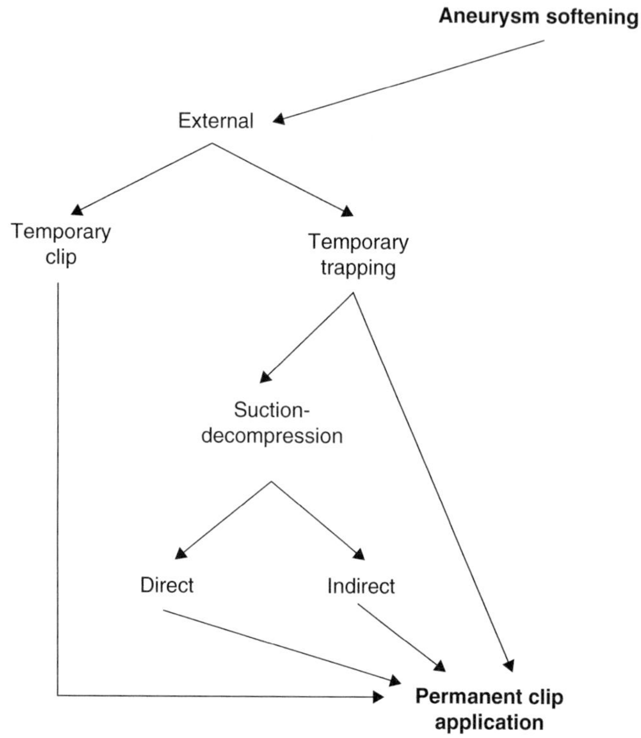

Fig. 2 Temporary clipping or trapping are modes for aneurysm softening during dissection and permanent clip application

Table 1 Modes of aneurysm softening

	Mechanism of action	Dose	Advantages	Disadvantages
Temporary clip	• Mechanical obstruction of blood flow through parent vessel	• Frequently one clip	• Ease of use	• No flow through parent vessel distal to occlusion during procedure
		• Occasionally multiple	• On-off demand • Can be repeated • Non-invasive procedure	• May require complex skull base procedures to gain proximal control
Cardiac arrest with deep hypothermia	• Decreases $CMRO_2$	• 15–17 °C	• Cerebral protection	• High-risk procedure with permanent morbidity/mortality of 14–18%
			• Controlled systemic hypotension	• Invasive procedure • Staff requirements
Rapid ventricular pacing	• Enforces ventricular tachycardia, compromising ventricular filling	• >150–160 BPM	• On-off demand	• Invasive procedure
	• Absence of AV synchrony		• Response more predictable than adenosine	• Need for external defibrillator pads
	• Reduces cardiac output		• Shorter hypotensive period than adenosine • Can be repeated • Some flow through parent vessel during procedure	• Need for cardiologist

Table 1 (continued)

	Mechanism of action	Dose	Advantages	Disadvantages
Adenosine	• An i.v. bolus blocks the AV-node dose-dependently • Asystole is transient and very short • Plasma half-life of <10 s	• 0.5 mg per kg body mass	• Controlled systemic hypotension • No need for complex logistic coordination • Non-invasive procedure • Can be repeated • Does not cause rebound hypertension or tachyphylaxis • Some flow through parent vessel during procedure	• Prolonged hypotension • Effect duration unpredictable • Need for external defibrillator pads

AV Atrioventricular, *BPM* beats per min, *CMRO2* cerebral metabolic rate of oxygen consumption

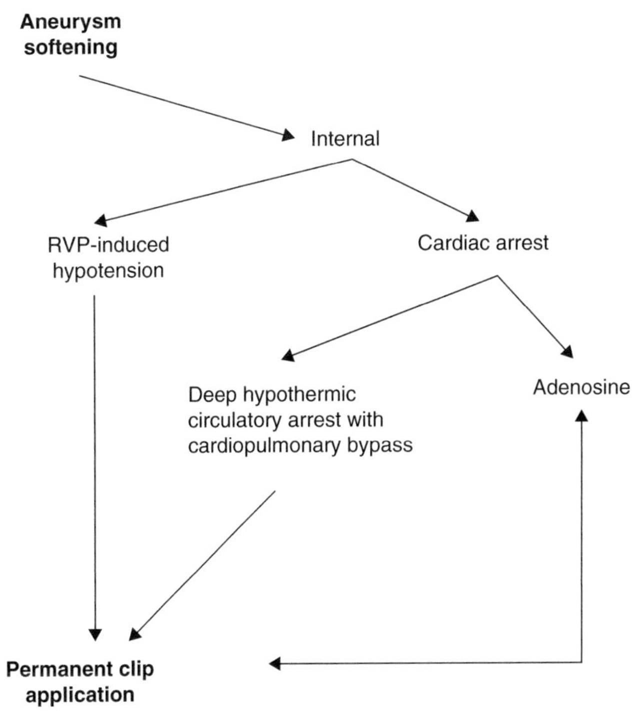

Fig. 3 Techniques for internal aneurysm softening during dissection and permanent clip application

[7] reported on the use of rapid ventricular pacing (RVP) in intracerebral aneurysm surgery. Cardiac pacing wires were advanced into the right ventricle to generate ventricular tachycardia and near circulatory arrest in order to facilitate clipping (Fig. 3, Table 1). However, RVP never gained much attention and was replaced, in select centers, by cardiac standstill during deep hypothermia (Fig. 3) [8–10]. The premise for deep hypothermia is that this treatment lowers the cerebral metabolic rate of oxygen consumption. The complexity involved in extracorporeal circulation and the high complication rates associated with this approach prevented its widespread application and later restricted its use (Table 1). More recently, the RVP method has resurfaced in cerebrovascular surgery [11, 12].

In 1999, Groff et al. introduced adenosine to induce rapidly reversible cardiac arrest, and hence arterial hypotension, during cerebral aneurysm surgery (Fig. 3, Table 1) [13]. Adenosine is commonly used to treat paroxysmal supraventricular tachyarrhythmia. After a bolus injection, the heart rate is dose-dependently reduced until a complete atrioventricular-node (AV-node) blockade is reached. However, this effect on the AV node is transient and very short acting. In patients with normal sinus rhythm, the administration of adenosine gradually slows the heart rate for about 20–30 s before asystole is reached, for a mean time of 15 s, after which the heart rate spontaneously begins to increase until it returns to baseline, in about 20–30 s [14, 15]. Adenosine has a very short plasma half-life of less than 10 s and, unlike other hypotensive agents, it does not cause rebound hypertension or tachyphylaxis. Therefore, multiple administrations during a single procedure are possible [15–17]. Furthermore, adenosine use does not require the same amount of preparation and equipment, or the same staff numbers, as required for RVP or deep hypothermic circulatory arrest with cardiopulmonary bypass (Table 1), making it suitable for situations of sudden aneurysmal rupture [17]. In addition, experimental data suggest that adenosine may be a potent endogenous neuroprotective agent in both acute and long-lasting ischemia [18, 19].

We have found adenosine to be a very useful adjunct to temporary clipping during intracranial aneurysm surgery in a number of scenarios, and therefore we decided to review the use of adenosine in our clinical practice.

Patients and Methods

We reviewed our prospectively collected clinical database to identify all patients for whom adenosine was used during surgery between September 2011 and July 2014. We reviewed operative reports, imaging results, and clinical charts. The following data were recorded: sex; age; Hunt and Hess grade; rupture status; aneurysm location and size; reason for adenosine use, number of adenosine injections, dose used, and whether it was successful; and postoperative complications. Patients' clinic follow-up visits were also reviewed, as were the postoperative angiographic results. Neurological status at follow-up was assessed with the modified Rankin Scale (mRS).

In all cases the use of adenosine was anticipated and all the patients had transcutaneous pacemakers placed as a precaution for prolonged bradycardia or asystole. Patients with a history of severe asthma, symptomatic asthma, or sick sinus syndrome/heart block were excluded from undergoing this procedure. Adenosine was injected via a central venous catheter so that a high dose would reach its major site of action, the AV node.

Results

Fourteen patients (8 females, 6 males) underwent surgical clipping; 7 procedures were elective and 7 were performed after subarachnoid hemorrhage (Table 2). The patients' mean age was 54.4 years (range, 39–70 years).

Sixteen craniotomies were performed in the 14 patients; two patients had two craniotomies each during the same procedure, because not all the aneurysms could be reached via one opening (Table 2). A total of 16 aneurysms were clipped under adenosine-induced asystole (8 in basilar arteries [BAs], 7 in internal carotid arteries [ICAs], and 1 in the middle cerebral artery [MCA]). The average aneurysm size was 7.7 mm (range, 2–36 mm) (Table 2).

The main indication for using adenosine was for proximal control as an adjunct to temporary clipping in narrow surgical corridors (Table 3), the majority of which were BA aneurysms (Fig. 4). Adenosine was also used for aneurysm softening in four cases; for instance in a tiny ICA-posterior communicating artery (PCOM) aneurysm in a patient with very fragile vessels (Fig. 5). Intraoperative aneurysm rupture occurred in one patient, with a BA aneurysm, requiring two rounds of adenosine-induced cardiac arrest during clipping (Table 3).

A single adenosine dose was used in 12 patients, whereas 2 patients had repeat injections, 1 patient for intraoperative rupture and 1 patient for further dissection. The median total dose was 30 mg, with a range of 18 to 60 mg (Table 3). Adenosine immediately induced transient bradycardia with concomitant arterial hypotension in all patients, and the majority also had a short-lasting, self-limiting asystole for 20 s (range 5–30 s) per dose.

Some of the patients had multiple aneurysms clipped *en passant*, but not using adenosine, resulting in an additional 16 aneurysms being clipped during these surgeries (11 MCAs, 4 ICAs, and 1 anterior communicating artery [ACOM]) (Table 3).

Transient cardiac arrhythmia was noted in one patient, who went into atrial fibrillation after the second adenosine bolus. He received electroconversion at the end of the surgery while still under general anesthesia, using the transcutaneous pacemaker pads already in place, without noticeable complications.

Postoperatively, the patients' clinical condition at last follow-up was generally good (mean mRS score, 1.6;

Table 2 Patient characteristics

Patient	Sex	Age (years)	SAH	Hunt and Hess scale	Aneurysm location	Size (mm)	Follow-up (days)	mRS at follow-up
1	Female	70	Yes	5	BA (tip)	4	69	6
2	Male	42	Yes	2	BA (tip)	5	849	1
3	Female	55	Yes	1	BA (tip)	4	936	1
4	Female	64	Yes	1	ICA (PCOM)	3	814	2
5	Female	50	No	0	ICA (top)	2	200	1
6-1	Male	57	No	0	ICA (top)	6	192	1
6-2	Male	57	No	0	MCA	4	192	1
7	Female	56	Yes	2	ICA (PCOM)	14	115	0
8	Male	71	Yes	4	BA (blister-like)	12	5	6
9	Female	39	No	5	BA (tip, previously coiled)	36	87	6
10	Female	54	No	0	ICA (top)	6	245	0
11-1	Male	48	No	0	BA (SCA)	3	146	0
11-2	Male	48	No	0	ICA (PCOM)	3	146	0
12	Female	57	No	1	ICA (PCOM, previously coiled)	10	218	2
13	Male	54	No	0	BA (tip)	6	243	0
14	Female	49	Yes	1	BA (tip)	5	26	2

BA basilar artery, *ICA* internal carotid artery, *MCA* middle cerebral artery, *PCOM* posterior communicating artery, *SCA* superior cerebellar artery, *mRS* modified Rankin scale, *SAH* subarachnoid hemorrhage

Table 3 Results

Patient	Aneurysm location	Indication	Adenosine bolus	Adenosine dose (mg)	Duration of asystole (s)	Adenosine effect	Comments
1	BA (tip)	Temporary clip in narrow corridor	1	20	10	Bradyc—10 s asystole—spontaneous	
2	BA (tip)	Temporary clip in narrow corridor	1	18	20	Bradyc—20 s asystole—spontaneous	
3	BA (tip)	Temporary clip	1	20	20	Bradyc—20 s asystole—spontaneous	MCA *en passant*
4	ICA (PCOM)	Aneurysm softening	1	20	3	Bradyc—3 s asystole—spontaneous	MCA *en passant*
5	ICA (top)	Temporary clip	1	20	3	Bradyc—3 s asystole—spontaneous	MCA *en passant*
6-1	ICA (top)	Temporary clip	1	30	10	Bradyc—10 s asystole—spontaneous	MCA *en passant*
6-2	MCA*	Temporary clip	2	60	20s per dose	Bradyc—20 s asystole—spontaneous	*Heavily calcified M1 with inherent risk of emboli with temporary clipping. Short AFib after last dose of adenosine, ectroconversion
7	ICA (PCOM)	Aneurysm softening	1	40	20	Bradyc—20 s asystole—spontaneous	2 MCA aneurysms *en passant*
8	BA (tip)	Intraoperative rupture	2	60	30s per dose	Bradyc—30 s asystole—spontaneous	
9	BA (tip)	Aneurysm softening	1	40	10	Bradyc—10 s asystole—spontaneous	
10	ICA (top)	Temporary clip	1	40	10	Bradyc—10 s asystole—spontaneous	
11-1	BA (SCA)	Temporary clip in narrow corridor	1	20	5	Bradyc—20 s asystole—spontaneous	MCA *en passant*
11-2	ICA (PCOM)	Temporary clip	1	20	5	Bradyc—5 s asystole—spontaneous	MCA *en passant*
12	ICA (PCOM, previously coiled)	Aneurysm softening	1	30	20	Bradyc—20 s asystole—spontaneous	
13	BA (tip)	Temporary clip	1	45	10	Bradyc—10 s asystole—spontaneous	ACOM, 2 ICA and 3 MCA aneurysms *en passant*
14	BA (tip)	Temporary clip	1	45	10	Bradyc—10 s asystole—spontaneous	

[*] *AFib* Atrial fibrillation, *ACOM* anterior communicating artery, *Bradyc* bradycardia, *M1* is the first segment of the MCA

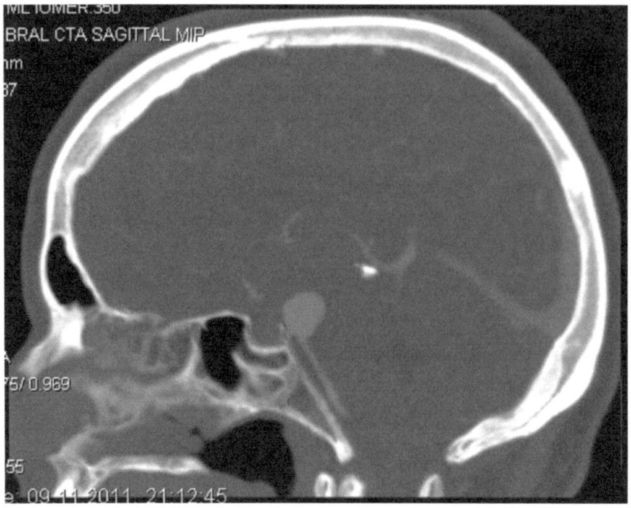

Fig. 4 Patient 3, with a basilar tip aneurysm

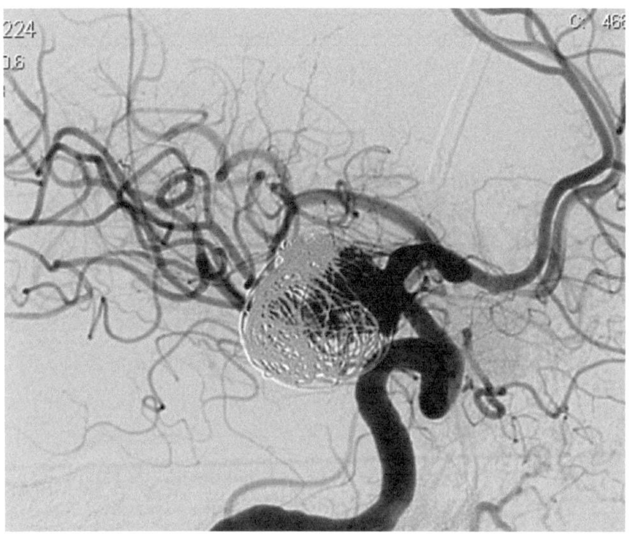

Fig. 5 Patient 12, with a previously coiled posterior communicating artery *PCOM* aneurysm

Table 2), but there were three deaths, all attributed to SAH (all three of these patients were Hunt and Hess grade 4 or 5 on admission; Table 2).

Discussion

In this study, the author's experience using adenosine-induced cardiac arrest to facilitate permanent clip application during surgery for 16 intracranial aneurysms was reviewed (Table 2). The main indication for adenosine use was the softening of posterior circulation aneurysms in a narrow surgical corridor (Table 3). It should be noted that the majority of the BA aneurysms were small (Table 2), making the dissection of the perforators relatively easy to perform without a temporary clip. Hence, it was possible to use adenosine only for the final softening of the aneurysm when the permanent clip was to be placed. It was used pre-emptively in 15 cases, and was used for an intraoperative rupture in only one patient (Table 3).

In all patients, adenosine induced bradycardia with concomitant arterial hypotension, and the majority also had asystole for 5–15 s, allowing for application of the permanent clip to a very soft aneurysm (Table 3). Induction of cardiac arrest was associated with significant reductions in arterial pressure. No significant overshoot in the course of arterial pressure was observed after cardiac activity had fully recovered, even with the higher adenosine doses. However, one patient developed transient atrial fibrillation that needed intraoperative electroconversion, but otherwise this patient had an uneventful recovery.

Safe microsurgical exposure and permanent clipping of an aneurysm relies on proximal and distal control of the parent artery, circumferential exposure of the aneurysm neck and its branches and perforators, and, lastly, complete exposure of the aneurysm sac (Fig. 1) [4]. Temporary clipping allows for the softening of an aneurysm in the final stages of aneurysm neck and perforator dissection, as well as during permanent clip application (Fig. 2) [4]. Aneurysm trapping can be followed by suction-decompression to facilitate clip reconstruction [5]. Lastly, temporary clipping is important for dealing with intraoperative aneurysm rupture [6]. However, temporary clipping may have limitations. In cases of early aneurysm rupture, the application of a temporary clip can be extremely difficult and potentially dangerous, owing to poor visualization of the relevant vessels and even the cranial nerves [16]. In the paraclinoid region, temporary clipping can be difficult owing to the skull base bone covering the ICA proximal to the aneurysm [20]. Although exposure of the cavernous ICA can be performed via an intra- or extradural clinoidectomy, either of these approaches may put cranial nerves at risk [21]. In the posterior circulation, temporary clipping may be challenging, owing to the very narrow surgical corridors, irrespective of which approach is used [22, 23]. Although most neurosurgeons feel more comfortable with a transsylvian approach, this approach may require the technically demanding drilling of both the anterior clinoid process and the posterior clinoid process (PCP), depending on the height of the BA tip relative to the PCP [24, 25]. The temporary clipping time is limited by the potential for ischemic complications. Complete trapping of BA aneurysms requires the temporary clipping of not only the BA trunk, but also the posterior cerebral artery (PCA) bilaterally, to avoid retrograde filling. If the first PCA segment is adherent to the aneurysm dome, temporary clipping of the PCOM and the second PCA segment bilaterally is necessary for trapping. All these clips must be applied after the temporary clipping of the BA trunk, and these maneuvers consume the

Table 4 Scenarios in which adenosine was found to be useful

• For intraoperative aneurysm rupture
• To reduce or avoid dangerous drilling of ACP
• To reduce or avoid dangerous drilling of PCP
• To reduce temporary clipping time in order to limit the potential for ischemic complications
• To reduce risk of cranial nerve damage
• For particularly atherosclerotic parent vessels
• For particularly fragile parent vessels (blood-blister aneurysms)
• For previously coiled aneurysms
• For previously stented or flow-diverted aneurysms

ACP Anterior clinoid process, *PCP* posterior clinoid process

temporary clipping time. There is also an inherent risk to cranial nerves, specifically the oculomotor nerves, when applying the temporary clips. Similarly, complete trapping of ACOM aneurysms requires the application and subsequent removal of four temporary clips on both the first and the second segment of the anterior cerebral artery bilaterally, maneuvers that also consume the temporary clipping time.

As temporary clipping may not always be feasible or advisable, aneurysm softening can be obtained by reducing the systemic blood pressure by the application of brief cardiac arrest using adenosine; several authors have found this procedure to be a useful adjunct (Table 4) [15–17, 26, 27]. A recent study by the Northwestern University Feinberg School of Medicine has shown that adenosine-induced flow arrest implemented to facilitate intracranial aneurysm clip ligation does not worsen neurologic outcomes [28]. The same group also found that adenosine-assisted intracranial aneurysm surgery was not associated with an increase in perioperative cardiac complications or mortality in patients with a low risk of coronary artery disease [29]. Lastly, a large case series (n = 98) describing adenosine-induced asystole for endovascular aortic aneurysm repair reported a 2% incidence of self-limited ST-segment depression on electrocardiography and a 4% incidence of temporary heart block requiring <30 s of pacing [30].

Conclusions

Adenosine-induced temporary cardiac arrest appears to be a safe and effective method for achieving transient deep hypotension and asystole during the microsurgical clipping of intracranial aneurysms.

Financial Disclosure The authors do not have any personal or institutional financial interest in the drugs, materials, or devices described in the article.

Grant Information/Other Acknowledgments No grants have been received by the authors.

References

1. Rodriguez-Hernandez A, Lawton MT. Management of a recurrent coiled giant posterior cerebral artery aneurysm with trapping and thrombectomy: 3-dimensional operative video. Neurosurgery. 2012;71:ons191. https://doi.org/10.1227/NEU.0b013e3182732081.
2. Sughrue ME, Saloner D, Rayz VL, Lawton MT. Giant intracranial aneurysms: evolution of management in a contemporary surgical series. Neurosurgery. 2011;69:1261–70; discussion 1270–1. https://doi.org/10.1227/NEU.0b013e31822bb8a6.
3. Waldron JS, Halbach VV, Lawton MT. Microsurgical management of incompletely coiled and recurrent aneurysms: trends, techniques, and observations on coil extrusion. Neurosurgery. 2009;64:301–15; discussion 315–7. https://doi.org/10.1227/01.NEU.0000335178.15274.B4.
4. Lawton MT. Seven aneurysms: tenets and techniques for clipping. New York: Thieme; 2011.
5. Batjer HH, Samson DS. Retrograde suction decompression of giant paraclinoidal aneurysms. Technical note. J Neurosurg. 1990;73:305–6. https://doi.org/10.3171/jns.1990.73.2.0305.
6. Batjer H, Samson DS. Management of intraoperative aneurysm rupture. Clin Neurosurg. 1990;36:275–88.
7. Small JM, Stephenson SC, Campkin TV, Davison PH, McIlveen JS. Elective circulatory arrest by artificial pacemaker. Lancet. 1966;1:570–2.
8. Ponce FA, Spetzler RF, Han PP, Wait SD, Killory BD, Nakaji P, Zabramski JM. Cardiac standstill for cerebral aneurysms in 103 patients: an update on the experience at the Barrow Neurological Institute. Clinical article. J Neurosurg. 2011;114:877–84. https://doi.org/10.3171/2010.9.JNS091178.
9. Taki W, Sakai N, Nakahara I, Osaka N, Koshiji T, Matsuda K, Enoki Y, Kikuchi H. Circulatory arrest with profound hypothermia during the surgical treatment of large internal carotid artery aneurysm–case report. Neurol Med Chir (Tokyo). 1998;38:725–9.
10. Young WL, Lawton MT, Gupta DK, Hashimoto T. Anesthetic management of deep hypothermic circulatory arrest for cerebral aneurysm clipping. Anesthesiology. 2002;96:497–503.
11. Saldien V, Menovsky T, Rommens M, Van der Steen G, Van Loock K, Vermeersch G, Mott C, Bosmans J, De Ridder D, Maas AI. Rapid ventricular pacing for flow arrest during cerebrovascular surgery: revival of an old concept. Neurosurgery. 2012;70:270–5. https://doi.org/10.1227/NEU.0b013e318236d84a.
12. Whiteley JR, Payne R, Rodriguez-Diaz C, Ellegala DB, Reeves ST. Rapid ventricular pacing: a novel technique to decrease cardiac output for giant basilar aneurysm surgery. J Clin Anesth. 2012;24:656–8. https://doi.org/10.1016/j.jclinane.2012.04.013.
13. Groff MW, Adams DC, Kahn RA, Kumbar UM, Yang BY, Bederson JB. Adenosine-induced transient asystole for management of a basilar artery aneurysm. Case report. J Neurosurg. 1999;91:687–90. https://doi.org/10.3171/jns.1999.91.4.0687.
14. Bebawy JF, Gupta DK, Bendok BR, Hemmer LB, Zeeni C, Avram MJ, Batjer HH, Koht A. Adenosine-induced flow arrest to facilitate intracranial aneurysm clip ligation: dose-response data and safety profile. Anesth Analg. 2010;110:1406–11. https://doi.org/10.1213/ANE.0b013e3181d65bf5.
15. Guinn NR, McDonagh DL, Borel CO, Wright DR, Zomorodi AR, Powers CJ, Warner DS, Lam AM, Britz GW. Adenosine-induced transient asystole for intracranial aneurysm surgery: a retrospective review. J Neurosurg Anesthesiol. 2011;23:35–40. https://doi.org/10.1097/ANA.0b013e3181ef2b11.
16. Bendok BR, Gupta DK, Rahme RJ, Eddleman CS, Adel JG, Sherma AK, Surdell DL, Bebawy JF, Koht A, Batjer HH. Adenosine for temporary flow arrest during intracranial aneurysm surgery: a single-center retrospective review. Neurosurgery. 2011;69:815–20; discussion 820–1. https://doi.org/10.1227/NEU.0b013e318226632c.

17. Luostarinen T, Takala RS, Niemi TT, Katila AJ, Niemela M, Hernesniemi J, Randell T. Adenosine-induced cardiac arrest during intraoperative cerebral aneurysm rupture. World Neurosurg. 2010;73:79–83; discussion e79. https://doi.org/10.1016/j.surneu.2009.06.018.
18. Li J, Zeng Z, Viollet B, Ronnett GV, McCullough LD. Neuroprotective effects of adenosine monophosphate-activated protein kinase inhibition and gene deletion in stroke. Stroke. 2007;38:2992–9. https://doi.org/10.1161/STROKEAHA.107.490904.
19. Plaschke K, Grant M, Weigand MA, Zuchner J, Martin E, Bardenheuer HJ. Neuromodulatory effect of propentofylline on rat brain under acute and long-term hypoperfusion. Br J Pharmacol. 2001;133:107–16. https://doi.org/10.1038/sj.bjp.0704061.
20. Golshani K, Ferrell A, Zomorodi A, Smith TP, Britz GW. A review of the management of posterior communicating artery aneurysms in the modern era. Surg Neurol Int. 2010;1:88. https://doi.org/10.4103/2152-7806.74147.
21. Sanai N, Caldwell N, Englot DJ, Lawton MT. Advanced technical skills are required for microsurgical clipping of posterior communicating artery aneurysms in the endovascular era. Neurosurgery. 2012;71:285–94; discussion 294–5. https://doi.org/10.1227/NEU.0b013e318256c3eb.
22. Hernesniemi J, Ishii K, Niemela M, Kivipelto L, Fujiki M, Shen H. Subtemporal approach to basilar bifurcation aneurysms: advanced technique and clinical experience. Acta Neurochir Suppl. 2005;94:31–8.
23. Hernesniemi J, Korja M. At the apex of cerebrovascular surgery—basilar tip aneurysms. World Neurosurg. 2013. https://doi.org/10.1016/j.wneu.2013.07.112.
24. Figueiredo EG, Zabramski JM, Deshmukh P, Crawford NR, Preul MC, Spetzler RF. Anatomical and quantitative description of the transcavernous approach to interpeduncular and prepontine cisterns. Technical note. J Neurosurg. 2006;104:957–64. https://doi.org/10.3171/jns.2006.104.6.957.
25. Krisht AF, Krayenbuhl N, Sercl D, Bikmaz K, Kadri PA. Results of microsurgical clipping of 50 high complexity basilar apex aneurysms. Neurosurgery. 2007;60:242–50; discussion 250–2. https://doi.org/10.1227/01.NEU.0000249265.88203.DF.
26. Benech CA, Perez R, Faccani G, Trompeo AC, Cavallo S, Beninati S, Berardino M. Adenosine-induced cardiac arrest in complex cerebral aneurysms surgery: an Italian single-center experience. J Neurosurg Sci. 2014;58:87–94.
27. Powers CJ, Wright DR, McDonagh DL, Borel CO, Zomorodi AR, Britz GW. Transient adenosine-induced asystole during the surgical treatment of anterior circulation cerebral aneurysms: technical note. Neurosurgery. 2010;67:461–70. https://doi.org/10.1227/NEU.0b013e3181f7ef46.
28. Bebawy JF, Zeeni C, Sharma S, Kim ES, DeWood MS, Hemmer LB, Ramaiah VK, Bendok BR, Koht A, Gupta DK. Adenosine-induced flow arrest to facilitate intracranial aneurysm clip ligation does not worsen neurologic outcome. Anesth Analg. 2013;117:1205–10. https://doi.org/10.1213/ANE.0b013e3182a6d31b.
29. Khan SA, McDonagh DL, Adogwa O, Gokhale S, Toche UN, Verla T, Zomorodi AR, Britz GW. Perioperative cardiac complications and 30-day mortality in patients undergoing intracranial aneurysmal surgery with adenosine-induced flow arrest: a retrospective comparative study. Neurosurgery. 2014;74:267–71; discussion 271–2. https://doi.org/10.1227/NEU.0000000000000258.
30. Kahn RA, Moskowitz DM, Marin ML, Hollier LH, Parsons R, Teodorescu V, McLaughlin M. Safety and efficacy of high-dose adenosine-induced asystole during endovascular AAA repair. J Endovasc Ther. 2000;7:292–6. https://doi.org/10.1583/1545-1550(2000)007<0292:SAEOHD>2.3.CO;2.

Endoscope-Assisted Microneurosurgery for Intracranial Aneurysms: Operative Technique, Reliability, and Feasibility Based on 14 Years of Personal Experience

Massimo Gallieni, Mattia Del Maestro, Sabino Luzzi, Donatella Trovarelli, Alessandro Ricci, and Renato Galzio

Abstract Endoscope-assisted microneurosurgery (EAM) combines endoscopic and microsurgical techniques for the treatment of deeply located intracranial lesions. During aneurysm surgery, endoscopic assistance may aid in the visualization of perforating arteries, especially when minimally invasive approaches are used. Between 2002 and 2015, a total of 183 patients with 208 intracranial aneurysms were surgically treated in our department. EAM was performed in 191 procedures. In all, 159 aneurysms were located in the anterior circulation and 49 in the posterior circulation. Of these, 135 aneurysms were ruptured. Lesions were exposed through standard skull base microsurgical approaches. The endoscope was employed during three steps: initial inspection, true operative time, and final inspection. Complications directly related to endoscopic procedures were rare; no surgical mortality was observed in this series. A retrospective analysis of each procedure showed that the usefulness of EAM depended on the anatomical location and size of the lesions. Its advantages were especially evident when dedicated scopes and holders were used.

Keywords Intracranial aneurysms · Sub-arachnoid hemorrhage · Clip ligation · Microneurosurgery · Endoscope-assisted microsurgery

M. Gallieni, M.D. (✉) · M. Del Maestro, M.D.
Department of Life, Health and Environmental Sciences (MESVA), University of L'Aquila, L'Aquila, Italy

S. Luzzi, M.D. · A. Ricci, M.D.
Department of Neurosurgery, San Salvatore City Hospital, L'Aquila, Italy

D. Trovarelli, M.D.
Department of Anesthesiology, San Salvatore City Hospital, L'Aquila, Italy

R. Galzio, M.D.
Department of Life, Health and Environmental Sciences (MESVA), University of L'Aquila, L'Aquila, Italy

Department of Neurosurgery, San Salvatore City Hospital, L'Aquila, Italy

Introduction

During operative approaches to treat deep-seated intracranial lesions, an endoscope may be used to assist with microsurgical maneuvers and control their efficacy. This technique is usually referred to as endoscope-assisted microneurosurgery (EAM). In the late 1970s, Apuzzo and Halves first reported the use of the endoscope as a technical adjunct during microsurgical resection of pituitary lesions with suprasellar involvement [1, 2]. Indeed, endoscope use was intended to optimize the visualization of the neurovascular structures located beyond the line of sight of the microscope. In 1995, Matula et al. introduced the concept of EAM as an adjunct tool for the treatment of intracranial lesions, mainly in the posterior fossa and parasellar region [3]. In 1998, Perneczky ultimately pioneered and popularized the use of the endoscope in cranial neurosurgery, giving life to the revolutionary concept of "minimally invasive neurosurgery" [4].

During EAM procedures, the endoscope is used to look around corners in an effort to overcome some intrinsic limits related to a basic microscopic view of the operative field. Furthermore, the endoscope provides clearer vision while also allowing for a less traumatic dissection of the structures located in a deeper level of the operative field. In aneurysm surgery, the introduction of the endoscope has led to improved visualization of perforating arteries, especially those arising from the posterior wall of the internal carotid artery (ICA), anterior communicating artery (ACoA), and basilar artery (BA). Endoscopic vision also is direct, which has reduced the need for brain retraction and manipulation of the aneurysm before clipping. Endoscope assistance has even allowed for the implementation of some minimally invasive approaches, such as the eyebrow ("supraciliary") keyhole approach and its variants [5–7]. The main goal of this retrospective study was to evaluate the usefulness, reliability, feasibility, advantages, and limitations of EAM in a personal institutional series of 208 surgically treated intracranial aneurysms.

G. Esposito et al. (eds.), *Trends in the Management of Cerebrovascular Diseases*, Acta Neurochirurgica Supplement, Vol. 129, https://doi.org/10.1007/978-3-319-73739-3_3, © Springer International Publishing AG, part of Springer Nature 2018

Materials and Methods

Patients Cohort

Between 2002 and 2015, 183 patients with 208 intracranial aneurysms were surgically treated by the senior author (R.G.). One hundred and ninety-one were EAM procedures. Eighty-one patients were males and 102 females, aged from 13 to 82 years (mean 50.3 years). Forty-eight patients (26.2%) presented with one or more unruptured aneurysms, whereas 135 (73.8%) had a sub-arachnoid hemorrhage (SAH) (Table 1). Twenty patients had multiple aneurysms. Eight patients with multiple aneurysms underwent multiple surgical procedures. Patients in Hunt–Hess (HH) grade 4–5 were excluded from the study. Aneurysm sizes, as maximal diameter ranged between 4 and 42 mm (mean 9.2 mm). One hundred and fifty-nine procedures were carried out on 1 or more anterior circulation aneurysms, whereas 49 were carried out on 1 or more posterior circle aneurysms (Table 2).

Table 1 Clinical onset and HH grade of treated patients

Clinical onset	SAH	135	73.8%
	Incidental	48	26.2%
Hunt–Hess Grade	I	56	41.5%
	II	58	43%
	III	21	15.5%
Timing of surgery (for ruptured aneurysms)	*<48 h*	89	65.9%
	3rd–7th days	21	15.5%
	>7th day	25	18.6%

Table 2 Aneurysms site

Aneurysms site		No.
Anterior circulation	ICA-Opht[a]	18
	ICA-PCoA	22
	ICA-AChA	25
	ICA bifurcation	21
	MCA[b]	40
	ACoA	33
Posterior circulation	BA	13
	MBT	4
	VBJ	6
	VA[c]	16
	Distal arteries	10
Total		208

[a]*Opht* ophthalmic artery
[b]*MCA* middle cerebral artery
[c]*VA* vertebral artery

Operative Technique

At the end of each selected approach, the opening of the basal cisterns and the dissection of the aneurysm, is performed under microscopic vision whereupon the endoscope is introduced into the operative field. All EAM procedures are performed with two different endoscopes: a straightforward telescope, 0° viewing angle, 2.7 mm in diameter, and 15 cm working length (Karl Storz GmbH and Co. KG, Tuttlingen, Germany, Hopkins Galzio Endoscope), and a forward-oblique telescope, 30° viewing angle, 2.7 mm in diameter, 15 cm working length, with a viewing direction at 6 and 12o'clock (Karl Storz GmbH and Co. KG, Tuttlingen, Germany, Hopkins Galzio Endoscope) (Fig. 1). A xenon light illuminates the field and the light intensity is usually set at an output up to 20% of the maximum power to avoid thermal injuries. Endoscopic and microscopic images are combined in a picture and both are seen together on a 7-in. high-resolution LCD screen assembled with the microscope and mounted above the binocular headpiece, and on a further 21-in. high-resolution monitor outside the operative field (Karl Storz GmbH and Co. KG, Tuttlingen, Germany) (Fig. 2). EAM involves three different steps: initial inspection, true operative time, and final inspection. During the initial inspection, a 0° endoscope is introduced freehand under microscopic view, a 30° endoscope often being used.

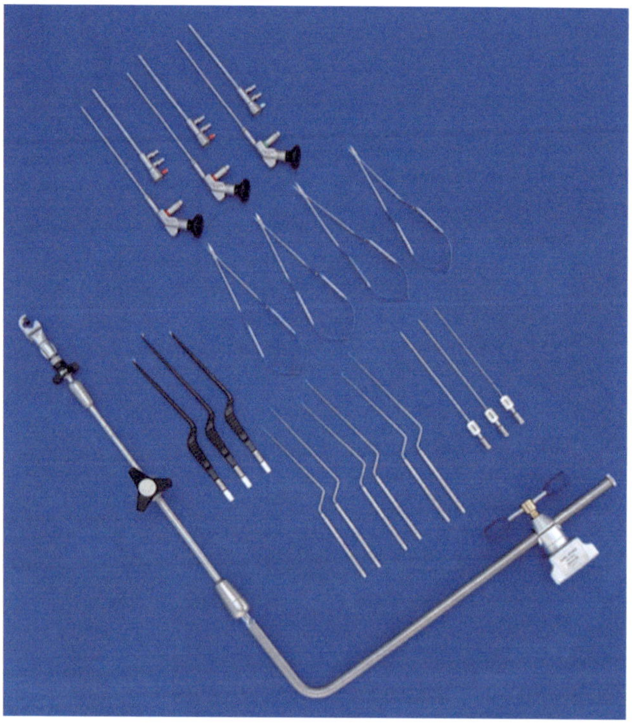

Fig. 1 Endoscopic instrumentation with mechanical holder

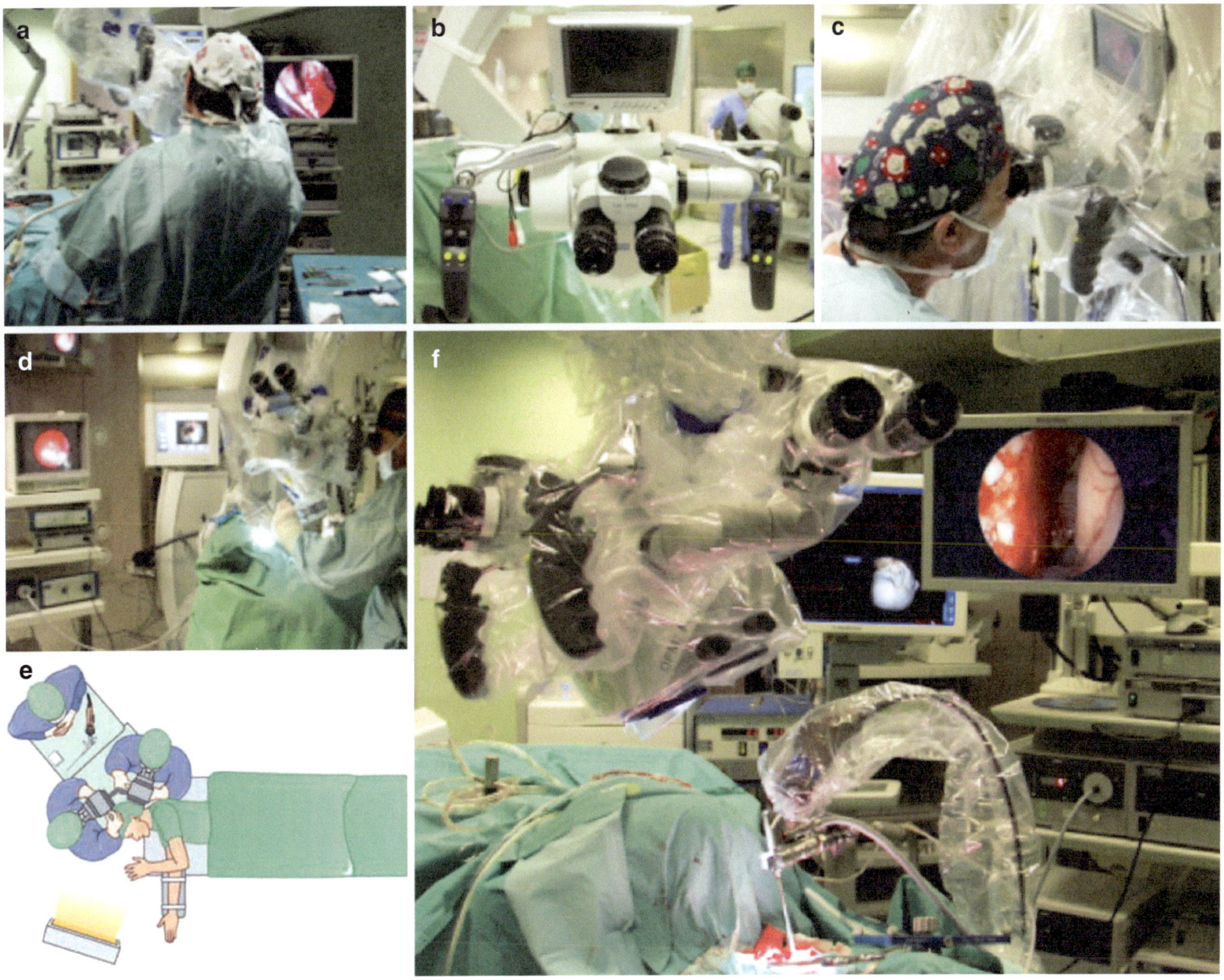

Fig. 2 Schematic drawing (**e**) and pictures illustrating the ideal position of the endoscopic monitor (**a**, **d**), placed in front of the surgeon. The 7-in. monitor mounted above the binocular headpiece allows the surgeon to maintain simultaneous control of the microscopic and endoscopic views by minimal ergonomic eye movements (**b**, **c**). Endoscope fixed in the operative field with mechanical holder (**f**)

This initial maneuver permits full inspection of the blind spot of the aneurysm and, at the same time, an early and clearer visualization of perforating branches. After the initial inspection, the endoscope is fixed to the operative table by a mechanical holder. Positioning of each clip during the true operative time is performed under a simultaneous microscopic-endoscopic view, the real time endoscopic visualization of the hidden perforating branches allowing them to be spared from any inadvertent and dangerous occlusion. Conversely, the microscopic view enables full control of the endoscope and avoids injuries to the surrounding neurovascular structures. The last step of the technique, the final inspection, is a freehand endoscopic final check of the parent artery, perforating branches, and the surrounding structures after the definitive clipping (Table 3).

Results

A successful clipping was achieved in all treated cases. In 71 aneurysms (34.2%) the adjunct of the endoscope offered extra important information about the presence of tiny perforating arteries hidden in the blind spot of aneurysms at a specific site at the ICA posterior wall, backside of the ACoA complex, and superior or posterior aspects of basilar top and midbasilar trunk (MBT). EAM also enabled clearer visualization of the posterior aspect of the aneurysm neck before the clip ligation in the same sites. In 42 cases (20.2%), the endoscope allowed for very early detection of a suboptimal or incorrect clip positioning, leading to re-positioning of the definitive clip. Most cases of incorrect clip positioning involved an inadvertent occlusion of one or more perforators.

Table 3 Endoscopic findings resulting in intraoperative clip repositioning

Aneurysms site		No.	Neck remnant	Branch occlusion	Perforator occlusion
Anterior circulation	ICA-Opht[a]	18	2	–	–
	ICA-PCoA	22	4	2	1
	ICA-AChA	25	2	4	2
	ICA bifurcation	21	3	–	–
	MCA[b]	40	–	–	–
	ACoA	33	8	4	4
Posterior circulation	BA	13	3	1	2
	MBT	4	–	–	–
	VBJ	6	—	—	—
	VA[c]	16	—	—	—
	Distal arteries	10	—	—	–
Total		208	22	11	9

[a]*Opht* ophthalmic artery
[b]*MCA* middle cerebral artery
[c]*VA* vertebral artery

The overall complication rate was of 2.4%. In three cases, impingement of the cerebral parenchyma by the endoscope was seen, despite the microscopic control. In two further cases, transient third nerve palsy caused by incomplete damage or encroachment by the endoscope or clip was seen. No aneurysm rupture was caused by the endoscope. Excellent to good recovery (GOS 4–5) was achieved in 166 patients (90%). Table 3 details the intra-operative endoscopic findings resulting in intraoperative clip repositioning.

Discussion

Although Perneczky was among the first major contributors to the field of EAM [4, 8], also advocating using the endoscope in intracranial aneurysms' surgery [9, 10], others have reported on the successful use of EAM for aneurysms surgery [11–14]. It remains today a matter of debate whether the adjunct of the endoscope is advantageous in this specific subset of pathology. In the contemporary era of minimal invasive or keyhole, skull base approaches, some non-negligible limits related to the mere microscopic view are emerging, specifically the rigid line of sight to the operative target that imposes restrictions for a certain number of specific lesions. Indeed, the smaller the extension of craniotomy, the lower the working angles to the lesion. For aneurysms, this concept is more meaningful, especially for selected sites where perforating arteries are generally hidden within the blind spot of the aneurysm itself or within the back wall of the parent vessel. The rationale of the addition of the endoscope in this surgery is linked to the attempt to overcome these limits. Although rigid, the endoscopes commonly employed for this purpose are very thin (2.7 mm) and easily adapt to the working space with little interference with the surgical maneuvers. Furthermore, the introduction of the endoscope provides a further and nearer source of light to both the operative field and the lesion, with all the related advantages. If the forward-oblique telescope is useful during the simultaneous microscopic-endoscopic view, the 30° line of sight of the angled optic is essential to inspect fully and widely the backside of the aneurysm parent artery, branches, and perforatings. In selected cases, clip ligation of the aneurysm may be performed under a full endoscopic view to obtain a "real time" sparing of the perforating arteries, thus avoiding any inadvertent stop flow into these tiny and less tolerant vessels (Fig. 3). The same advantage is obtained in the preservation of those cranial nerves located behind or very close to the aneurysm, parent vessel, or branch, but hidden by the aneurysm itself. In the present series, endoscopic assistance has been very useful as an adjunct tool to the microsurgical treatment of selected aneurysms of ICA, posterior communicating artery (PCoA), anterior choroidal artery (AChA), ACoA, and BA. In more than 20% of these aneurysms the endoscopic inspection allowed changing or repositioning of the clip or sparing one or more perforating branches, thus benefitting the surgery. Conversely, based on the authors' experience, EAM has no indication for aneurysms other than the aforementioned more superficial or far from perforating branches. EAM is not beneficial and may even become injurious in terms of the overall outcome for vertebrobasilar junction (VBJ), proximal posterior inferior cerebellar artery (PICA), distal superior cerebellar artery (SCA), and anterior inferior cerebellar artery (AICA)

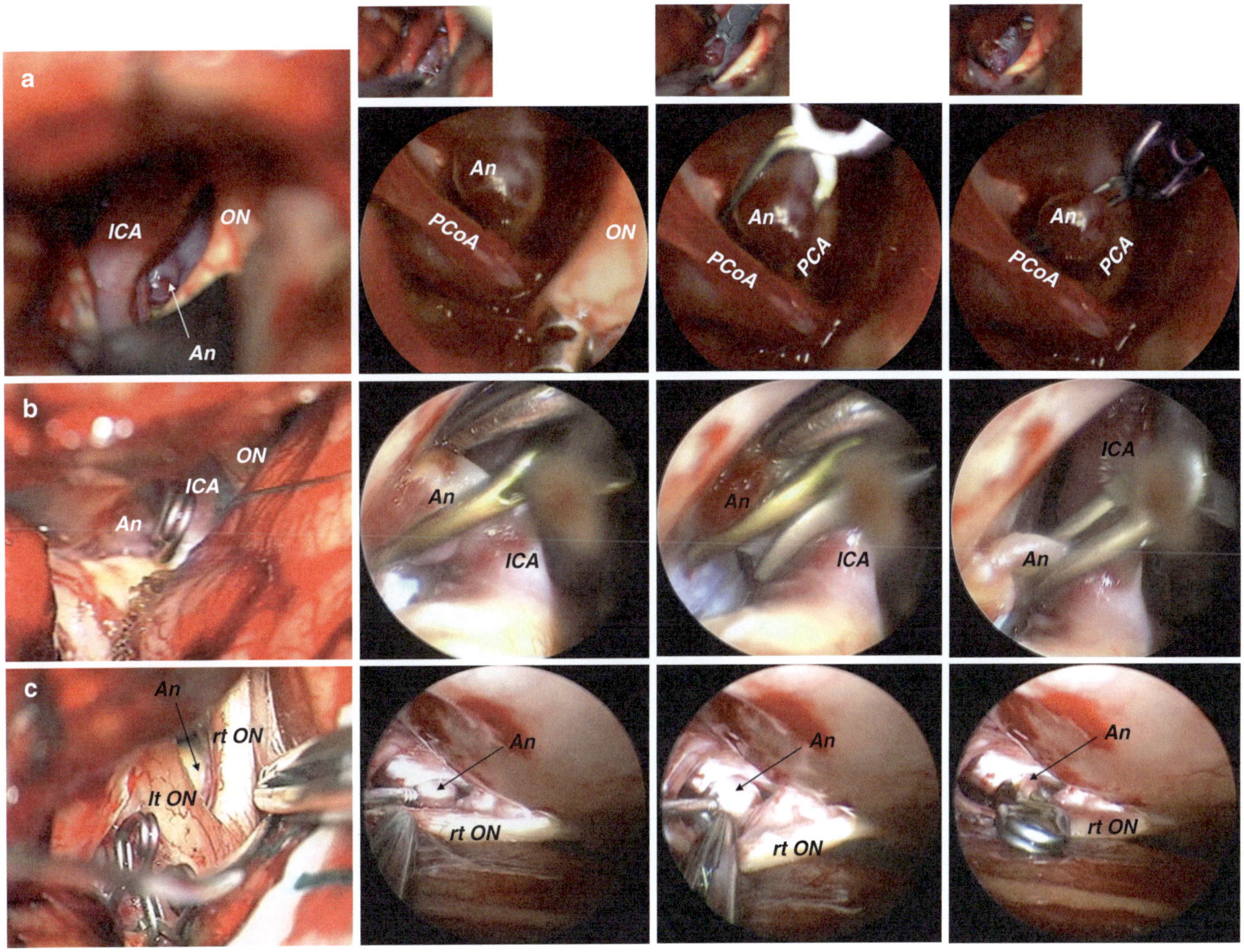

Fig. 3 Microsurgical vision of aneurysm (An) of the left PCA-SCA junctional portion of the basilar artery, lying in the corridors between optic nerve (ON) and ICA. The aneurysm was clipped through the corridor between ON and ICA, with the endoscope fixed to a mechanical holder. The final endoscopic control allowed to confirm patency of the left PCA not clearly visible under the microscope (**a**). Microsurgical view of a left ICA-PCoA aneurysm (An) after microsurgical clipping. Endoscopic inspection reveals incomplete clipping of the aneurysm. Application of an additional clip, removal of the previously released clip under endoscopic vision. Final control reveals complete aneurysm occlusion (**b**). Microscopic vision of a contralateral right ICA-PCoA aneurysm (An) through the left (lt ON) and right (rt ON) optic nerves. Endoscopic inspection of the aneurysm through the optic chiasm. Clipping of the aneurysm and final control in endoscopic view (**c**)

aneurysms, where the need to work through narrowed corridors beyond the posterior fossa cranial nerves may lead to severe sequelae by accidental cranial nerves injuries. Very large and giant aneurysms benefit less from EAM compared to the smaller ones, both because these lesions are usually exposed through larger skull base approaches, and because the larger volume of these aneurysms makes the insertion and fixation of the endoscope more difficult, which may then become dangerous.

Technically, the authors have found that the best way to obtain a complementary rather than co-axial view between microscope and endoscope and, at the same time avoid interferences with the instruments and surgical maneuvers, is to choose complementary corridors to the aneurysm. The initial endoscopic inspection of the aneurysm, parent artery, and perforating branches aids in an early understanding of the anatomy and in constructing mentally the final clipping before application of the clip but, obviously, it cannot assist in the dissection of the aneurysm, which must be performed by conventional microneurosurgical techniques. Care must be taken that all the surgical maneuvers during the *true operative time* are conducted with the endoscope firmly and mechanically fixed to the operative field. The fixation of the endoscope also allows for two-handed surgery. During the endoscopic post-clipping inspection, the usefulness of this technique may be combined with other fundamental and well-established techniques such as intraoperative neurophysiological monitoring, Doppler flowmetry, and indocyanine green videoangiography to evaluate the complete exclusion of the aneurysm and the preserved patency of the parent vessel, branches, and perforatings. Generous washing of the basal cisterns and continuous irrigation of the endoscope lens during EAM has also made this technique useful and versatile for ruptured aneurysms with a high Fisher grade in the present series. Unfortunately, the most important limit of endoscope assistance, including for aneurysms, is the 2D view of most of the endoscopes commonly used today, and this may pose some problems in terms of spatial orientation during the clipping. Although recently 3D endoscopes have been introduced for diagnostic purposes, they are generally larger in diameter than 2D ones, and this limits their use for EAM. An adequate selection of the aneurysms, the use of specific dedicated endoscopes, and the implementation of some technical tips and precautions are as mandatory as an appropriate endoscopic training to obtain the best results from endoscopic assistance during aneurysm surgery.

The data of the present personal 14-years experience have shown EAM to be a useful, reliable, and versatile technique during microneurosurgical treatment of selected aneurysms, offering some important advantages to obtain the best patients' overall outcome.

Conflict of Interest Statement The authors declare that they have no conflict of interest.

References

1. Apuzzo ML, Heifetz MD, Weiss MH, Kurze T. Neurosurgical endoscopy using the side-viewing telescope. J Neurosurg. 1977;46(3):398–400.
2. Halves E, Bushe KA. Transsphenoidal operation on craniopharyngiomas with extrasellar extensions. The advantage of the operating endoscope [proceedings]. Acta Neurochir Suppl. 1979; 28(2):362.
3. Matula C, Tschabitscher M, Day JD, Reinprecht A, Koos WT. Endoscopically assisted microneurosurgery. Acta Neurochir. 1995;134(3–4):190–5.
4. Perneczky A, Fries G. Endoscope-assisted brain surgery: part 1—evolution, basic concept, and current technique. Neurosurgery. 1998;42(2):219–24.
5. Kim Y, Yoo C-J, Park CW, Kim MJ, Choi DH, Kim YJ, Park K. Modified supraorbital keyhole approach to anterior circulation aneurysms. J Cerebrovasc Endovasc Neurosurg. 2016; 18(1):5–11.
6. Ormond DR, Hadjipanayis CG. The supraorbital keyhole craniotomy through an eyebrow incision: its origins and evolution. Minim Invasive Surg. 2013;2013:296469.
7. Reisch R, Perneczky A, Filippi R. Surgical technique of the supraorbital key-hole craniotomy. Surg Neurol. 2003;59(3):223–7.
8. Fries G, Perneczky A. Endoscope-assisted brain surgery: part 2—analysis of 380 procedures. Neurosurgery. 1998;42(2): 226–31.
9. Fischer G, Oertel J, Perneczky A. Endoscopy in aneurysm surgery. Neurosurgery. 2012;70(2 Suppl Operative):184–90.
10. Perneczky A, Boecher-Schwarz HG. Endoscope-assisted microsurgery for cerebral aneurysms. Neurol Med Chir. 1998;38(Suppl):33–4.
11. Fischer J, Mustafa H. Endoscopic-guided clipping of cerebral aneurysms. Br J Neurosurg. 1994;8(5):559–65.
12. Kalavakonda C, Sekhar LN, Ramachandran P, Hechl P. Endoscope-assisted microsurgery for intracranial aneurysms. Neurosurgery. 2002;51(5):1119–26.
13. Kato Y, Sano H, Nagahisa S, Iwata S, Yoshida K, Yamamoto K, Kanno T. Endoscope-assisted microsurgery for cerebral aneurysms. Minim Invasive Neurosurg. 2000;43(2):91–7.
14. Taniguchi M, Takimoto H, Yoshimine T, Shimada N, Miyao Y, Hirata M, Maruno M, Kato A, Kohmura E, Hayakawa T. Application of a rigid endoscope to the microsurgical management of 54 cerebral aneurysms: results in 48 patients. J Neurosurg. 1999;91(2):231–7.

Giant and Very Large Intracranial Aneurysms: Surgical Strategies and Special Issues

Sabino Luzzi, Massimo Gallieni, Mattia Del Maestro, Donatella Trovarelli, Alessandro Ricci, and Renato Galzio

Abstract Giant intracranial aneurysms (GIAs) and very large intracranial aneurysms (VLAs) have a poor natural history because of a high incidence of bleeding and strokes. These lesions always represent a great challenge for neurosurgeons and interventional neuroradiologists because of some peculiar intrinsic features such as size, angioarchitecture, wide neck, mass effect, intraluminal thrombosis, atherosclerotic changes, involvement of branches and perforators, and a frequent need to perform revascularization procedures. The results of a cumulative surgical series of 75 VLAs and GIAs are reported. Thirty-three aneurysms were unruptured. Sixty aneurysms underwent direct surgical treatment consisting of 56 direct clippings, 3 trappings w/o revascularization, and 1 wrapping. Fifteen aneurysms were treated by means of extracranial to intracranial (EC-IC) high-flow bypass. An mRS score ranging between 0 and 2 was observed in 54 patients, whereas an mRS of 3 was seen in 5 patients. Four patients had a severe disability (mRS 4–5) and six patients died. Aneurysm's fragmentation, with stacking and seating clips, thrombectomy, and aneurysmorrhaphy were the techniques most frequently employed. Revascularization options involving EC-IC high-flow bypass were used in cases not amenable for direct treatment. Some technical tips and special issues related to the surgical management of these complex lesions are discussed.

Keywords Intracranial aneurysms · Giant intracranial aneurysms · Clipping · By-pass surgery · Revascularization techniques · Subarachnoid hemorrhage

S. Luzzi, M.D. · A. Ricci, M.D.
Department of Neurosurgery, San Salvatore City Hospital, L'Aquila, Italy

M. Gallieni, M.D. (✉) · M. Del Maestro, M.D.
Department of Life, Health and Environmental Sciences (MESVA), University of L'Aquila, L'Aquila, Italy

D. Trovarelli, M.D.
Department of Anesthesiology, San Salvatore City Hospital, L'Aquila, Italy

R. Galzio, M.D.
Department of Neurosurgery, San Salvatore City Hospital, L'Aquila, Italy

Department of Life, Health and Environmental Sciences (MESVA), University of L'Aquila, L'Aquila, Italy

Introduction

Despite the tremendous advances in the understanding of their pathophysiology and surgical management, GIAs (giant intracranial aneurysms) and VLAs (very large intracranial aneurysms) still remain among the most demanding challenges for both the neurosurgeon and the interventional neuroradiologist. In their classical definition, GIAs have at least one diameter larger than 2.5 cm, with an irregular geometric configuration and a broad neck. GIAs often incorporate efferent vessels and have thick arachnoid adhesion to the surrounding structures. A massive intraluminal thrombosis is often present with atherosclerotic changes frequently involving the sac, the neck, and even the parent artery. Although theoretically the flow pulsatility may also produce a progressive enlargement of the smaller aneurysms that may become giant [1], recently GIAs formation and enlargement have proved to be completely different from those of the smaller aneurysms. Indeed, they seem to be related to a massive degeneration of the elastic lamina with a lack of the muscular layer caused by repeated sub-adventitial hemorrhages by vasa vasorum. Therefore, GIAs should be considered as a "*proliferative disease of the vessel wall induced by extravascular activity*" [2]. Regarding the intraluminal thrombosis, it occurs in approximately 60% of cases and is strictly related to the high turbulence of the jet flow. Compared with that of the smaller ones, the natural history of GIAs is extremely dismal because of their higher tendency to bleed and a higher incidence of related strokes, with consequent severe disability and death ultimately. The estimated risk of rupture is six times higher for GIAs, and a mortality rate at 2 years greater than 60% has been reported for those untreated [3, 4]. All these intrinsic features, as well as the mass effect they cause to the neighboring neurovascular structures, make VLAs and GIAs a specific subset of lesions where an aggressive treatment must be considered mandatory, as reported in a large series of publications [5–13]. Although endovascular techniques, especially with the advent of flow-diverters, flow-disruptors, and stents, are increasing their efficacy, microneurosurgery still remains the unique curative option for most of these aneurysms, especially for those with a complex angioarchitecture, involvement of efferent branches, and a massive intraluminal thrombosis. Furthermore, microsurgery is the only treatment option possible in all cases where a revascularization procedure is need.

The aim of this retrospective study is to report the decision-making process, the surgical strategies, and the special issues related to the management of VLAs and GIAs in a personal series of 75 aneurysms consecutively treated.

Materials and Methods

Between 2000 and 2015, a cohort of 428 patients, harboring 510 intracranial aneurysms, was surgically treated by the senior author (R.G.). Among these, 75 VLAs and GIAs aneurysms in 71 patients were selected and retrospectively analyzed. A further 31 VLAs (n. 19) and GIAs (n. 12), were treated by endovascular techniques. In the surgical series, 41 patients were females and 30 were males, with ages ranging between 14 and 80 years (mean 53 years). Forty-eight patients suffered from hypertension, 34 from diabetes, 16 from hypercholesterolemia, and 14 from obesity. Twenty-seven patients were smokers. In two patients, a familiar history of aneurysms was found. Fifty-six aneurysms (74.67%) were located in the anterior circle, whereas the remaining 19 (25.33%) involved the posterior circulation (Table 1). Thirty-eight aneurysms presented with a subarachnoid hemorrhage (SAH) and 33 were taken into charge to our Department because of incidental findings or symptoms attributable to the mass effect or stroke. Cranial nerve neuropathies were observed in nine patients, three with an internal carotid artery (ICA) posterior wall giant aneurysm (all with a third cranial nerve palsy). The remaining six patients suffered from a third to sixth cranial nerve impairment in various combinations. All the elective patients underwent 3D CT angiography; T1 and T2 weighted MRI, to reveal an eventual intra-aneurysmal thrombus, and six-vessels brain digital subtraction angiography (DSA) with 3D volume rendering. A detailed study of both superficial temporal artery (STA) and occipital artery (OA) was carried out in all cases where a revascularization procedure was planned or presumed. STAs and OAs larger than 3 mm were considered as suitable

Table 1 Description of aneurysms site, clinical onset, and surgical methods of treatment

Aneurysms site		No.	Clinical onset SAH	Clinical onset Not SAH	Surgical methods of treatment Clipping	Wrapping	Trapping	Trapping + EC-IC	EC-IC
Anterior circulation	Intracavernous ICA	6	0	6	0	0	0	6	0
	Para-clinoidal ICA	5	4	1	4	1	0	0	0
	ICA-ophthalmic	12	6	6	11	0	0	1	0
	ICA siphon	9	5	4	4	0	1	4	0
	ICA bifurcation	5	3	2	5	0	0	0	0
	MCA	13	7	6	11	0	0	2	0
	ACA/ACoA	5	4	1	5	0	0	0	0
	ACA2	1	1	0	1	0	0	0	0
Posterior circulation	PCA (P2-P3)	3	1	2	2	0	1	0	0
	PCA (P1-P2)	1	0	1	0	0	0	0	1
	BA tip	5	4	1	5	0	0	0	0
	BA/SCA	2	2	0	2	0	0	0	0
	BA/AICA	1	1	0	1	0	0	0	0
	AICA (proximal)	1	0	1	0	0	1	0	0
	VBJ	1	1	0	1	0	0	0	0
	VA/PICA	2	1	1	2	0	0	0	0
	Distal PICA	2	2	0	2	0	0	0	0
	VA	1	0	1	0	0	0	1	0
Total		75	42	33	56	1	3	14	1

potential donors for selected cases where the putative need for a revascularization of a distal middle cerebral artery (MCA) or posterior cerebral artery (PCA) branches might be anticipated. Moreover, in those cases where a high flow bypass was planned, the Allen test was performed in both forearms to evaluate the suitability of the radial artery as conduit. Both saphenous veins and radial arteries were traced with Doppler sonography in these cases. In all cases of aneurysms involving ICA, balloon test occlusion (BTO) was performed. For BTO, occlusion of the ICA was performed as near as possible to the aneurysms by means of a 5 Fr balloon inflated for 10 min in the first step, after which the patient was neurologically evaluated and underwent DSA. In all the cases where the patient passed the first step, an intravenous administration of labetalol (200 mL; 1 mg/mL in 2 min) was given to decrease the mean arterial pressure to a level of 20% of the baseline. The patient was then evaluated for a further 20 min and, after the induction of the relative hypotension, a final angiogram was performed. Additionally, in all the elective cases, a preoperative neurophysiological baseline assessment was performed based upon trans cranial motor-evoked potentials (TES-MEPs), somatosensory-evoked potentials (SSEPs), and brainstem-evoked potential (BAEPs), the latter only for posterior circulation aneurysms. Computerized visual field evaluation and hormonal assessment were decided case by case according to the site of the lesion. All the patients with ruptured aneurysms underwent 3D CT angiography and DSA. In selected hemorrhagic cases, MRI ruled out an intra-aneurysmal partial thrombosis.

Results

Sixty aneurysms were judged suitable for direct surgical treatment. In the remaining 15 aneurysms, a flow replacement of the parent artery or a branch was needed. In the surgical cases, the pterional trans-sylvan was the most used approach for the anterior circulation aneurysms. As a general rule, a wide drilling of the superior aspect of the greater sphenoid wing with or w/o anterior clinoidectomy, as well as a wide opening of the sylvian fissure (extended pterional approach), allowed one to maximize the exposure of the sac and to shallow the surgical field for most of the GIAs. More complex antero-lateral approaches were performed in selected cases. A cranio-orbitary approach, sometimes involving the mobilization of the zygomatic arch (fronto-temporo-orbito-zygomatic FTOZ approach), was performed in selected cases of giant superior or superior-posterior projecting anterior communicating (ACoA) aneurysms and high riding basilar top aneurysms. An intradural, rather than extradural, anterior clinoidectomy was performed when needed, especially in selected cases of ICA-ophthalmic aneurysms. The Sonopet ultrasonic aspirator (Stryker Portage, MI, USA) was frequently employed for this purpose to avoid any thermal injury to the optic nerve. Distal A2-pericallosal aneurysms were approached by an anterior interhemispheric route. P2-P3 PCA aneurysms were treated through a subtemporal transtentorial approach, whereas a case of a giant P1-P2 aneurysm was approached via an extended pterional approach with a trans-sylvan and pre-temporal combined access route. All the high-riding basilar top aneurysms were approached by an FTOZ approach involving a wide opening of the sylvan fissure. A posterior transcavernous clinoidectomy was performed in two cases of low-riding and superior-posterior projecting basilar top aneurysms. A combined supra-infratentorial transtentorial route was employed for mid-basilar trunk aneurysms. In only one case of very large low basilar aneurysm was a pure posterior petrosectomy, involving a retrolabyrinthine exposure, performed. A retrosigmoid approach was rarely used to clip distal very large superior cerebellar artery (SCA), anterior inferior cerebellar artery (AICA), and posterior inferior cerebellar artery (PICA) aneurysms. The postero-lateral far lateral approach proved to be very useful for the treatment of vertebro-basilar junction aneurysms and proximal PICA aneurysm. In a rare case of a distal very large PICA aneurysm, a suboccipital craniotomy was performed. A direct clipping was possible in most cases (56 aneurysms). A stacking and seating technique was used with most GIAs. In 21 aneurysms, an intra-aneurysmal thrombectomy was performed to reconstruct the profile of the parent vessel and definitively clip the aneurysms at the neck. Frequently, for ICA-posterior communicating artery (PCoA) aneurysms, multiple fenestrated clips were used to draw a clip line at the level of the posterior wall of the ICA, at the same time sparing PCoA, anterior choroidal artery (AChA), and perforating branches. Temporary occlusion of the parent artery was necessary in some cases of giant MCA bifurcation or trifurcation aneurysms. Temporary clipping was also applied to dissect and reshape the sac in selected cases of ACoA GIAs. In these circumstances, temporary occlusion more frequently encountered a dominant A1. Seldom was a complete trapping of the ACoA necessary. Temporary clipping was always performed under propofol-induced burst suppression and EEG, SSEPs, and TES-MEPs neurophysiological monitoring. Simple trapping was done in three giant thrombosed ICA aneurysms where patients passed BTO. Wrapping with muscle was the only treatment possible in one aneurysm. Fifteen patients underwent a revascularization procedure. In eight of these, an extracranial to intracranial (EC-IC) high flow by-pass was performed before to trap the aneurysm, whereas high flow EC-IC by-pass was the only treatment performed for all the giant intracavernous aneurysms and a further giant P1-P2 PCA aneurysm (Table 1). Elective patient candidates for a high flow bypass started aspirin (325 mg/day)

Table 2 Overall data about revascularization procedures

Aneurysms site		No.	Surgical methods of treatment		Type of graft		Patent graft at last follow-up	
			Trapping + EC-IC	EC-IC	RAG	SVG	RAG	SVG
Anterior circulation	Intracavernous ICA	6	6	0	4	2	4	1
	ICA-ophthalmic	1	1	0	1	–	1	–
	ICA siphon	4	4	0	3	1	3	0
	MCA	2	2	0	1	1	1	1
Posterior circulation	PCA (P1-P2)	1	0	1	1	–	1	–
	VA	1	1	0	1	–	1	–
Total		15	14	1	11	4	11	2

Table 3 Overall patient outcome

Modified Rankin scale (mRS)	0–1	2	3	4–5	6
Hemorrhagic 38	22 (57.89%)	4 (10.53%)	3 (7.89%)	3 (7.89%)	6 (15.79%)
Not hemorrhagic 33	25 (75.75%)	3 (9.09%)	2 (6.06%)	1 (3.03%)	2 (6.06%)
Total patients 71	47 (66.20%)	7 (9.86%)	5 (7.05%)	4 (5.63%)	8 (11.27%)

the day before surgery at least, and continued for 6 months after surgery. A radial artery graft (RAG) was the conduit in 11 patients and the saphenous vein (SVG) in 4 cases. The overall rate of the graft patency was 86% (Table 2). Both during direct clipping and during revascularization procedures, the combination of intraoperative indocyanine green videoangiography (ICG), microdoppler ultrasound (MDU), and neurophysiological monitoring were paramount to check constantly the complete exclusion of the aneurysm, the adequacy of the flow into the parent artery, branches, perforators, and by-passes, as well as to recognize promptly any warning sign of ischemia in a real time modality. In five cases, a combined simultaneous endovascular and surgical treatment was performed. In no cases was a deep hypothermia adenosine-induced circulatory arrest considered necessary in the present series.

A good overall outcome (mRS 0–2) was achieved in 54 patients, 26 of whom suffered from an SAH. The best outcome was obtained in all the anterior circulation aneurysms and in eight aneurysms involving the posterior circle. A moderate disability (mRS 3) was seen in five patients, three of whom were hemorrhagic. Severe disability (mRS 4–5) was the final outcome in four patients and six patients died (Table 3).

Discussion

VLAs and GIAs are challenging lesions where an aggressive treatment must be consider mandatory because of their poor natural history and bad prognosis [3]. The complex decision-making process related to these aneurysms should always take into account factors such as patient age and comorbidities, neurological status, Hunt–Hess and Fisher grades, aneurysm site and angioarchitecture, eventual intra-aneurysmal thrombosis, previous endovascular treatments, adequacy of cross-flow, caliber of PCoAs, BTO results, and the need for revascularization procedures. In the acute phase, endovascular treatment was reserved for older patients (age > 70 years) in severe neurological condition at admission (Hunt–Hess 4–5; Fisher 4). Except for these cases, an endovascular option was almost never considered for ruptured GIAs. The advent of pipeline embolization devices (PED) in the last few years has instead made a "first-line" endovascular approach more rational in selected elective cases of giant non-thrombosed aneurysms involving the intracavernous and paraclinoid ICA. Mid-basilar trunk large and fusiform non-thrombosed aneurysms were also considered as good candidates for flow diversion, as well as selected cases of basilar top aneurysms. Nevertheless, the DSA finding of a slow and turbulent flow into the aneurysm, with the consequent high likelihood of early thrombosis, was always considered a *conditio sine qua non* for flow diversion. Conversely, one of the most important exclusion criteria for the endovascular treatment was the presence of an intra-aneurysmal thrombus because of the related mass effect and the high incidence of strokes caused by distal embolization of atherosclerotic material. The literature reports a series of severe complications related to both balloon-assisted coiling and PED for GIAs [14]. The intrinsic features of a very complex angioarchitecture of these lesions, which frequently involves the need for a thrombectomy and a possible distal flow replacement, make microneurosurgery still the best treatment option today for most ruptured and unruptured

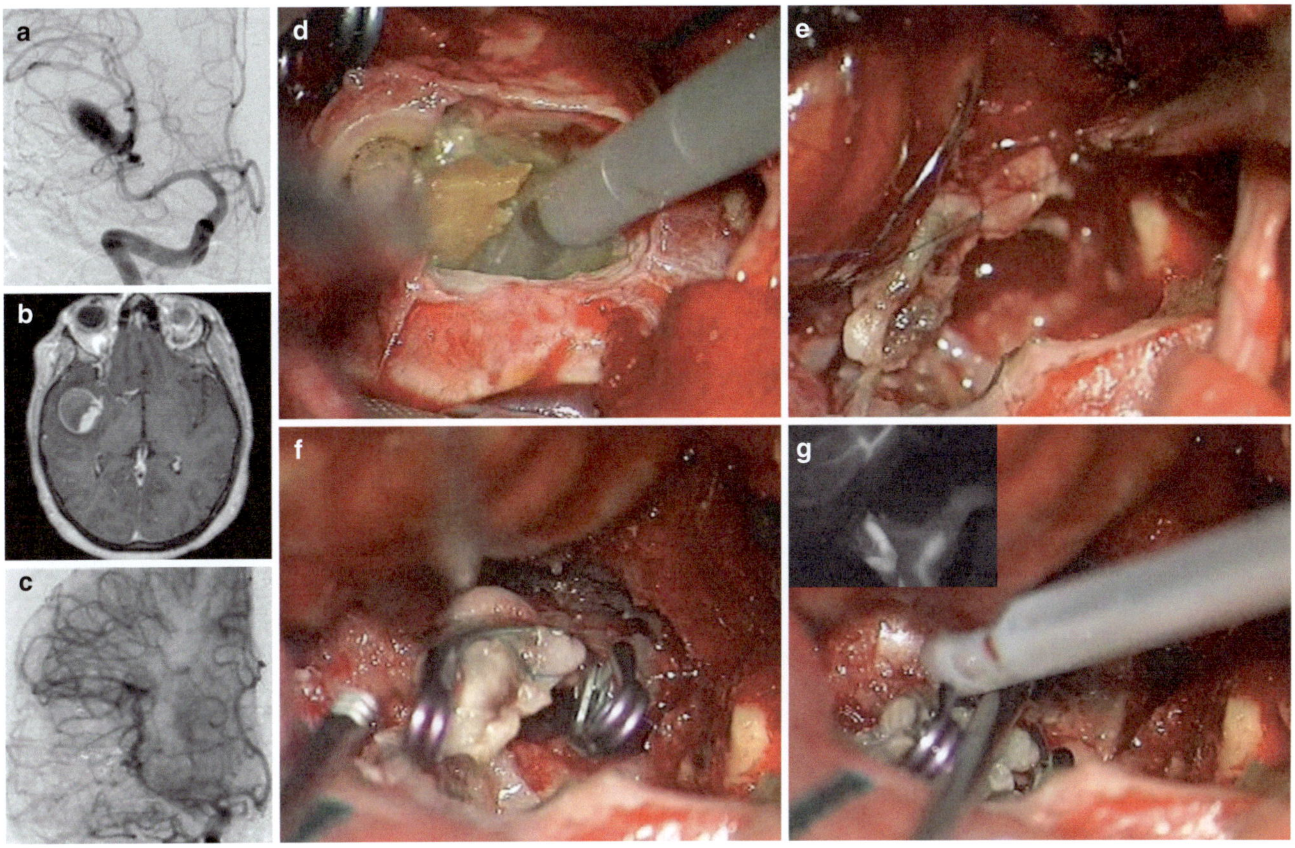

Fig. 1 Pre-operative DSA showing a very large partially thrombosed aneurysm of the right MCA (**a**). T1-weighted MRI showing intra-aneurysmal thrombus (**b**). Aneurysmal thrombectomy with ultrasonic aspirator (**d**). Aneurysmorraphy (**e**) with tandem clipping reinforcement (**f**). MDU and ICG flow check of the parent artery and branches (**g**). Post-operative DSA showing the complete exclusion of the aneurysm (**c**)

VLAs and GIAs. Angiographic and clinical results of the present series confirm that a direct treatment of the aneurysm is advisable whenever possible, whereas more complex revascularization procedures, stand-alone or associated with proximal ligation or trapping of the aneurysm, should be reserved for limited cases not amenable to direct clipping and burdened with mass effect. Technically, giant thrombosed aneurysms always require a deliberate opening of the sac, an intra-aneurysmal thrombectomy, and a subsequent aneurysmorrhaphy that is more often performed under proximal temporary clipping of the parent artery (Fig. 1). Seldom, and generally for distal ICA aneurysms in patients with a valuable contralateral cross-flow, a trapping of the parent artery is required during aneurysmorrhaphy. Even in burst suppression, SSEPs and BAEPs monitoring add paramount information to distinguish between those tolerated and those not tolerated by stop flow conditions. An important surgical tip during thrombectomy is always to check for a complete freeing of the proximal and distal parent artery ostium from the thrombus to dramatically decrease the risk of distal embolization of atherosclerotic material. A generous washing of the parent artery with heparin solution is recommended before aneurysmorrhaphy and before temporary clips release. Running suture with prolene or ethilon is generally used for aneurysmorrhaphy and, in most of conditions, a tandem clipping with angulated clips is performed to reinforce the site of the suture line. A constant intraoperatively check of the flow is elegantly obtained in these cases thanks to ICG and MDU. The stacking and seating technique with multiple clips is frequently employed to clip these aneurysms, both thrombosed and non-thrombosed. Fenestrated clips are useful to spare branching vessels, especially in posterior wall giant ICA aneurysms. Fenestrated clips are also frequently employed as boost clips to reinforce the clip blades closure of standard clips. The latter technical tip applies mainly to those cases characterized by the presence of severe atherosclerotic changes involving the aneurysm neck and the parent artery.

The literature suggests that surgical or endovascular proximal Hunterian occlusion of the parent artery harboring a large to giant aneurysm should be avoided because of a high incidence of stroke, even in those non-thrombosed aneurysms where the patient passed BTO [11, 15–22].

Regarding the revascularization procedures (Fig. 2), the rationale for a bypass for GIAs may include the need for flow replacement of the parent artery or one or more branches in

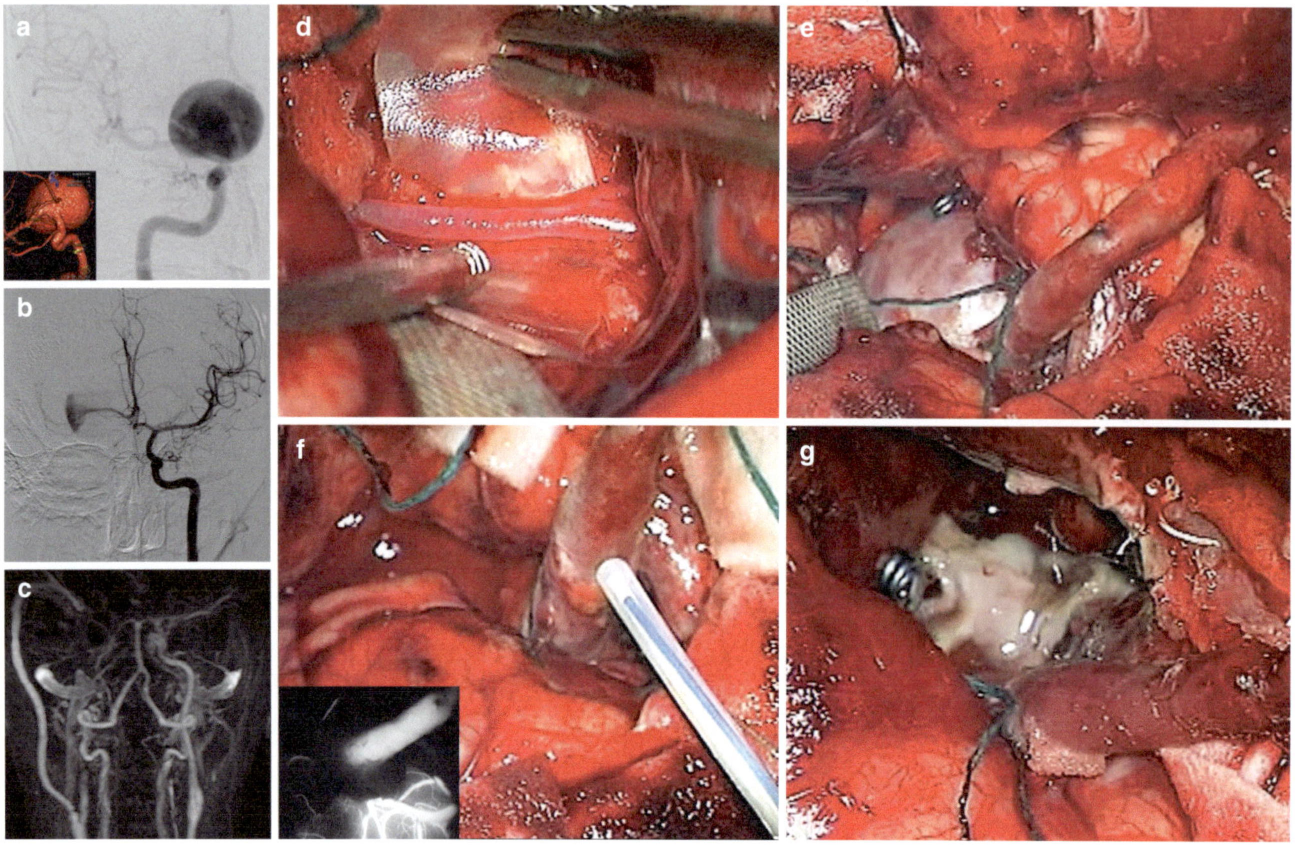

Fig. 2 Pre-operative DSA with 3D volume rendering showing a giant partially thrombosed aneurysm of the right iuxta-clinoidal ICA with huge mass effect (**a**). BTO showing an unsatisfactory cross-flow. The patient also failed BTO clinically (**b**). Initial step of EC-IC involving the superior frontal branch of post-bifurcation MCA (**d**). Saphenous vein graft EC-IC bypass (**e**). Intra-operative MDU and ICG flow check showing the patency of the bypass (**f**). Final clipping of the aneurysm achieved after thrombectomy (**g**). Post-operative MRI angiography at 6th month follow-up showing the complete exclusion of the aneurysm and the patency of the high flow bypass (**c**)

those cases where they cannot be preserved, but also the prevention of a post-operative stroke in selected cases requiring a prolonged temporary parent vessel occlusion (temporary bypass), especially in patients with a reduced cerebrovascular reserve. In the personal series, the authors preferred to proceed to bypass whenever in doubt because of the detection of TES-MEPs or SSEPs modifications not exceeding the threshold considered predictive of ischemia, or in rare cases of contradictory findings between TES-MEPs and SSEPs. RAG high-flow bypass is the most frequently performed to replace ICA and proximal MCA. RAG seems to be associated with a lower incidence of long-term graft occlusion [9], being therefore considered as the best conduit for high-flow bypasses, as also confirmed by the present data. Revascularization procedures aimed at replacing distal ACA or PICA involve side-to-side in situ bypasses. A further bypass option, especially in rare cases of large fusiform M1 MCA aneurysms, is the interposition-graft bypass, where the radial artery or STA should be preferentially used.

Microneurosurgery is still, to date, the best treatment option for most very large and giant complex intracranial aneurysms. The surgical treatment of these lesions always requires detailed and careful preoperative planning and specific surgical skills, including extensive experience in the management of direct clipping of intracranial aneurysms and dexterity with micro suturing techniques. The preoperative planning of these aneurysms should also take into account the selection of the most suitable approach among a large number of skull base approaches in which the neurovascular surgeon must have great confidence. Neuronavigation, intraoperative neurophysiological monitoring, ICG videoangiography, and MDU are essential and unavoidable tools in the surgical armory needed to treat these extremely complex and challenging lesions.

Conflict of Interest Statement The authors declare that they have no conflict of interest.

References

1. Barth A, de Tribolet N. Growth of small saccular aneurysms to giant aneurysms: presentation of three cases. Surg Neurol. 1994;41(4):277–80.
2. Krings T, Piske RL, Lasjaunias PL. Intracranial arterial aneurysm vasculopathies: targeting the outer vessel wall. Neuroradiology. 2005;47(12):931–7.
3. Barrow DL, Alleyne C. Natural history of giant intracranial aneurysms and indications for intervention. Clin Neurosurg. 1995;42:214–44.
4. International Study of Unruptured Intracranial Aneurysms Investigators. Unruptured intracranial aneurysms—risk of rupture and risks of surgical intervention. N Engl J Med. 1998;339(24):1725–33.
5. Drake CG. Giant intracranial aneurysms: experience with surgical treatment in 174 patients. Clin Neurosurg. 1979;26:12–95.
6. Hosobuchi Y. Direct surgical treatment of giant intracranial aneurysms. J Neurosurg. 1979;51(6):743–56.
7. Lawton MT, Spetzler RF. Surgical management of giant intracranial aneurysms: experience with 171 patients. Clin Neurosurg. 1995;42:245–66.
8. Lawton MT, Spetzler RF. Surgical strategies for giant intracranial aneurysms. Neurosurg Clin N Am. 1998;9(4):725–42.
9. Sekhar LN, Tariq F, Mai JC, Kim LJ, Ghodke B, Hallam DK, Bulsara KR. Unyielding progress: treatment paradigms for giant aneurysms. Clin Neurosurg. 2012;59:6–21.
10. Sousa A, Sousa Filho J, Dellaretti Filho M. Treatment of giant intracranial aneurysms: a review based on experience from 286 cases. Arq Bras Neurocir. 2015;34(4):295–303.
11. Spetzler RF, Schuster H, Roski RA. Elective extracranial-intracranial arterial bypass in the treatment of inoperable giant aneurysms of the internal carotid artery. J Neurosurg. 1980;53(1):22–7.
12. Sundt TM, Piepgras DG. Surgical approach to giant intracranial aneurysms. Operative experience with 80 cases. J Neurosurg. 1979;51(6):731–42.
13. Symon L, Vajda J. Surgical experiences with giant intracranial aneurysms. J Neurosurg. 1984;61(6):1009–28.
14. Jahromi BS, Mocco J, Bang JA, Gologorsky Y, Siddiqui AH, Horowitz MB, Hopkins LN, Levy EI. Clinical and angiographic outcome after endovascular management of giant intracranial aneurysms. Neurosurgery. 2008;63(4):662–74.
15. Diaz FG, Ausman JI, Pearce JE. Ischemic complications after combined internal carotid artery occlusion and extracranial-intracranial anastomosis. Neurosurgery. 1982;10(5):563–70.
16. Hacein-Bey L, Connolly ES, Duong H, Vang MC, Lazar RM, Marshall RS, Young WL, Solomon RA, Pile-Spellman J. Treatment of inoperable carotid aneurysms with endovascular carotid occlusion after extracranial-intracranial bypass surgery. Neurosurgery. 1997;41(6):1225–31.
17. Heros RC. Thromboembolic complications after combined internal carotid ligation and extra- to-intracranial bypass. Surg Neurol. 1984;21(1):75–9.
18. Heros RC, Nelson PB, Ojemann RG, Crowell RM, DeBrun G. Large and giant paraclinoid aneurysms: surgical techniques, complications, and results. Neurosurgery. 1983;12(2):153–63.
19. Ibrahim TF, Jahromi BR, Miettinen J, Raj R, Andrade-Barazarte H, Goehre F, Kivisaari R, Lehto H, Hernesniemi J. Long-term causes of death and excess mortality after carotid artery ligation. World Neurosurg. 2016;90:116–22.
20. Niiro M, Shimozuru T, Nakamura K, Kadota K, Kuratsu J. Long-term follow-up study of patients with cavernous sinus aneurysm treated by proximal occlusion. Neurol Med Chir. 2000;40(2):88–96.
21. Polevaya NV, Kalani MYS, Steinberg GK, Tse VCK. The transition from hunterian ligation to intracranial aneurysm clips: a historical perspective. Neurosurg Focus. 2006;20(6):E3.
22. Steinberg GK, Drake CG, Peerless SJ. Deliberate basilar or vertebral artery occlusion in the treatment of intracranial aneurysms. Immediate results and long-term outcome in 201 patients. J Neurosurg. 1993;79(2):161–73.

Modified Extradural Temporopolar Approach for Paraclinoid Aneurysms: Operative Nuance and Surgical Result

Naoki Otani, Terushige Toyooka, Satoru Takeuchi, Arata Tomiyama, Yasuaki Nakao, Takuji Yamamoto, Kojiro Wada, and Kentaro Mori

Abstract *Background.* Extradural temporopolar approach can provide extensive exposure of the anterior clinoid process, which can prevent intraoperative neurovascular injury in anterior clinoidectomy for paraclinoid aneurysms. The present study investigates the usefulness of this modified technique, and operative nuances are discussed here.

Methods. We retrospectively reviewed the medical charts of 30 consecutive patients with paraclinoid aneurysms who underwent treatment with this modified extradural temporopolar approach between September 2009 and March 2016.

Results. Worsening of visual acuity was documented postoperatively in three patients (10.0%), and visual field function worsened in three patients (10.0%). Postoperative outcome was good recovery in all patients. No operation-related mortality occurred in the series.

Conclusion. Extradural anterior clinoidectomy via the modified extradural temporopolar approach is safe and may be recommended for surgical treatment of paraclinoid aneurysms to reduce the risk of intraoperative optic neurovascular injury.

Keywords Extradural temporopolar approach · Paraclinoid anevurysm · Skull base surgery · Microneurosurgery

N. Otani, M.D. (✉) · T. Toyooka · S. Takeuchi · A. Tomiyama
K. Wada · K. Mori
Department of Neurosurgery, National Defense Medical College, Tokorozawa, Japan
e-mail: naotani@ndmc.ac.jp

Y. Nakao · T. Yamamoto
Department of Neurosurgery, Juntendo University Shizuoka Hospital, Izunokuni, Japan

Introduction

Paraclinoid aneurysms present great difficulties for complete clipping, which may require removal of the anterior clinoid process (ACP). The extradural technique for complete removal of the ACP was introduced by Dolenc in 1983 [1]. The extradural temporopolar approach (EDTPA) is a variant of Dolenc's technique and provides a surgical corridor to the central skull base [2]. The disadvantage of the EDTPA is the risk of injuring the neurovascular structures passing through the superior orbital fissure (SOF) during dissection [3]. Therefore, we recently modified EDTPA to be less invasive [4, 5]. Here we show the feasibility and usefulness of this modified approach for direct clipping of paraclinoid aneurysms and suggest that modified EDTPA can be safely performed and this procedure may improve the surgical outcome for paraclinoid aneurysms.

Patients and Methods

Patient Characteristics

This retrospective analysis included 30 consecutive patients (27 women and 3 men) aged 30–75 years (mean 53.5 years) with paraclinoid aneurysms who underwent modified EDTPA with mini-peeling of the dura propria at the National Defense Medical College Hospital and Juntendo University Shizuoka Hospital between September 2009 and March 2016. Medical charts, radiological findings, surgical techniques, complications, and the final results of anterior clinoidectomy were retrospectively reviewed. All patients underwent detailed preoperative and postoperative evaluation of visual function, which involved testing visual acuity with optimum correction lenses for both eyes, visual field examinations, and funduscopy.

G. Esposito et al. (eds.), *Trends in the Management of Cerebrovascular Diseases*, Acta Neurochirurgica Supplement, Vol. 129, https://doi.org/10.1007/978-3-319-73739-3_5,

Surgical Procedure

After induction of general anesthesia, the patient is placed in the supine position, and the head is rotated away from the operative side at about 30°. A semi-coronal skin incision is performed followed by interfascial dissection. The cervical common carotid artery, the internal carotid artery (ICA), and the external carotid artery are routinely exposed for proximal control, suction decompression, intraoperative angiography, and high-flow bypass if necessary. A standard frontotemporal craniotomy is performed. The temporal squama is rongeured out until the floor of the middle cranial fossa is exposed. The lesser wing of the sphenoid is flattened until the meningo-orbital band (MOB) is exposed. The middle fossa dura is dissected until the SOF and the foramen rotundum (FR) are exposed (Fig. 1a). The roof of the SOF is skeletonized and opened to expose the junction between the dura propria of the temporal lobe and the periosteal dura (Fig. 1a; arrowheads). The bone around the MOB is drilled (Fig. 1a; arrow) and the MOB is incised. The dura between SOF and FR, where no neuronal structure is present, is partially incised (Fig. 1a; red dashed line). Peeling of the dura propria is continued until the ACP is exposed epidurally (Fig. 1b). Drilling of the ACP with a high-speed drill using cold saline irrigation is started from the lateral part of the ACP, and the optic canal is then partially opened (Fig. 1b). After removal of the ACP, the clinoid segment (C3) of the ICA can be seen (Fig. 1b). The remainder of the optic strut can be removed with a micro-punch to provide space for the clip blade. The dura mater is opened along the sylvian fissure, and continued inferomedially to the level of the optic nerve (Fig. 1b; red dashed line). Additional wide opening of the sylvian fissure is helpful for minimal retraction of the frontal lobe to expose the ICA and the optic nerve. The posterior communicating artery, anterior choroidal artery, and their branches are identified. In addition, the horizontal portion of the anterior cerebral artery (ACA) is dissected. An incision from the falciform ligament to the optic sheath helps to mobilize the optic nerve. An additional incision is made across the distal dural ring to expose and identify the origin of the ophthalmic artery and to mobilize the ICA. After temporary clips are applied to the proximal ICA, under suction decompression, aneurysm dissection and clipping are performed.

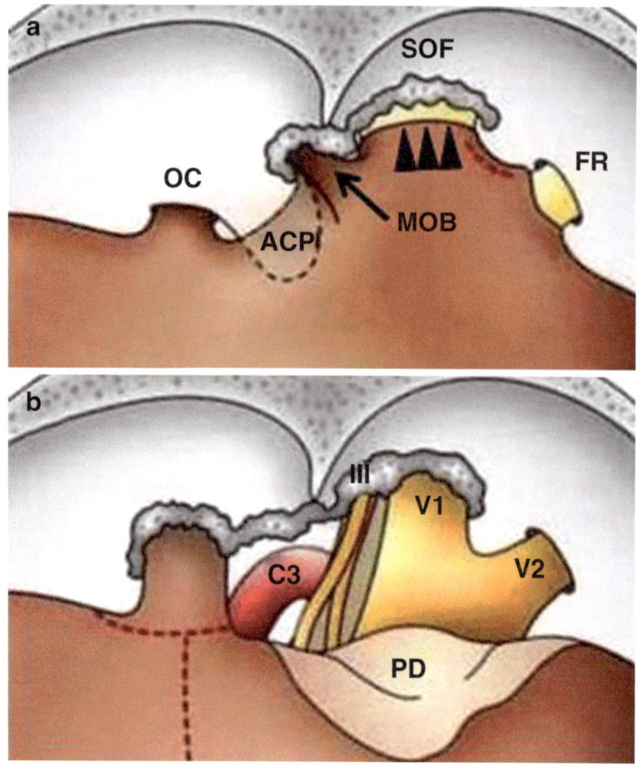

Fig. 1 Surgical procedures for clipping of paraclinoid aneurysms using the modified EDTPA technique. The middle fossa dura is dissected until the superior orbital fissure (SOF) and the foramen rotundum (FR) are exposed (**a**). The roof of the SOF is skeletonized and opened to expose the junction between the dura propria and the periosteal dura (**a**; arrowheads). The dura between the SOF and FR, where no neuronal structure is present, is partially incised (**a**; red dashed line). Peeling of the dura propria is continued until the anterior clinoid process (ACP) is exposed epidurally, and then the optic canal (OC) is opened (**b**). After removal of the ACP, the clinoid segment (C3) of the internal carotid artery can be seen through carotid-oculomotor membrane (**b**). Then the dura mater is opened along the sylvian fissure, and continued inferomedially to the level of the optic nerve (**b**; red dashed line). *SOF* superior orbital fissure, *FR* foramen rotundum, *MOB* meningo-orbital band, *PD* periosteal dura, *V1* first division of the trigeminal nerve, *V2* second division of the trigeminal nerve, OC optic canal, *III* oculomotor nerve

Results

The aneurysm was small (<6 mm) in 10 cases, medium (6–11 mm) in 13, and large (>12 mm) in 7. Twenty-six patients were asymptomatic, and four presented with symptoms including visual disturbance. Spinal drainage was induced in all patients. Orbito-zygomatic craniotomy was additionally performed in two patients. Total removal of the ACP was performed in all patients. The optic canal was opened widely in 28 patients and partially in 2. The falciform ligament was cut in 28 patients. The dural ring was incised in 28 patients. Suction decompression was used for clipping of aneurysms in 15. The cervical ICA was secured in all patients for proximal control of the ICA, and high-flow bypass was needed in one.

Direct clipping of the aneurysm neck was successfully achieved in all cases. Postoperative 3DCTA or DSA revealed no major branch occlusion or residual aneurysm. There was no surgical mortality related to EDTPA.

Overall visual acuity after surgery was unchanged in 27, and worsened in 3 (10.0%) postoperatively. These

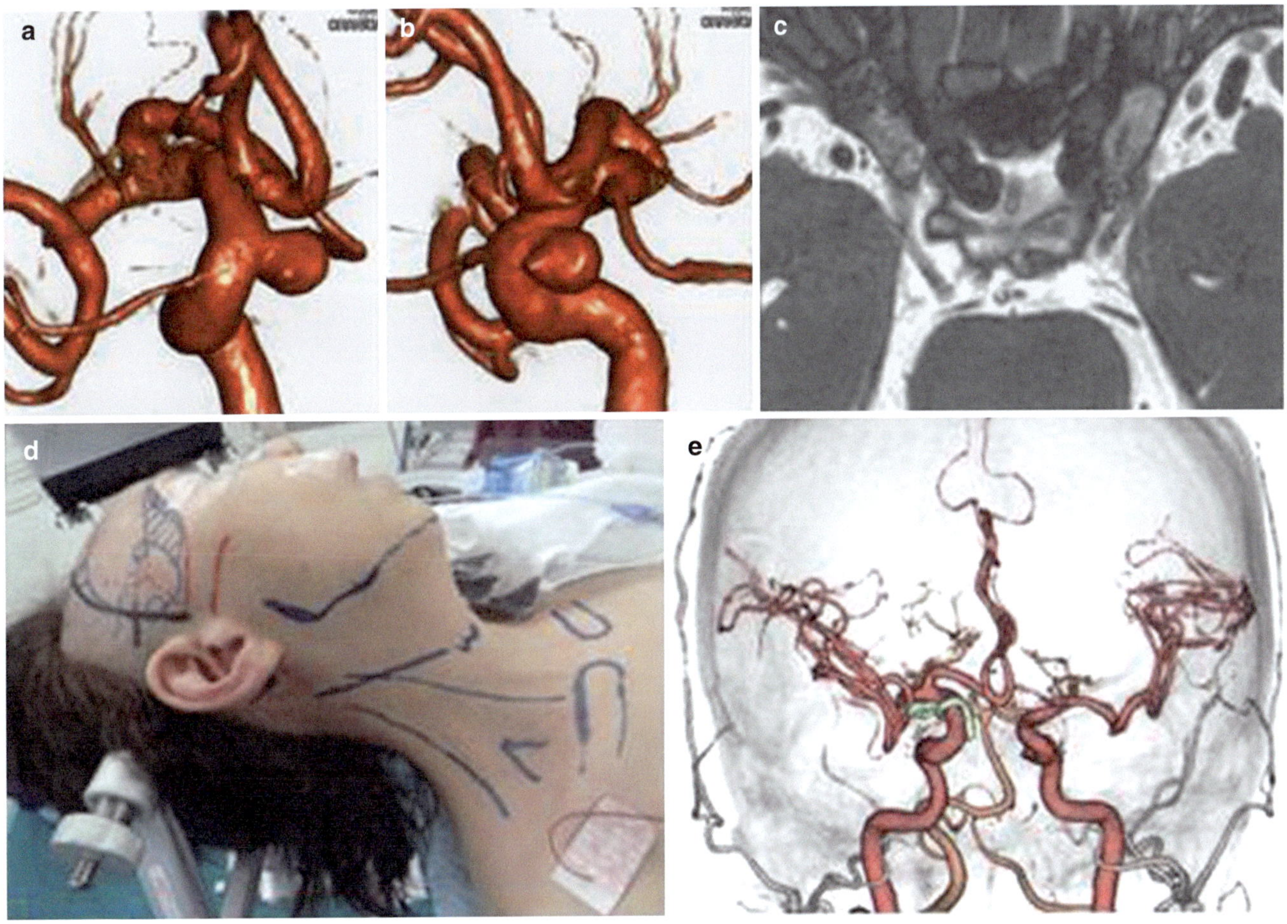

Fig. 2 A 67-year-old female presented with mild headache. 3DCTA and MR imaging incidentally discovered carotid cave aneurysm on the right. (**a–c**) The modified EDTPA was performed. (**d**) Complete clipping was achieved and (**e**) the postoperative course was uneventful

postoperative visual disturbances were usually confirmed as transient unilateral lower-nasal quadrantanopsia, which was definitely detected using a quantitative visual examination without subjective visual symptoms. One patient suffered transient brain swelling caused by sphenoparietal sinus injury during peeling of the dural layers. One patient experienced postoperative acute epidural hematoma which was evacuated immediately. No permanent neurological deficits were encountered. Postoperative outcome was good recovery in all patients.

Case Presentation

Case 1 A 67-year-old female presented with mild headache. 3DCTA and MR imaging incidentally discovered a carotid cave aneurysm on the right (Fig. 2a–c). The modified EDTPA was performed (Fig. 2d). Complete clipping was achieved (Fig. 2e) and the postoperative course was uneventful.

Case 2 A 71-year-old male presented with left hemiquadrantanopsia and decreased visual acuity. 3DCTA showed a small paraclinoid aneurysm originating from the C2 of the ICA and projecting medial-superiorly. Modified EDTPA was used. Under suction decompression, aneurysmal dissection and complete clipping was performed (Fig. 3a–d), and the postoperative course was uneventful. Postoperative visual examination showed that his visual disturbance had normalized.

Discussion

Removal of the ACP is one of the essential skull base techniques for treating paraclinoid aneurysms [6, 7]. Anterior clinoidectomy can be performed through the intradural approach or extradural approach [2, 8]. Extradural anterior clinoidectomy is more extensive than the intradural procedure and requires a clear understanding of the anatomical background of the ACP and its surrounding neurovascular structures. In particular, the surgeon must have good knowledge of the osseous structure of the SOF, the neurovascular structures passing through the SOF, and the membranous

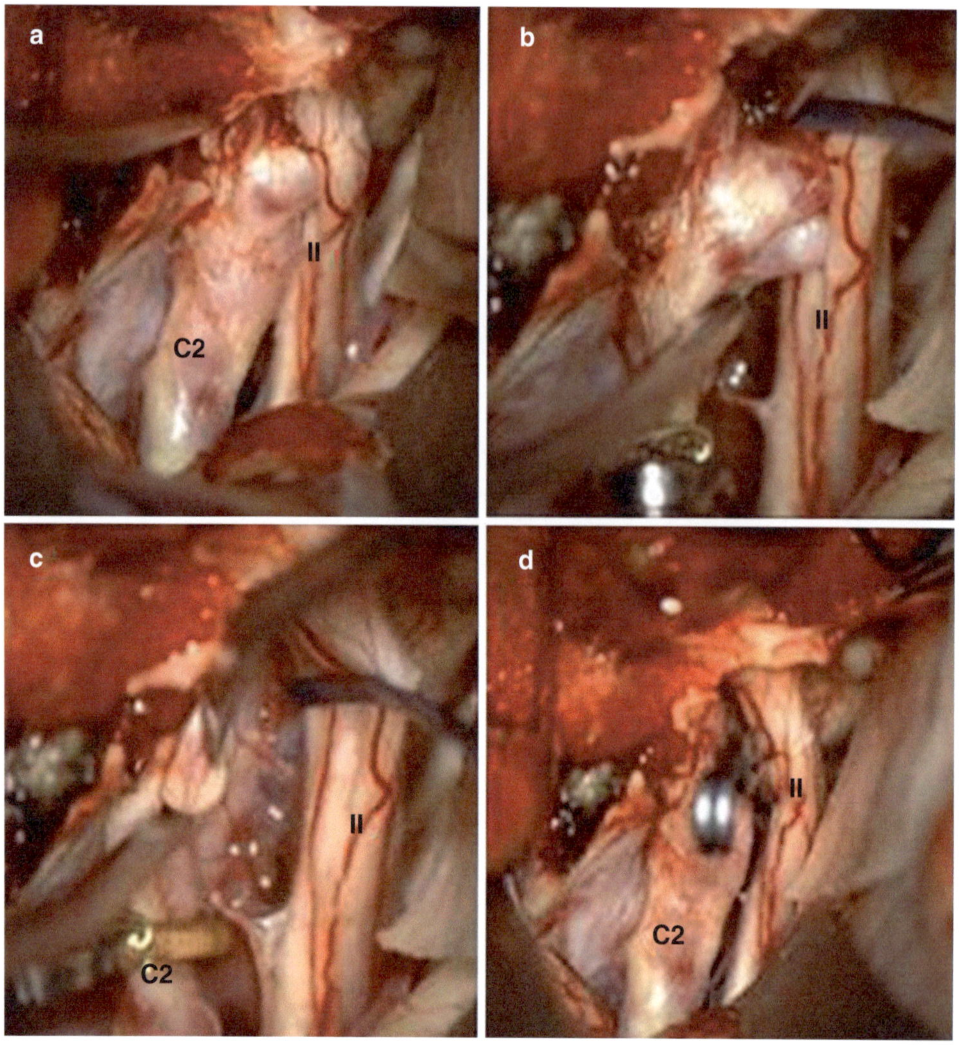

Fig. 3 A 71-year-old male presented with left hemi-quadrantanopsia and decreased visual acuity. 3DCTA showed a small paraclinoid aneurysm originating from the C2 of the ICA and projecting medial-superiorly. The modified EDTPA was performed. Under suction decompression, aneurysmal dissection and complete clipping was performed (**a–d**) and the postoperative course was uneventful. Postoperative visual examination showed visual disturbance had normalized

structures including the MOB and walls of the Cavernous Sinus (CS). Extradural anterior clinoidectomy was originally described in 1983 by Dolenc [1]. This technique was then developed, as Selective Extradural Anterior Clinoidectomy (SEAC) without peeling of the lateral wall of the CS requires opening of the optic canal and en bloc removal of the ACP [8, 9]. Recently, the latter method has been refined by minimizing the area of peeling in the lateral wall of the SOF, including the anterior part of the CS that requires extradural exposure of the ACP [10, 11]. In addition, this extradural procedure has been developed as a trans-SOF approach with mini-peeling of the SOF [12–14]. These techniques promote exposure of the entire ACP with safe drilling. Compared to previous surgical procedures, our trans-SOF approach caused fewer surgical complications, such as visual disturbance, oculomotor nerve disturbance, and poor surgical outcome [4, 5]. This modified technique requires peeling of the dura propria of the temporal lobe from the SOF. Otani et al. [4] suggested that the junction between the dura propria, which consists of the cranial nerve perineurium, and the periosteal dura was invaginated under the SOF. In contrast, no such invagination of the periosteal dura was present at the levels of the FR and Foramen Rotundum (FO). Therefore, SOF skeletonization is mandatory just before peeling of the dura propria at the SOF level. The original Dolenc's procedure requires dural incision at the SOF and may carry the risk of injury to the cranial nerves. Our modified method requires skeletonization of the SOF to expose this junction and needs only minimal dural incision between the SOF and FR where no cranial nerves are present. The dura propria peeling can be safely performed from these junctions until the ACP is totally exposed epidurally.

Cadaveric studies have shown that the anterior clinoidectomy technique can double the exposure and mobilization of the optic nerve and ICA, as well as triple or quadruple the optico-carotid triangle width and oculomotor triangle size [15, 16]. Subsequently, the medial tentorium should be carefully shaved off from the anterior petroclinoid ligament to avoid injury to the extradural part of the oculomotor nerve. After tentorial cutting, the temporal lobe with dura mater can be retracted posteriorly. We have not experienced any temporal lobe contusion caused by such retraction. The extent of dura propria peeling into the CS depends on the individual pathology. Consequently, the ETA technique was useful for maximal resection of tumors involving the retrochiasmatic space. In the present study, one patient suffered transient brain swelling caused by sphenoparietal sinus injury during peeling of the dural layers. The sphenoparietal sinus should be carefully dissected and spared at the dura propria. Care should be taken to maintain the sphenoparietal sinus at the dura propria and to stop the peeling at the point where the sphenoparietal sinus drains into the CS to prevent problems of venous congestion.

Conclusion

A series of 30 patients with paraclinoid aneurysms who underwent ETA was analyzed. Clipping of the aneurysms was achieved with minimal surgical complications in the majority of the patients. The modified EDTPA technique, which leads to excellent improvement of the visual function and overall clinical outcomes, can be a useful and safe surgical technique.

Conflict of Interest Statement There is no potential COI which should be disclosed.

References

1. Dolenc VV. Direct microsurgical repair of intracavernous vascular lesions. J Neurosurg. 1983;58:824–31.
2. Day JD, Giannotta SL, Fukushima T. Extradural temporopolar approach to lesions of the upper basilar artery and infrachiasmatic region. J Neurosurg. 1994;81:230–5.
3. Yoon BH, Kim HK, Park MS, Kim SM, Chung SY, Lanzino G. Meningeal layers around anterior clinoid process as a delicate area in extradural anterior clinoidectomy: anatomical and clinical study. J Korean Neurosurg Soc. 2012;52:391–5.
4. Otani N, Wada K, Toyooka T, Fujii K, Kobayashi Y, Mori K. Operative surgical nuances of modified extradural temporopolar approach with mini-peeling of dura propria based on cadaveric anatomical study of lateral cavernous structures. Surg Neurol Int. 2016;7(Suppl 16):S454–8.
5. Otani N, Wada K, Toyooka T, Fujii K, Ueno H, Tomura S, Tomiyama A, Nakao Y, Yamamoto T, Mori K. Usefulness of suction decompression method combined with extradural temporopolar approach during clipping of complicated internal carotid artery aneurysm. World Neurosurg. 2016;90:293–9.
6. Day AL. Aneurysms of the ophthalmic segment. A clinical and anatomical analysis. J Neurosurg. 1990;72:677–91.
7. Nutik SL. Removal of the anterior clinoid process for exposure of the proximal intracranial carotid artery. J Neurosurg. 1988;69:529–34.
8. Yonekawa Y, Ogata N, Imhof HG, Olivecrona M, Strommer K, Kwak TE, Roth P, Groscurth P. Selective extradural anterior clinoidectomy for supra- and parasellar processes. Technical note. J Neurosurg. 1997;87:636–42.
9. Otani N, Muroi C, Yano H, Khan N, Pangalu A, Yonekawa Y. Surgical management of tuberculum sellae meningioma: role of of selective extradural anterior clinoidectomy. Br J Neurosurg. 2006;20:129–38.
10. Coscarella E, Bakaya MK, Morcos JJ. An alternative extradural exposure to the anterior clinoid process: the superior orbital fissure as a surgical corridor. Neurosurgery. 2003;53:162–6.
11. Noguchi A, Balasingam V, Shiokawa Y, McMenomey SO, Delashaw JB Jr. Extradural anterior clinoidectomy. Technical note. J Neurosurg. 2005;102:945–50.
12. Mori K, Yamamoto T, Oyama K, Ueno H, Nakao Y, Honma K. Modified three-dimensional skull base model with artificial dura mater, cranial nerves, and venous sinuses for training in skull base surgery: technical note. Neurol Med Chir (Tokyo). 2008;48: 582–7.
13. Mori K. Dissectable modified three-dimensional temporal bone and whole skull base models for training in skull base approaches. Skull Base. 2009;19:333–44.
14. Mori K, Yamamoto T, Oyama K, Nakao Y. Modification of three-dimensional prototype temporal bone model for training in skull-base surgery. Neurosurg Rev. 2009;32:233–8.
15. Evans JJ, Hwang YS, Lee JH. Pre- versus post-anterior clinoidectomy measurements of the optic nerve, internal carotid artery and opticocarotid triangle. A cadaveric morphometric study. Neurosurgery. 2000;46:1018–23.
16. Sade B, Kweon CY, Evans JJ, Lee JH. Enhanced exposure of caroticooculomotor triangle following extradural anterior clinoidectomy: a comparative anatomical study. Skull Base. 2005;15:157–61.

Extradural Anterior Clinoidectomy and Optic Canal Unroofing for Paraclinoid and Basilar Aneurysms: Usefulness of a No-Drill Instrumental Method

Koichi Iwasaki, Hiroki Toda, Hirokuni Hashikata, Masanori Goto, and Hitoshi Fukuda

Abstract The authors describe extradural anterior clinoidectomy without the use of a high-speed drill or ultrasonic device to clip paraclinoid and basilar aneurysms, which can eliminate potential complications related to traditional power drilling or ultrasonic device use. This method involves four steps: (1) partial osteotomy of the sphenoid wing at the superior orbital fissure (SOF); (2) peeling of the dura propria of the temporal lobe from the inner cavernous membrane of the SOF; (3) isolation and resection of the exposed meningo-orbital band to expose the superolateral aspect of the anterior clinoid process (ACP); and (4) piecemeal rongeuring of ACP and the roof of the optic canal. The entire procedure was performed using surgical instruments, including micro-rongeurs, a fine Kerrison punch, and micro-dissectors. Subsequently, intradural neck clipping was performed. Twenty consecutive patients with paraclinoid and basilar aneurysms successfully underwent clipping after this non-drill extradural clinoidectomy. Minor morbidity was noted in two patients (cerebrospinal fluid leakage in one and transient oculomotor palsy in the other). The non-drill method is a simple, easy, safe, and quick alternative to traditional power drilling in extradural clinoidectomy, and this method can avoid morbidity related to direct mechanical/thermal injury of important neurovascular structures.

Keywords Skull base surgery · Paraclinoid aneurysm · Extradural anterior clinoidectomy · No-drill method · Surgical complication

K. Iwasaki, M.D. (✉) · H. Toda, M.D. · H. Hashikata, M.D.
M. Goto, M.D.
Department of Neurosurgery, Kitano Medical Research Institute and Hospital, Osaka, Japan

H. Fukuda, M.D.
Department of Neurosurgery, Amagasaki General Medical Center, Amagasaki, Japan

Introduction

Anterior clinoidectomy combined with optic canal unroofing, which was originally introduced by Dolenc [1], is a difficult but essential part of the surgical procedure for paraclinoid lesions, including aneurysms and skull base tumors [2–4]. This method has the following advantages: (1) a wider surgical view and less brain retraction; (2) early decompression and mobilization of the optic nerve; and (3) enhanced visualization of the ophthalmic artery and the proximal neck of the aneurysm [5, 6]. A high-speed drill has been traditionally used in this method; however, its use may cause mechanical and/or heat injury to important underlying neurovascular structures, leading to catastrophic sequelae [2, 3, 7]. In addition ultrasonic bone removal has recently been suggested to reduce potential complications related to the traditional power-drilling technique. However, ultrasound-related neuropathies have also been recognized as possible morbidities [8]. Due to these complications, we have avoided the use of a high-speed drill or ultrasonic device in our method.

Materials and Methods

Patient Profile: Between January 2006 and January 2016, 20 consecutive patients with paraclinoid and basilar aneurysms were successfully treated using no-drill extradural anterior clinoidectomy (5 men and 15 women; age range 32–74 years). Of the 20 patients, 19 had paraclinoid aneurysms and 1 had a basilar aneurysm. Additionally, four patients had large or giant aneurysms, and the retrograde suction decompression method [9] was used for safe clipping. The clinical details of the 20 patients are shown in Table 1.

Surgical technique: The no-drill clinoidectomy method includes six steps: (1) the sphenoid ridge is rongeured flat to the base of ACP, after a standard frontotemporal craniotomy; (2) the lateral wall of the SOF is partially removed; (3) the

G. Esposito et al. (eds.), *Trends in the Management of Cerebrovascular Diseases*, Acta Neurochirurgica Supplement, Vol. 129,
https://doi.org/10.1007/978-3-319-73739-3_6, © Springer International Publishing AG, part of Springer Nature 2018

Table 1 Clinical details of the 20 study patients with paraclinoid and basilar aneurysms undergoing no-drill, instrumental extradural anterior clinoidectomy

Case no.	Sex	Age	Aneurysm size (mm)	Symptom	Morbidity	Combined method
1	M	41	5	No	No	
2	F	42	5	SAH	No	
3	F	51	5	No	No	
4	F	73	25	Visual disturbance	No	Suction decompression
5	F	71	18	No	No	
6	M	72	5	SAH	No	
7	F	39	5	No	No	
8	F	55	6	No	No	
9	F	57	7	No	No	
10	F	55	15	No	No	Suction decompression
11	F	59	6	No	No	
12	F	65	5	SAH	No	
13	M	73	4	No	CSF leakage	
14	F	32	7	No	No	
15[a]	F	63	21	Visual disturbance	No	Suction decompression
16	F	48	15	SAH	Transient oculomotor palsy	Suction decompression
17	F	74	18	Oculomotor palsy	No	
18	M	33	5	No	No	
19	M	47	8	No	No	
20	F	49	5	No	No	

[a]Patient had basilar aneurysm

dura propria of the temporal lobe is peeled off from the inner cavernous membrane; (4) the MOB is fully isolated and resected to expose the superolateral aspect of ACP; (5) ACP and the roof of the optic canal are rongeured in a piecemeal fashion; and (6) the clinoid tip is removed en bloc after detaching it from the optic strut, and the optic strut is rongeured away, if necessary (Fig. 1). The entire method is performed using surgical instruments (micro-rongeurs, fine Kerrison punch, micro-dissectors, and a micro-curette; Fig. 2), without the use of a power drill or ultrasonic device.

Results

Neck clipping was successfully performed in all patients after sufficient exposure of the neck and parent arteries. Mechanical and/or heat injury to the underlying important neurovascular structures, such as the carotid artery and optic nerve, did not occur. Minor morbidity was seen in only two patients (CSF leakage in one and transient oculomotor palsy in the other).

Representative case: A 63-year-old woman (Case 15) presented to our hospital with a 6-month history of progressive blurred vision of the left eye. Neurological examination revealed decreased left visual acuity (right 1.0, left 0.3). Neuroradiological examination showed a large left paraclinoid aneurysm (21 mm in diameter) with compression of the left optic nerve (Fig. 3). This aneurysm was successfully clipped via extradural clinoidectomy and the suction decompression method [9].

Discussion

The most serious complication during anterior clinoidectomy using a power drill is mechanical damage to the carotid artery under ACP, which may result in mortality [2, 7]. Another serious complication is heat damage to the optic nerve, which may result in severe morbidity [2]. Our non-drill method can avoid such serious complications. Allowing the surgeon to use safer instruments such as a fine Kerrison punch and micro-rongeurs instead of a high-power drill essentially creates a sufficient surgical corridor around ACP. Based on a cadaveric study, we emphasize that sufficient detachment of the MOB to expose the superolateral aspect of ACP is the key step in no-drill, instrumental cli-

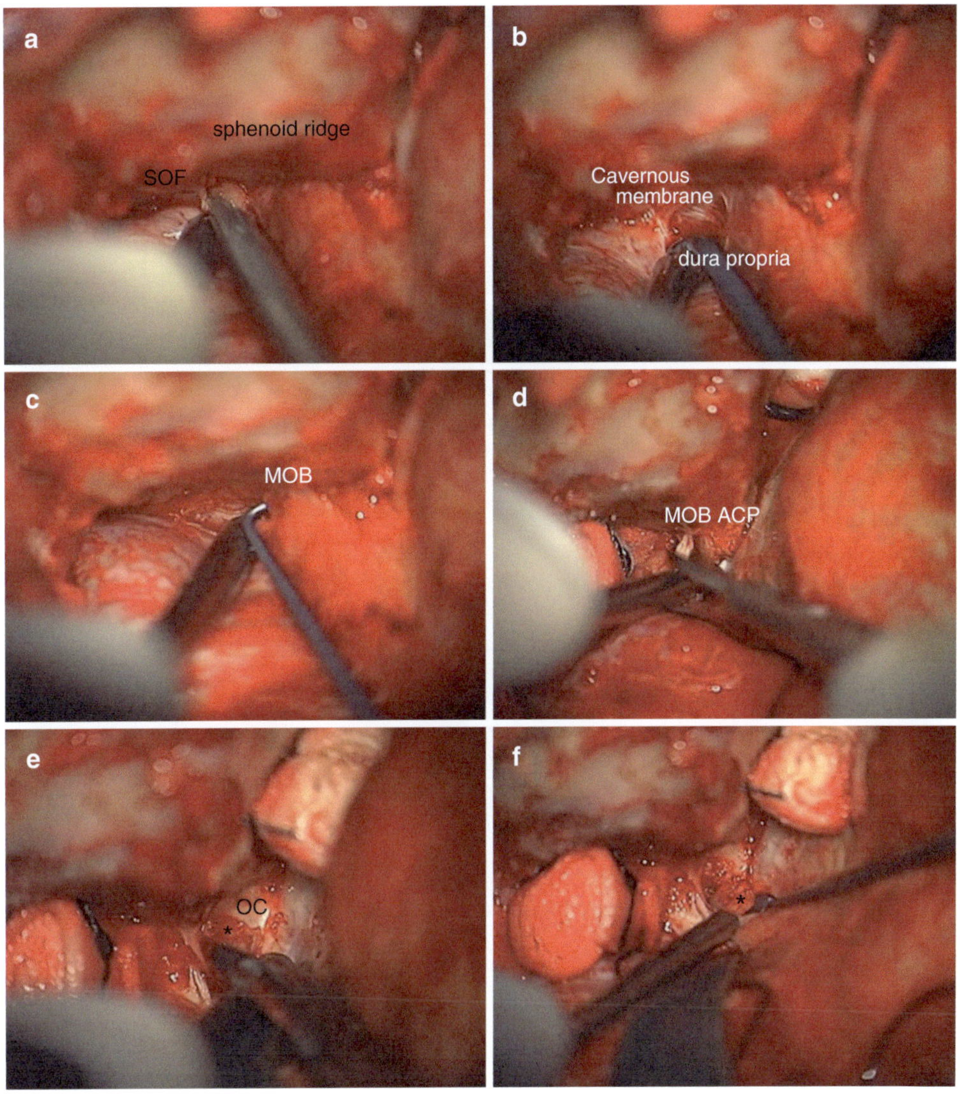

Fig. 1 Intraoperative photographs of no-drill extradural anterior clinoidectomy (left side craniotomy). (**a**) After standard left frontotemporal craniotomy, the sphenoid ridge is rongeured flat to the base of ACP, and then, the lateral wall of the SOF is partially removed using a fine Kerrison punch. (**b**) The dura propria of the temporal lobe is peeled off from the inner cavernous membrane using a Rhoton® micro-dissector. (**c**, **d**) The MOB is fully isolated and resected to expose the superolateral aspect of ACP using micro-scissors. (**e**) ACP (asterisk) and the roof of the OC are rongeured in a piecemeal fashion using a micro-rongeur. (**f**) The clinoid tip (asterisk) is removed en bloc after detaching it from the optic strut using a Rhoton® micro-dissector. *ACP* anterior clinoid process, *MOB* meningo-orbital band, *OC* Optic canal, *SOF* Superior orbital fissure

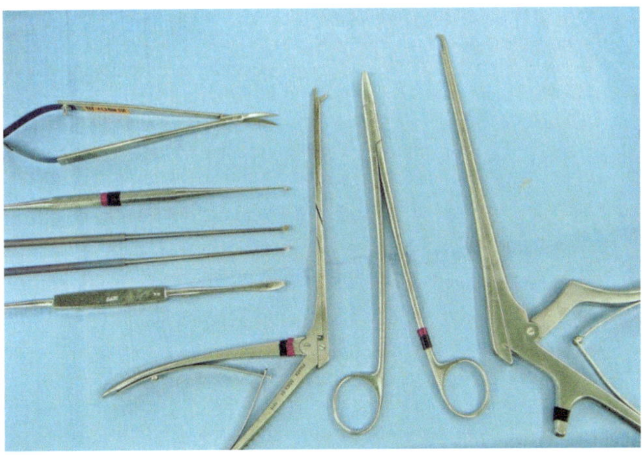

Fig. 2 The surgical instruments used for no-drill extradural anterior clinoidectomy include micro-rongeurs, a fine Kerrison punch, Rhoton® micro-dissectors, a micro-curette, and micro-scissors

noidectomy [3]. The complex microanatomy of the MOB with its neighboring structures and the surgical details for stepwise detachment of the MOB have been reported elsewhere [3]. In addition to aneurysmal clipping, we have applied this method to treat more than 50 cases of skull base tumors, without complications.

Conclusion

Power drilling is generally not necessary for the process of removal of the anterior clinoid, optic canal roof, and optic strut. Our no-drill technique is an easy, safe, and quick alternative to power drilling in extradural clinoidectomy. This method can avoid power drill-related and ultrasound-related mechanical/thermal injury of neighboring neurovascular structures.

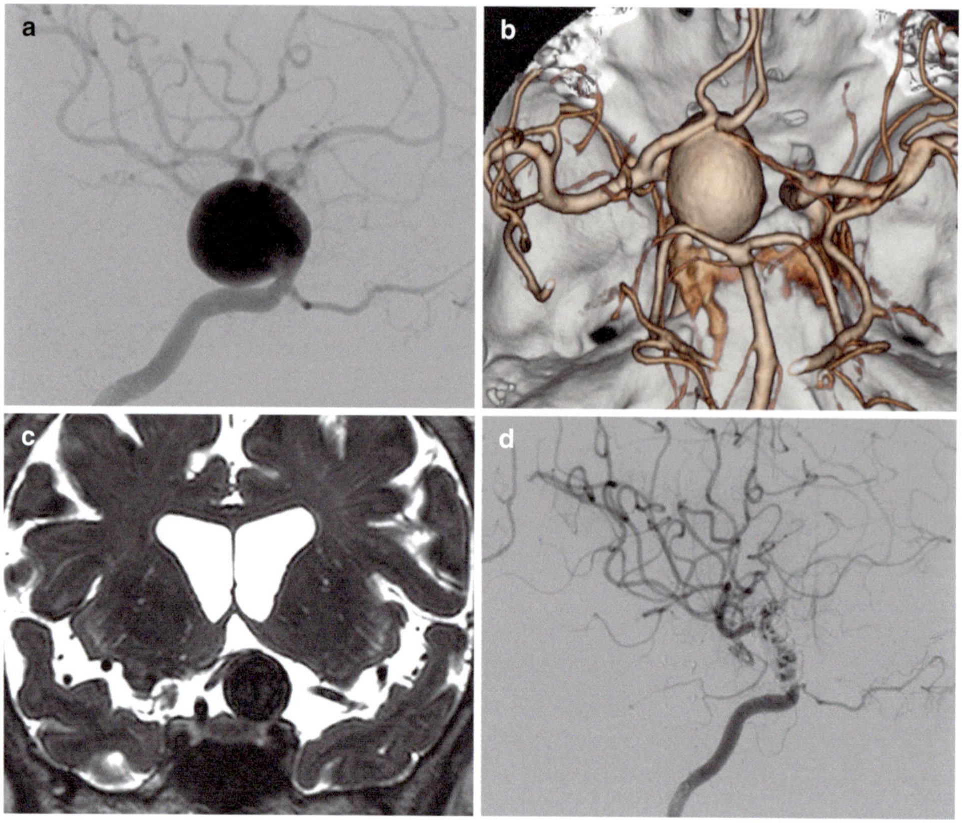

Fig. 3 Neuroradiological examination of a representative case. A preoperative angiogram (**a**) and 3D computed tomography angiogram (**b**) show a left paraclinoid large aneurysm (21 mm in diameter). A coronal T2-weighted magnetic resonance image (**c**) shows severe compression of the left optic nerve by the aneurysm. A postoperative angiogram (**d**) shows successful clipping

All Sources of Financial Support The authors report no conflicts.

References

1. Dolenc VV. A combined epi- and subdural direct approach to carotid-ophthalmic artery aneurysms. J Neurosurg. 1985;62:667–72.
2. Chang DJ. The "no-drill" technique of anterior clinoidectomy: a cranial base approach to the paraclinoid and parasellar region. Neurosurgery. 2009;94:ons96–ons106.
3. Fukuda H, Evins AI, Burrell JC, Iwasaki K, Stieg KP, Bernardo A. The meningo-orbital band: microsurgical anatomy and surgical detachment of the membranous structures through a frontotemporal craniotomy with removal of the anterior clinoid process. J Neurol Surg B Skull Base. 2014;75:125–32.
4. Lee JH, Jeun SS, Evans J, Kosmorsky G. Surgical management of clinoidal meningiomas. Neurosurgery. 2001;48:1012–21.
5. Evans JJ, Hwang YS, Lee JH. Pre- versus post-anterior clinoidectomy measurements of the optic nerve, internal carotid artery, and opticocarotid triangle: a cadaveric morphometric study. Neurosurgery. 2000;46:1018–23.
6. Nutik SL. Removal of the anterior clinoid process for exposure of the proximal intracranial carotid artery. J Neurosurg. 1988;69:529–34.
7. Korosue K, Heros RC. "Subclinoid" carotid aneurysm with erosion of the anterior clinoid process and fatal intraoperative rupture. Neurosurgery. 1992;31:356–60.
8. Ridderheim PA, von Essen C, Zetterlund B. Indirect injury to cranial nerves after surgery with cavitron ultrasonic surgical aspirator (CUSA). Case report. Acta Neurochir. 1987;89:84–6.
9. Batjer HH, Samson DS. Retrograde suction decompression of giant paraclinoidal aneurysms. Technical note. J Neurosurg. 1990;73:305–6.

Intraoperative Measurement of Arterial Blood Flow in Aneurysm Surgery

Alberto Pasqualin, Pietro Meneghelli, Angelo Musumeci, Alessandro Della Puppa, Giacomo Pavesi, Giampietro Pinna, and Renato Scienza

Abstract Intraoperative flowmetry (IF) has been recently introduced during cerebral aneurysm surgery in order to obtain a safer surgical exclusion of the aneurysm. This study evaluates the usefulness of IF during surgery for cerebral aneurysms and compares the results obtained in the joined surgical series of Verona and Padua to the more recent results obtained at the neurosurgical department of Verona.

In the first surgical series, between 2001 and 2010, a total of 312 patients were submitted to IF during surgery for cerebral aneurysm at the neurosurgical departments of Verona and Padua: 162 patients presented with subarachnoid hemorrhage (SAH) whereas 150 patients harbored unruptured aneurysms. In the second series, between 2011 and 2016, 112 patients were submitted to IF during surgery for cerebral aneurysm at the neurosurgical department of Verona; 24 patients were admitted for SAH, whereas 88 patients were operated on for unruptured aneurysms.

Comparison of the baseline values in the two surgical series and the baseline values between unruptured and ruptured aneurysms showed no statistical differences between the two clinical series. Analysis of flowmetry measurements showed three types of loco-regional flow derangements: hyperemia after temporary arterial occlusion, redistribution of flow in efferent vessels after clipping, and low flow in patients with SAH-related vasospasm.

IF provides real-time data about flow derangements caused by surgical clipping of cerebral aneurysm, thus enabling the surgeon to obtain a safer exclusion; furthermore, it permits the evaluation of other effects of clipping on the loco-regional blood flow. It is suggested that—in contribution with intraoperative neurophysiological monitoring—IF may now constitute the most reliable tool for increasing safety in aneurysm surgery.

Keywords Intraoperative flowmetry · Cerebral aneurysm · Clipping · Surgery · Temporary arterial occlusion (TAO)

Introduction

Aneurysm surgery remains a challenging section of neurosurgery because of the high risks and the possible dramatic consequences of inappropriate aneurysm clipping. The complete exclusion of the aneurysm bears the risk of inadvertent stenosis or even occlusion of the distal branches and subsequent clipping-related ischemia. Thus, the efferent and parent vessels have to be dissected carefully in order to obtain adequate visualization of the aneurysm's neck and morphology. These delicate maneuvers may require the use of temporary arterial occlusion (TAO) to reduce the risk of bleeding caused by intraoperative aneurysmal rupture and also to reduce the tension of the aneurysm walls, with a subsequent safer dissection of the neck and sac from the surrounding structures.

In the past few years, many techniques have been introduced to help the surgeon because, even in experienced hands, visual examination alone does not identify all instances of vessel compromise. The use of intraoperative angiography [1–3] and, more recently, of indocyanine green videoangiography [4, 5] permits an anatomical investigation of the surgical field, enabling the surgeon to detect vessel compromise and incomplete exclusion of the aneurysm. The ability to detect these anomalies is, however, limited to the visualization of the intensity of the contrast medium, without any quantitative evaluation of flow. Measurement of vascular

A. Pasqualin, M.D. (✉)
Section of Vascular Neurosurgery, Institute of Neurosurgery, Verona City and University Hospital, Verona, Italy

P. Meneghelli, M.D. · A. Musumeci, M.D. · G. Pinna, M.D.
Institute of Neurosurgery, Verona City and University Hospital, Verona, Italy

A. Della Puppa, M.D. · R. Scienza, M.D.
Division of Neurosurgery, Padua City Hospital, Padova, Italy

G. Pavesi, M.D.
Division of Neurosurgery, Baggiovara Hospital, Modena, Italy

https://doi.org/10.1007/978-3-319-73739-3_7,

flow velocity with the microvascular Doppler probe gives an indirect evaluation of the vessel's patency and of the exclusion of the aneurysm [6, 7].

Charbel et al. [8] introduced the use of the Micro-Flow Probe in 1998: this technique permits a direct and real time evaluation of flow in mL/min on the efferent vessels in order to avoid their compromise during the surgical clipping; the comparison between the pre-clipping and post-clipping flow values gives an immediate feedback about the patency of the efferent vessels.

The aims of this study were (1) to evaluate the usefulness of intraoperative flowmetry (IF) during surgery for cerebral aneurysms; (2) to compare the results obtained with Charbel Micro-Flow Probe in two surgical series, namely, the joined series of the neurosurgical departments of Verona and Padua and the more recent surgical series of the neurosurgical department of Verona; and (3) to report and analyze blood flow derangements caused by clipping.

Materials and Methods

Patient Populations

Data regarding patients submitted to aneurysm surgery at the two neurosurgical departments of Verona and Padua from July 2001 to 2010 and at the neurosurgical department of Verona from January 2011 to September 2016 were prospectively collected and subsequently identified via a retrospective review.

The first surgical series comprehended 312 patients (26% of the patients operated on in the same period for intracranial aneurysm) that were submitted to aneurysm surgery with the aid of IF; there were 203 females and 109 males with a mean age of 55.4 years (range 18–78); 162 patients presented a subarachnoid hemorrhage (SAH) on admission, whereas 150 patients were operated on for unruptured aneurysms. Multiple aneurysms were found in 25 patients, with a total of 345 aneurysms clipped. The aneurysm locations for ruptured and unruptured aneurysms are reported in Table 1; overall, the mean diameter of the aneurysm was 11 mm (range 3–40 mm); there were 65 large aneurysms (>15 mm in diameter) and 15 giant aneurysms (≥25 mm in diameter). SAH patients were submitted to early surgery (<72 h after bleeding) in 84% of cases. TAO was applied in 113 patients (36%); the mean occlusion time was 6.7 min (range 1–20 min).

The recent surgical series of the Verona neurosurgical department comprehends 112 patients submitted to IF-assisted aneurysm surgery (47% of the patients operated on in the same period and more specifically 22% of all SAH patients and 75% of all patients treated for unruptured aneurysms).

Table 1 Intraoperative flowmetry for cerebral aneurysms; treated in Verona and Padua (2001–2010)

	Ruptured	Unruptured	Total
MCA	83	94	177
ACoA	66	27	93
ICA	19	35	54
Distal ACA	9	5	14
Posterior circulation	2	5	7
TOTAL	179	166	345

MCA Middle cerebral artery, *ACoA* Anterior communicating artery, *ICA* Internal carotid artery, *ACA* Anterior cerebral artery

Table 2 Intraoperative flowmetry for cerebral aneurysms; treated in Verona (2011–2016)

	Ruptured	Unruptured	Total
MCA	9	67	76
ACoA	8	17	25
ICA	3	9	12
Distal ACA	4	2	6
Posterior circulation	–	–	–
TOTAL	24	95	119

MCA Middle cerebral artery, *ACoA* Anterior communicating artery, *ICA* Internal carotid artery, *ACA* Anterior cerebral artery

There were 73 females and 39 males with a mean age of 54.4 years (range 17–78); 24 patients showed SAH at the admission, whereas 88 patients were operated on for unruptured aneurysms. Multiple aneurysms were found in 6 patients for a total of 119 aneurysms clipped. The aneurysm location for ruptured and unruptured aneurysms is reported in Table 2; the mean diameter of the aneurysms was 10.2 mm (range 3–32 mm); there were 12 large aneurysms (>15 mm in diameter) and 5 giant aneurysms (≥25 mm in diameter). SAH patients were submitted to early surgery (<72 h after bleeding) in 87% of cases. TAO was applied to 56 patients (50%); the mean occlusion time was 6.2 min (range 1–20 min).

Intraoperative Flowmetry Technique

IF measurements were performed using a 1.5- and 2.0-mm tip Charbel Micro-Flow Probe (HQN 1.5 MB, HQN 2 MB and HQN 3 MB respectively) connected to the electronic flow detection unit (Transonic Flowmeter HT331 series, Transonic, USA).

The measurement procedure started with the accurate circumferential dissection of the vessel at risk in order to allow the correct position of the probe that should encircle the artery; then the appropriate tip was chosen according to the vessel's size. After simple connection and calibration of the

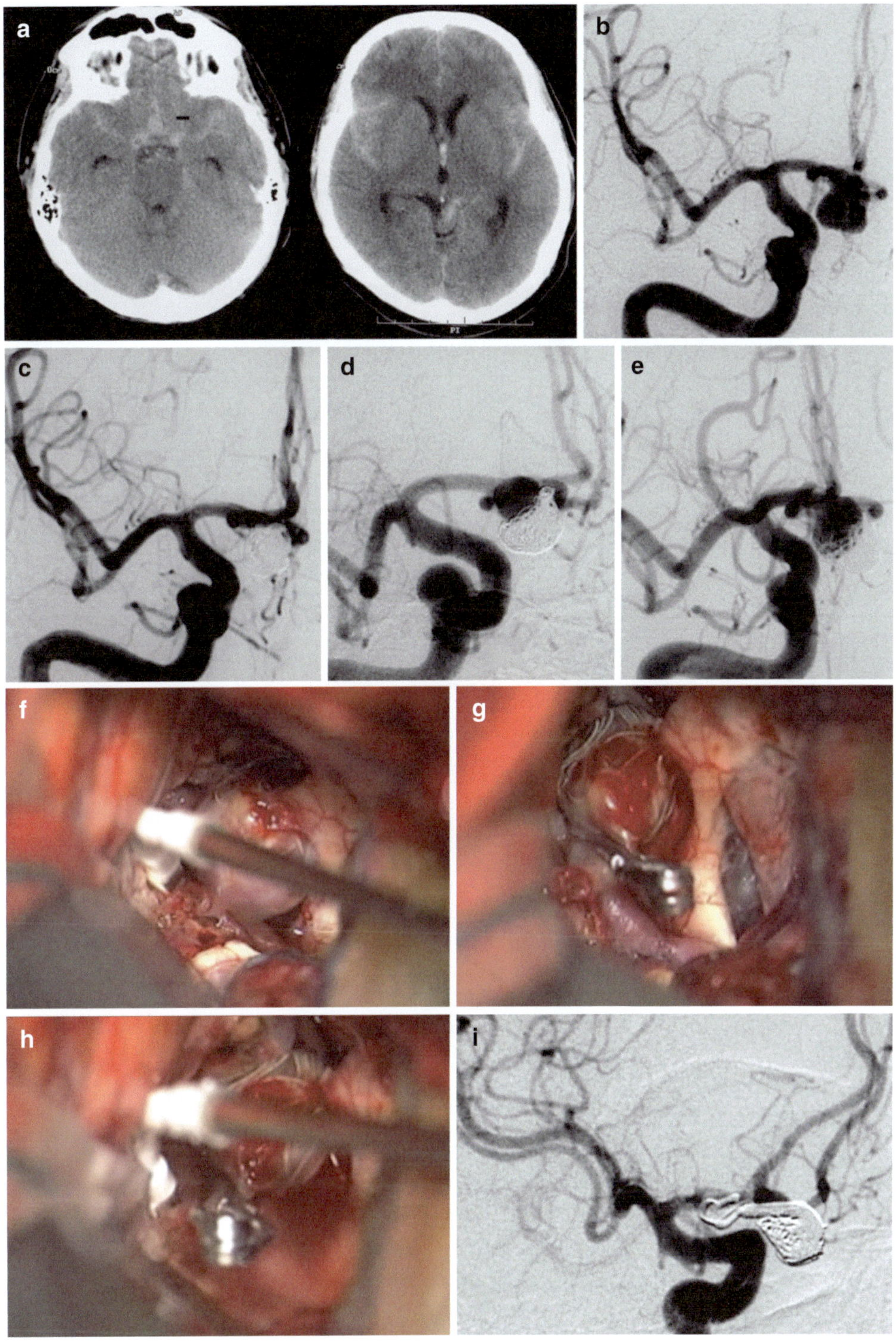

Fig. 1 A 49-year-old man presenting with subarachnoid hemorrhage, Glasgow Coma Scale (GCS) 13 on admission, Fisher III on CT scan (**a**); digital subtraction angiography (DSA) showed a large (antero-inferiorly projecting) anterior communicating artery aneurysm (**b**), which was then submitted to endovascular occlusion with seven coils (**c**); follow-up DSA showed recanalization of the aneurysm at 11 months (**d**); progressive enlargement of the sac at 2 years (**e**). The patient was then submitted to surgery: flow was measured on the A2 segments before clipping (**f**) then the clip was placed on the neck of the aneurysm (**g**); the flow measured after clipping did not show any significant difference from the pre-clip values (**h**). Post-operative DSA showed the correct exclusion of the aneurysm and normal injection of both the A2 segments (**i**). The patient did not show neurological deficits after surgery

probe, recordings were obtained from the vessels at risk, completely immersed in topically irrigated Ringer's solution, before and after the surgical clipping (Fig. 1). Systemic blood pressure and PaCO2 levels were recorded at those times. The comparison between the basal and post-clip flow values identified the possible presence of flow derangement, with the consequent need for clip repositioning in order to restore normal perfusion (Fig. 2).

Data Collection, Clinical and Radiological Follow-Up

During the surgical procedure, data regarding the flow values measured before and after surgical clipping were recorded together with the mean arterial pressure (MAP) in mmHg and the end tidal (ET) CO_2; moreover, the following

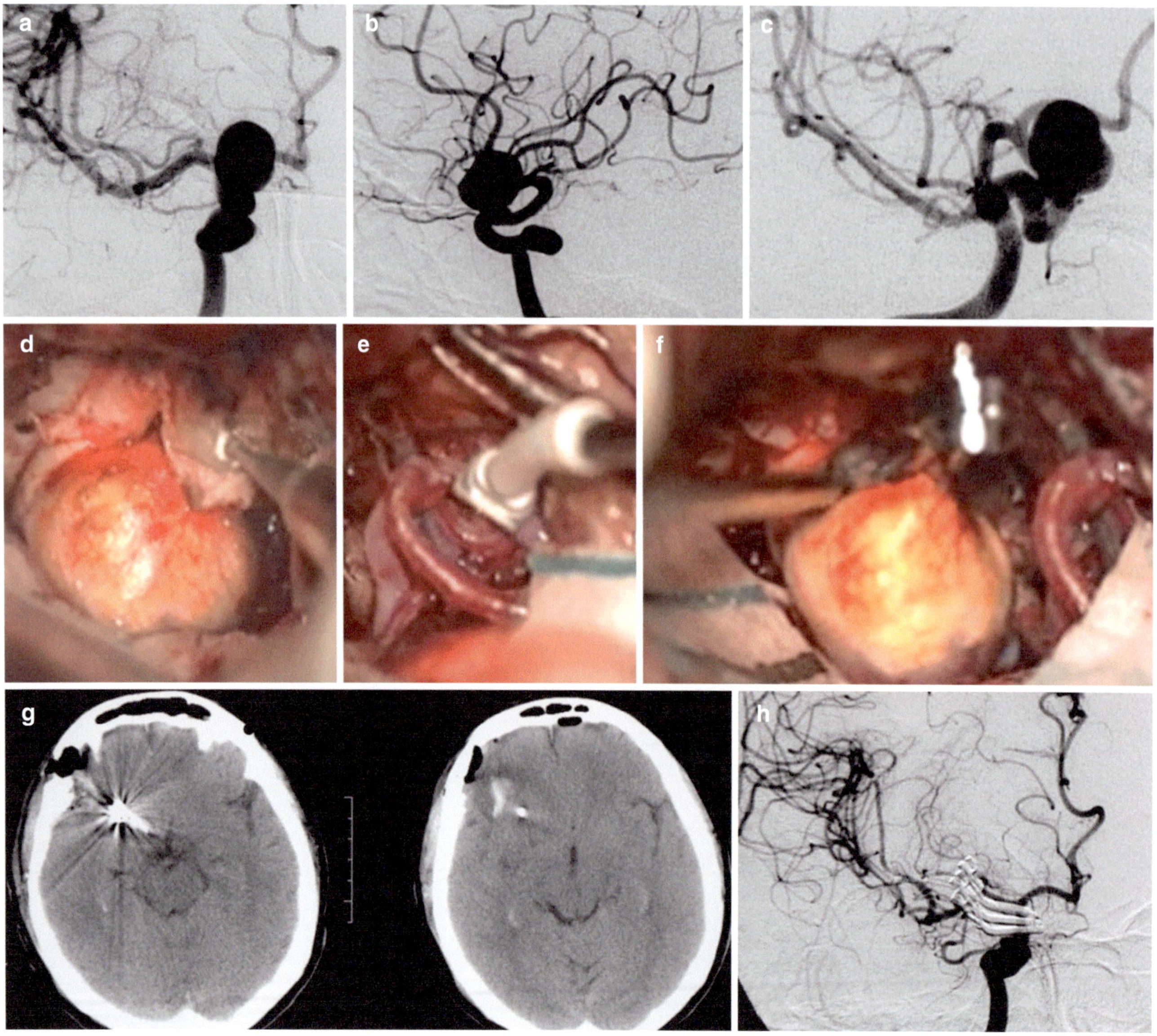

Fig. 2 A 64-year-old woman with incidental discovery of a partially calcific right carotid ophthalmic aneurysm, as it is shown in the preoperative DSA (**a–c**). The patient was submitted to surgery: after a partial clinoidectomy (**d**), flow was measured on the M1 tract before and after clipping (**e**), resulting in a safe surgical exclusion with multiple clips (**f**). Post-operative CT scan showed a minimal deposition of blood along the surgical corridor (**g**) and DSA (**h**) showed complete exclusion of the aneurysm and normal injection of both M1 and A1 segments. The patient did not show neurological deficits after surgery, and particularly had no visual impairment

parameters were recorded: the need for clip repositioning and its relationship with intraoperative flowmetry; the use of TAO, with the modality (continued or intermittent) and the overall duration of the temporary clipping; timing of surgery for patients with aneurysmal SAH; surgery within 72 h from aneurysm rupture was defined as early surgery. Patients were operated on under total intravenous anesthesia (TIVA) in normothermia or mild hypothermia. CT scans were generally obtained during the first day after surgery and then prior to discharge; any other CT scan was related to the onset of neurological deficit in order to evaluate the presence of ischemic regions with possible/certain relationship to the clipping procedure. All the CT scan images were evaluated by the senior authors (A.P., R.S.) in their departments.

Clinical evaluation of all the patients was recorded at discharge and 6 months after discharge; the clinical outcome was collected according to the modified Rankin Scale (mRS) and divided into favorable (1–2 mRS) and unfavorable (3–6). All the clinical and radiological data were collected in a specific sheet for each patient: data regarding blood flow measurements, TAO duration and modality, and clinical and radiological outcome were prospectively recorded in order to permit a post hoc analysis; all data were finally collected in a specific flowmetry database. A statistical analysis was carried out using the chi-square test, and the Fisher exact test if the sample size was too small.

Results

Intraoperative Flow Measurement

In the first clinical series, during the surgical procedure, 590 vessels were insonated with a total of 1307 flow measurements; in the second series, a total of 359 flow measurements were done on 190 vessels. The mean basal flow values for the main vessels (MCA, ACoA, ICA, pericallosal artery) recorded in the two surgical series are reported in Table 3; no statistical difference was demonstrated between the basal flow values of the two series. A comparison between ruptured and unruptured aneurysms basal flow values did not show any statistical difference for the same vessel in the first series ($p > 0.05$) (Table 4); no comparison was done between basal flow values in unruptured and ruptured aneurysms in the recent surgical series because of the small sample size of SAH patients.

Incidence of Vessel Compromise and Clipping Related Ischemia

In the first series, clip repositioning was needed in 53 patients (24 in ruptured and 29 in unruptured aneurysms) caused by the drop of the post-clip flow values in comparison with the basal flow. We considered a clip repositioning in the case of

Table 3 Basal flow values in mL/min detected on cerebral arteries in patients with cerebral aneurysms in the two surgical series (Verona-Padua 2001–2010 and Verona 2011–2016)

	Verona and Padua 2001–2010		Verona 2011–2016		
	Flow values (±SD)	Range	Flow values (±SD)	Range	*p* value
A1 tract	32.2 ± 19.3	9–68	33,2 ± 12.0	8–55	NS
A2 tract	23.5 ± 10.6	2–65	24.4 ± 12.2	9–45	NS
M1 tract	39.7 ± 17.3	29–80	58.2 ± 16.4	40–72	NS
M2 tract	21.8 ± 11.2	2–89	22.1 ± 11.4	6–70	NS
M3 tract	18.2 ± 10.4	3.8–45	15.8 ± 9.6	5–48	NS
Supraclinoid ICA	47.8 ± 21.7	13–100	–	–	–
Pericallosal A.	15.0 ± 5.3	9–27	11.1 ± 2.8	9–13	NS
PICA	11.1 ± 6.3	6–22	–	–	–

SD standard deviation, *NS* $p > 0.05$

Table 4 Basal flow values detected on cerebral arteries in patients with unruptured and ruptured aneurysms (Verona and Padua common experience, 2001–2010)

	Ruptured aneurysms	Unruptured aneurysms	
	Flow values ± SD	Flow values ± SD	*p* value
A1 tract	28.6 ± 10.9	30.9 ± 14.5	NS
A2 tract	24.7 ± 11.5	22.8 ± 10.3	NS
M1 tract	39.7 ± 14.5	39.2 ± 16.0	NS
M2 tract	21.7 ± 11.7	21.0 ± 10.6	NS
M3 tract	18.8 ± 11.0	13.5 ± 5.6	NS
Supraclinoid ICA	50.2 ± 23.0	42.0 ± 19.9	NS
Pericallosal A.	15.1 ± 4.6	14.9 ± 6.3	NS
PICA		12.2 ± 7.1	–

SD standard deviation, *NS* $p > 0.05$

a 40% decrease in flow values after clipping (Pasqualin et al., unpublished data). In the SAH group, 15 clip replacements were done on MCA (62%), 7 on ACoA, and 2 on ICA; no repositioning was needed for the pericallosal artery and posterior circulation artery aneurysms. In the unruptured aneurysms group, 24 clip replacements were done on MCA (82%), 1 on ACoA, 2 on ICA, and 2 on pericallosal artery aneurysms; no replacement was needed for posterior circulation artery aneurysms. In the two groups, complete flow restoration was obtained in 40 patients (75%); in the remaining patients, clip repositioning did not produce further changes of flow. A post hoc analysis between the intraoperative flow values and the postoperative CT scan images revealed 14 cases with clipping-related ischemia; the relationship between the flow values and postoperative ischemia are reported in Table 5. In the recent series, clip repositioning was needed in six patients (two in ruptured and four in unruptured aneurysms). In the unruptured aneurysms, clip repositioning was done in two cases for MCA aneurysms and in two cases for ACoA aneurysms; in the SAH patients it was needed in two cases for MCA aneurysms. Restoration of flow was obtained in five out of six patients. No post hoc analysis was done between intraoperative and postoperative data because of the small sample size of the recent series.

Intraoperative Clipping-Related Blood Flow Derangements

During surgery, three main phenomena of flow derangements were recorded: flow redistribution on efferent vessel after clipping, hyperemia after TAO, and low flow in distal branches in patients with aneurysmal SAH. In the first series,

Table 5 Relation between intraoperative flow values and clipping related ischemia

Aneurysm site	Ruptured/ unruptured	Size (mm)	Baseline flow (mL/min)	Flow after clip (mL/min)	Further changes	Clipping-related ischemia
MCA	Ruptured	16	20 (M_2)	9	15 (papav.)	Possible
MCA	Ruptured	10	45 (M_2)	12	32 (clip repos.)	Certain
ACoA	Ruptured	9	35 (A_2)	14	–	Possible
ACoA	Ruptured	15	18 (A_2)	4	–	Certain
MCA	Ruptured	20	19 (M_2)	2	–	Certain
MCA	Ruptured	40	21 (M_2)	3.8	–	Certain[a]
MCA + ACoA	Ruptured	10	23 (A_1)	8	–	Certain
ACoA	Ruptured	12	48 (A_2)	24	–	Certain
ACoA	Ruptured	18	27 (A_2)	18	–	Certain
ICA	Ruptured	18	40 (M_1)	10	–	Certain
MCA	Unruptured	25	8 (M_2)	2	–	Certain
PCA	Unruptured	15	24 (P_2)	4	–	Certain
MCA	Unruptured	15	0 (M_2)	0	–	Certain
MCA	Unruptured	18	49 (M_2)	12	–	Certain

[a]Artery occluded (verified at post-operative angiography)

Table 6 Post-occlusive hyperemia: pre- and post-occlusive flow values in the 2001–2010 series (13 cases with MCA aneurysms, 8 cases with ACoA aneurysms, 3 cases with ICA aneurysms, and 1 case with a pericallosal artery aneurysm)

	A1 tract (mL/min)	A2 tract (mL/min)	M1 tract (mL/min)	M2 tract (mL/min)
Pre-occlusion flow values	38.7	21.9	34.0	17.0
Post-occlusion flow values	51.2	35.4	87.0	35.9

Table 7 Post-occlusive hyperemia: pre- and post-occlusive flow values in the 2010–2016 series (seven cases with MCA aneurysms, one case with a ACoA aneurysm)

	A2 tract (mL/min)	M2 tract (mL/min)
Pre-occlusion flow values	9.1	22.1
Post-occlusion flow values	30.6	41.8

flow redistribution was reported in 14 patients: 11 patients with MCA aneurysm showed a decrease of flow in one of the efferent branches (mostly the temporal one) and increase of flow in the other after clipping; two patients with ICA bifurcation aneurysm showed redistribution of flow on M1 and A1 segments after clipping; and one patient with ACoA aneurysm showed decrease of flow on the right A2 segment and increase of flow on the left A2 segment after clipping.

TAO-related hyperemia was reported in 25 patients: 13 cases with MCA aneurysms, 8 cases with ACoA aneurysms, 3 cases with ICA aneurysms, and 1 case with a pericallosal aneurysm; flow values before and after TAO are reported in Table 6. In the second series, flow redistribution after clipping was noted in five cases: three patients with MCA aneurysm, one patient with ICA aneurysm and one patient with ACoA aneurysm. TAO hyperemia was recorded in eight cases: seven cases for MCA aneurysm and one case for ACoA aneurysm; flow values before and after TAO are reported in Table 7.

In the first surgical series, low flow in distal branches was reported in patients with SAH: the average basal flow measured on M3 was 11.2 mL/min in SAH patients whereas it was 16.1 mL/min in patients operated on for unruptured aneurysms. In the recent series, it was not possible to compare the flow values in distal branches because of the small sample size of the SAH patients.

Clinical Outcome

In the first surgical series, 132 patients (81%) operated on after SAH showed a favorable outcome (mRS 0–2), whereas 30 patients (19%) experienced an unfavorable outcome (mRS 3–6): 8 patients died after surgery due to the severity of bleeding at admission and another patient died 2 months after surgery due to medical complications during rehabilitation. A total of 142 patients (94%) operated on for unruptured aneurysms showed a favorable clinical outcome, whereas 7 patients (6%) experienced an unfavorable outcome. Two

Table 8 Unfavorable outcome according to the modified Rankin Score (mRS 3–6) at discharge

	Ruptured aneurysms				Unruptured aneurysms			
	mRS 3–4	mRS 5	mRS 6	Total	mRS 3–4	mRS 5	mRS 6	Total
Verona and Padua (2001–2010)	23 (14%)	2 (1%)	8 (5%)	162	6 (4%)	1 (0.6%)	2 (1.3%)	150
Verona (2011–2016)	2 (8%)	1 (4%)	1 (4%)	24	6 (7%)	–	–	88

Table 9 Unfavorable outcome according to the modified Rankin Score (mRS 3–6) at 6 months follow-up

	Ruptured aneurysms				Unruptured aneurysms			
	mRS 3–4	mRS 5	mRS 6	Total	mRS 3–4	mRS 5	mRS 6	Total
Verona and Padua (2001–2010)	20 (12%)	1 (0.6%)	9 (5.5%)	162	5 (3.3%)	–	2 (1.3%)	150
Verona (2011–2016)	2 (8%)	–	2 (8%)	24	4 (4.5%)	–	–	88

patients died after surgery: one from pulmonary embolism and the other from severe coagulopathy.

In the second surgical series, 20 patients (83%) operated on after SAH showed a favorable outcome whereas 4 patients (17%) presented an unfavorable outcome: 2 patients died due to the severity of bleeding at admission and another patient died months after surgery due to medical complications during rehabilitation. A total of 84 patients (95%) operated on for unruptured aneurysms achieved a favorable outcome whereas 4 patients (5%) showed an unfavorable outcome. There was no mortality. The unfavorable outcomes at discharge and 6 months after discharge of the two surgical series are reported in Tables 8 and 9.

Discussion

The quantitative measurement of flow in human arteries is based on the principle that the time taken for an ultrasound wave to move a defined distance against the blood flow takes longer than an ultrasound wave moving the same distance with blood flow. In the Charbel Micro-Flow Probe, two ultrasonic transducers are positioned at the tip of the probe with a fixed acoustic reflector in front of them: these structures define the sensing window. The two transducers emit and receive ultrasonic beams; once an ultrasonic beam starts from the first transducer, it reaches the reflector plate and subsequently the second transducer, and then the same happens from the second transducer to the first. Once the probe is placed around the vessel, the ultrasound beams have to intersect the vessel upstream or downstream to reach the transducers. The ultrasound transit time is affected by the motion of flow through the vessel, and the difference between the upstream and downstream transit time is used to obtain the volume of flow (in mL/min) through the vessel insonated, which is calculated by the electronic flow detection unit [8]. This technique does not rely on direct probe contact and the insonation angle is fixed within the probe. Furthermore, vessel wall thickness, hematocrit, and heart rate do not influence readings, as these factors cancel each other out in the upstream and downstream cycles. IF has been validated in laboratory and surgical practice [9, 10].

In surgery of cerebral aneurysms, IF is particularly useful, allowing a quantitative measurement of flow in the vessels adjacent to the aneurysm [8, 11–14] and detecting even a small difference between pre-clipping and post-clipping flow values; moreover, it enables the surgeon to replace/reposition the clip even when visual examination seems to exclude a flow impairment; in other words, in the majority of cases inadvertent stenosis (or even occlusion) of an efferent vessel can be avoided. In this regard, IF is superior to intraoperative Doppler, which does not give a quantitative information of flow [6, 7, 15–18]; the same can be said for indocyanine green videoangiography, which does not allow a quantitative information of flow, and visualizes only superficial vessels [4, 5, 12, 16, 19–24].

However, the minimum size of probes currently used for IF (1.5 mm) is still too large to record flow in small vessels, such as the perforators and the anterior choroidal artery, and this is a recognized limit of IF at the present time. Although technological advances could lead to the development of smaller probes in the near future, evaluation of flow in these small vessels can be done only using indocyanine green videoangiography [19, 25, 26] or indirectly through intraoperative neurophysiological monitoring [27–32].

Although, unlike indocyanine green videoangiography and intraoperative angiography [33–36], IF does not offer a morphological evaluation of aneurysm exclusion, we believe that its merit in the immediate detection of clipping-related ischemia is of overwhelming importance in aneurysm surgery. In theory, intraoperative neurophysiological monitoring (IOM) can also be used to indirectly detect ischemic changes, even if it does not allow a precise identification of the vessel at risk of ischemia. In practice, a moderate impairment of flow in an efferent vessel cannot lead to acute changes in evoked potentials during surgery, but could still cause subacute ischemic deterioration in the postoperative period, and this possibility is avoided with the use of flowmetry.

It must be stressed that, unlike IF, intraoperative neurophysiological monitoring gives precious information about the risk of ischemia during TAO, allowing to limit the period of occlusion whenever a change in evoked potentials occurs [37–41]. Considering that around 50% of radiological strokes occurring after TAO are in the distribution of perforating arteries [42–44], monitoring of motor-evoked potentials is especially important in this situation [27–29, 31, 32]. Moreover, as mentioned above, IOM allows an indirect recognition of flow impairment in small but crucial vessels, such as the perforators and the anterior choroidal artery, for which the actual size of the probe (1.5 mm) is too large to give an adequate signal. Considering these important points, we propose a combination of both techniques (IOM and IF) during surgery of cerebral aneurysms; in other words, these techniques should be considered complementary and very useful, especially when dealing with asymptomatic patients. The advantage of the complementary use of different intraoperative monitoring technologies in aneurysm surgery has been recognized by other authors [12, 36, 45, 46], although IF was not adopted and not even discussed in two of these studies [45, 46].

The current trend in our department is to use IF when even a small doubt remains regarding adequate maintenance of flow in the vessels adjacent to the aneurysm; in our recent surgical series (2011–2016), up to 75% of patients with unruptured aneurysms were submitted to IF, documenting our "obsession" for maintenance of flow in patients electively submitted to surgical exclusion of the aneurysm.

Regarding the flow values reported in this chapter, other neurosurgeons, using the same probe, found slightly different values, according to different modalities of anesthesia and different values of intraoperative CO_2 [13]. However, this is the first study to publish a large number of observations, giving reference values for the main intracranial arteries. Moreover, in our study, flow values were recorded in the vessels adjacent to the aneurysm before the first attempt to clip the aneurysm, and were considered as "control" values, easily comparable to post-clip values.

The validity of a comparison between basal and post-clip values is true in most—but not in all—cases, considering two phenomena that can occur after clipping, namely flow redistribution and postocclusive hyperemia. Flow redistribution, that is, decrease in flow in one efferent branch and increase in the other branch after clipping, is a rare phenomenon, observed in 5% of cases in our series; it is probably due to re-direction of flow caused by the position of the clip, or by spastic changes in one efferent vessel. In this situation, we have never observed ischemic postoperative deterioration, and we now consider the sum of the values detected in each efferent branch more important than the single value; in other words, if the sum of the post-clip values in the efferent branches is equal or similar to the sum of the pre-clip values, we do not try to reposition the clip.

Postocclusive hyperemia is a more interesting phenomenon, occurring in 15–20% of cases submitted to TAO in our experience. The occurrence of hyperemia immediately following experimental occlusion of a vessel has already been reported in the literature [47–49]; this phenomenon is probably short-lasting, roughly corresponding to the duration of the preceding ischemia [47]. To date, there are no reports of its occurrence in the clinical setting; this is the first study reporting the occurrence of quantitatively ascertained postocclusive hyperemia in aneurysm surgery. Since the measurement of flow in our patients is not always performed immediately after the end of temporary occlusion, this could explain the relatively low detection of hyperemia after temporary occlusion in this series. Our impression is that hyperemia occurs immediately after restoration of flow and can contribute to an overestimation of the real flow remaining in the efferent vessels after a period of TAO; when in doubt, we suggest that the flow values are recorded again, at least 10–15 min after the end of TAO.

In conclusion, IF constitutes a valuable adjunct in surgery of cerebral aneurysms, allowing a safer exclusion of the aneurysm by clip; its merits are particularly appreciated in surgery of MCA and ACoA aneurysms, particularly if the patient is operated on for an unruptured aneurysm. The association with IOM further increases the safety of surgery, especially during temporary arterial occlusion and whenever perforating arteries are close to the neck of the aneurysm.

References

1. Origitano TC, Schwartz K, Anderson D, Azar-Kia B, Reichman OH. Optimal clip application and intraoperative angiography for intracranial aneurysms. Surg Neurol. 1999;51:117–24.
2. Popadic A, Witzmann A, Amann T, Doringer W, Fleisch M, Hafel C, Hergan K, Langle M. The value of intraoperative angiography in surgery of intracranial aneurysms: a prospective study in 126 patients. Neuroradiology. 2001;43:466–71.
3. Tang G, Cawley CM, Dion JE, Barrow DL. Intraoperative angiography during aneurysm surgery: a prospective evaluation of efficacy. J Neurosurg. 2002;96:993–9.
4. Raabe A, Beck J, Gerlach R, Zimmermann M, Seifert V. Near-infrared indocyanine green video angiography: a new method for intraoperative assessment of vascular flow. Neurosurgery. 2003;52:132–9.
5. Raabe A, Nakaji P, Beck J, Kim LJ, Hsu FP, Kamerman JD, Seifert V, Spetzler RF. Prospective evaluation of surgical microscope-integrated intraoperative near-infrared indocyanine green videoangiography during aneurysm surgery. J Neurosurg. 2005;103:982–9.
6. Marchese E, Albanese A, Denaro L, Vignati A, Fernandez E, Maira G. Intraoperative microvascular Doppler in intracranial aneurysm surgery. Surg Neurol. 2005;63:336–42.

7. Stendel R, Pietila T, Al Hassan AA, Schilling A, Brock M. Intraoperative microvascular Doppler ultrasonography in cerebral aneurysm surgery. J Neurol Neurosurg Psychiatry. 2000;68:29–35.
8. Charbel FT, Hoffman WE, Misra M, Ostergren L. Ultrasonic perivascular flow probe: technique and application in neurosurgery. Neurol Res. 1998;20:439–42.
9. Hartman JC, Olszanski DA, Hullinger TG, Brunden MN. In vivo validation of a transit-time ultrasonic volume flow meter. J Pharmacol Toxicol Methods. 1994;31:153–60.
10. Lundell A, Bergqvist D, Mattsson E, Nilsson B. Volume blood flow measurements with a transit time flowmeter: an in vivo and in vitro variability and validation study. Clin Physiol. 1993;13:547–57.
11. Amin-Hanjani S, Meglio G, Gatto R, Bauer A, Charbel FT. The utility of intraoperative blood flow measurement during aneurysm surgery using an ultrasonic perivascular flow probe. Neurosurgery. 2006;58:ONS-305–12.
12. Della Puppa A, Volpin F, Gioffre G, Rustemi O, Troncon I, Scienza R. Microsurgical clipping of intracranial aneurysms assisted by green indocyanine videoangiography (ICGV) and ultrasonic perivascular microflow probe measurement. Clin Neurol Neurosurg. 2014;116:35–40.
13. Kirk HJ, Rao PJ, Seow K, Fuller J, Chandran N, Khurana VG. Intraoperative transit time flowmetry reduces the risk of ischemic neurological deficits in neurosurgery. Br J Neurosurg. 2009;23:40–7.
14. Nakayama N, Kuroda S, Houkin K, Takikawa S, Abe H. Intraoperative measurement of arterial blood flow using a transit time flowmeter: monitoring of hemodynamic changes during cerebrovascular surgery. Acta Neurochir. 2001;143:17–24.
15. Bailes JE, Tantuwaya LS, Fukushima T, Schurman GW, Davis D. Intraoperative microvascular Doppler sonography in aneurysm surgery. Neurosurgery. 1997;40:965–70.
16. Fischer G, Stadie A, Oertel JM. Near-infrared indocyanine green videoangiography versus microvascular Doppler sonography in aneurysm surgery. Acta Neurochir. 2010;152:1519–25.
17. Laborde G, Gilsbach J, Harders A. The microvascular Doppler—an intraoperative tool for the treatment of large and giant aneurysms. Acta Neurochir Suppl. 1988;42:75–80.
18. Siasios I, Kapsalaki EZ, Fountas KN. The role of intraoperative micro-Doppler ultrasound in verifying proper clip placement in intracranial aneurysm surgery. Neuroradiology. 2012;54:1109–18.
19. Abla AA, Lawton MT. Indocyanine green angiography for cerebral aneurysm surgery: advantages, limitations, and neurosurgeon intuition. World Neurosurg. 2014;82:e585–6.
20. Dashti R, Hernesniemi J. Intraoperative assessment of a quality of microneurosurgical clipping: role of indocyanine green videoangiography. World Neurosurg. 2014;82:e589–90.
21. Della Puppa A, Rustemi O, Rossetto M, Gioffre G, Munari M, Charbel FT, Scienza R. The "squeezing maneuver" in microsurgical clipping of intracranial aneurysms assisted by indocyanine green videoangiography. Neurosurgery. 2014;10(Suppl 2):208–12.
22. Lai LT, Morgan MK. Use of indocyanine green videoangiography during intracranial aneurysm surgery reduces the incidence of postoperative ischaemic complications. J Clin Neurosci. 2014;21:67–72.
23. Lane B, Bohnstedt BN, Cohen-Gadol AA. A prospective comparative study of microscope-integrated intraoperative fluorescein and indocyanine videoangiography for clip ligation of complex cerebral aneurysms. J Neurosurg. 2015;122:618–26.
24. Snyder LA, Spetzler RF. Current indications for indocyanine green angiography. World Neurosurg. 2011;76:405–6.
25. de Oliveira JG, Beck J, Seifert V, Teixeira MJ, Raabe A. Assessment of flow in perforating arteries during intracranial aneurysm surgery using intraoperative near-infrared indocyanine green videoangiography. Neurosurgery. 2007;61:63–72.
26. de Oliveira JG, Beck J, Seifert V, Teixeira MJ, Raabe A. Assessment of flow in perforating arteries during intracranial aneurysm surgery using intraoperative near-infrared indocyanine green videoangiography. Neurosurgery. 2008;62:1300–10.
27. Irie T, Yoshitani K, Ohnishi Y, Shinzawa M, Miura N, Kusaka Y, Miyazaki S, Miyamoto S. The efficacy of motor-evoked potentials on cerebral aneurysm surgery and new-onset postoperative motor deficits. J Neurosurg Anesthesiol. 2010;22:247–51.
28. Neuloh G, Pechstein U, Cedzich C, Schramm J. Motor evoked potential monitoring with supratentorial surgery. Neurosurgery. 2004;54:1061–70.
29. Quinones-Hinojosa A, Alam M, Lyon R, Yingling CD, Lawton MT. Transcranial motor evoked potentials during basilar artery aneurysm surgery: technique application for 30 consecutive patients. Neurosurgery. 2004;54:916–24.
30. Suzuki K, Kodama N, Sasaki T, Matsumoto M, Konno Y, Sakuma J, Oinuma M, Murakawa M. Intraoperative monitoring of blood flow insufficiency in the anterior choroidal artery during aneurysm surgery. J Neurosurg. 2003;98:507–14.
31. Szelenyi A, Langer D, Kothbauer K, De Camargo AB, Flamm ES, Deletis V. Monitoring of muscle motor evoked potentials during cerebral aneurysm surgery: intraoperative changes and postoperative outcome. J Neurosurg. 2006;105:675–81.
32. Yeon JY, Seo DW, Hong SC, Kim JS. Transcranial motor evoked potential monitoring during the surgical clipping of unruptured intracranial aneurysms. J Neurol Sci. 2010;293:29–34.
33. Alexander TD, Macdonald RL, Weir B, Kowalczuk A. Intraoperative angiography in cerebral aneurysm surgery: a prospective study of 100 craniotomies. Neurosurgery. 1996;39:10–7.
34. Chiang VL, Gailloud P, Murphy KJ, Rigamonti D, Tamargo RJ. Routine intraoperative angiography during aneurysm surgery. J Neurosurg. 2002;96:988–92.
35. Klopfenstein JD, Spetzler RF, Kim LJ, Feiz-Erfan I, Han PP, Zabramski JM, Porter RW, Albuquerque FC, McDougall CG, Fiorella DJ. Comparison of routine and selective use of intraoperative angiography during aneurysm surgery: a prospective assessment. J Neurosurg. 2004;100:230–5.
36. Morcos JJ. Editorial: indocyanine green videoangiography or intraoperative angiography? J Neurosurg. 2013;118:417–8.
37. Holland NR. Subcortical strokes from intracranial aneurysm surgery: implications for intraoperative neuromonitoring. J Clin Neurophysiol. 1998;15:439–46.
38. Kang D, Yao P, Wu Z, Yu L. Ischemia changes and tolerance ratio of evoked potential monitoring in intracranial aneurysm surgery. Clin Neurol Neurosurg. 2013;115:552–6.
39. Mizoi K, Yoshimoto T. Permissible temporary occlusion time in aneurysm surgery as evaluated by evoked potential monitoring. Neurosurgery. 1993;33:434–40.
40. Mooij JJ, Buchthal A, Belopavlovic M. Somatosensory evoked potential monitoring of temporary middle cerebral artery occlusion during aneurysm operation. Neurosurgery. 1987;21:492–6.
41. Wicks RT, Pradilla G, Raza SM, Hadelsberg U, Coon AL, Huang J, Tamargo RJ. Impact of changes in intraoperative somatosensory evoked potentials on stroke rates after clipping of intracranial aneurysms. Neurosurgery. 2012;70:1114–24.
42. Ferch R, Pasqualin A, Pinna G, Chioffi F, Bricolo A. Temporary arterial occlusion in the repair of ruptured intracranial aneurysms: an analysis of risk factors for stroke. J Neurosurg. 2002;97:836–42.
43. Ogilvy CS, Carter BS, Kaplan S, Rich C, Crowell RM. Temporary vessel occlusion for aneurysm surgery: risk factors for stroke in patients protected by induced hypothermia and hypertension and intravenous mannitol administration. J Neurosurg. 1996;84:785–91.

44. Samson D, Batjer HH, Bowman G, Mootz L, Krippner WJ Jr, Meyer YJ, Allen BC. A clinical study of the parameters and effects of temporary arterial occlusion in the management of intracranial aneurysms. Neurosurgery. 1994;34:22–8.
45. Gruber A, Dorfer C, Standhardt H, Bavinzski G, Knosp E. Prospective comparison of intraoperative vascular monitoring technologies during cerebral aneurysm surgery. Neurosurgery. 2011;68:657–73.
46. Raabe A, Seidel K. Prevention of ischemic complications during aneurysm surgery. J Neurosurg Sci. 2016;60:95–103.
47. Hossmann KA. Experimental models for the investigation of brain ischemia. Cardiovasc Res. 1998;39:106–20.
48. Macfarlane R, Moskowitz MA, Tasdemiroglu E, Wei EP, Kontos HA. Postischemic cerebral blood flow and neuroeffector mechanisms. Blood Vessels. 1991;28:46–51.
49. Sundt TM Jr, Waltz AG. Cerebral ischemia and reactive hyperemia. Studies of cortical blood flow and microcirculation before, during, and after temporary occlusion of middle cerebral artery of squirrel monkeys. Circ Res. 1971;28:426–33.

Clipping of Recurrent Cerebral Aneurysms After Coil Embolization

Shingo Toyota, Tetsuya Kumagai, Tetsu Goto, Kanji Mori, and Takuyu Taki

Abstract *Background and aims.* To assess the technical points of surgical clipping for recurrent aneurysms after coiling, we examine a consecutive series of 14 patients who underwent re-treatment.

Materials and methods. From 2009 to 2016, 27 recurrent aneurysms after coiling were re-treated with endovascular treatment or surgical clipping. Of these, 14 were re-treated surgically. In cases where the remnant neck was sufficiently large, neck clipping was chosen. Where the remnant neck was too small and the border between the thrombosed and non-thrombosed portion was distinct, partial clipping was chosen. Surgical clipping was attempted without removing the coils when technically feasible.

Results. Among the 14 cases, neck clipping was performed in 11, partial clipping in 2, and trapping with bypass in 1 case. Clipping without removal of coils was accomplished in all cases. No neurological deterioration occurred after surgical clipping in any case.

Conclusion. Clipping of recurrent aneurysms after coiling can compensate for the failure of initial endovascular therapy. For clipping without removal of coils, precise evaluation of the remnant neck is required. Bypass surgery is key to treatment in the case of aneurysm trapping.

Keywords Cerebral aneurysm · Clipping · Coil embolization · Recurrence · Retreatment

Introduction

Influenced by the good results of coil embolization in several clinical trials for ruptured aneurysms [1], endovascular treatment has often been selected as the first-choice treatment for ruptured aneurysms in Japan. Even in the treatment of unruptured aneurysms, excellent outcomes have been reported that are similar to those for surgical clipping [2]. However, an aneurysm may recur after coiling [3–5]. As a result of the increase in endovascular surgery, recurrence of aneurysms after coiling are diagnosed more frequently.

Many reports show that re-coil embolization is safe and efficient for the re-treatment of recurrent aneurysms after coiling [6–8]. On the other hand, surgical clipping is an alternative option for re-treatment, especially in cases unsuitable for coil embolization [9–13]. Microsurgical techniques for cerebral aneurysms have recently become well established with progress in intraoperative neuroendoscopy [14, 15], indocyanine green (ICG) videoangiography [16], and motor-evoked potential (MEP) monitoring [17]. Both endovascular techniques and well-established microsurgical techniques are available, and they play an important role even in the re-treatment of recurrent aneurysms [12].

We examine a consecutive series of 14 recurrent cerebral aneurysms after coil embolization, which were re-treated using surgical techniques, and focus on the technical points of clipping procedures.

Materials and Methods

From May 2009 to February 2016, 27 recurrent aneurysms after coil embolization were re-treated. All re-treatments were performed by the first author (S.T.). Re-treatment was considered in cases with a rapid increase in recurrent lesions, residuals greater than 30% of the original aneurysm, or blebs in the recurrent lesions.

Our re-treatment decision-making is discussed herein (Fig. 1). When the previous frames covered the aneurysms all around (Type 1) or almost around except for part of the neck (Type 2), coil embolization was chosen. In other cases, surgical clipping was chosen. In all, 14 cases were re-treated with surgical clipping. When the remnant neck was sufficiently tall, neck clipping was chosen (Type 3). When the remnant

S. Toyota (✉) · T. Kumagai · T. Goto · K. Mori · T. Taki
Department of Neurosurgery, Kansai Rosai Hospital, Amagasaki, Hyogo, Japan

https://doi.org/10.1007/978-3-319-73739-3_8,

neck was short and the border between the thrombosed and non-thrombosed portion was distinct, partial clipping of the non-thrombosed portion was chosen (Type 4). Surgical clipping was attempted without removal of embolized coils when technically feasible.

Results

Fourteen patients (7 males and 7 females) were re-treated using a microsurgical technique. As shown in Table 1, 12 aneurysms had ruptured. The affected artery was the internal carotid artery (ICA) in 10, anterior communicating artery (ACom A) in 2, anterior cerebral artery (ACA) in 1, and vertebral artery (VA) in 1. The average age at initial treatment was 50 ± 15 years. The average long diameter of the aneurysm was 5.1 ± 1.2 mm. The status of coil embolization at the initial treatment was 5 nearly complete occlusion cases, 7 neck remnant cases, and 2 partial embolization cases. The status of recurrence using our schema was 11 Type 3 cases, and 3 Type 4 cases. The average interval to re-treatment was 12 ± 9 months (Table 1).

In all 14 cases, surgical clipping was accomplished without the removal of coils. In 11 Type 3 cases, neck clipping was performed. In 2 Type 4 cases, partial clipping of the non-embolized portion was performed, but in 1 case, which was thought to be a Type 4 pseudoaneurysmal formation, trapping with bypass was performed. There was no neurological deterioration after surgical clipping in any case. No aneurysm required "re-retreatment" during the follow-up period.

Table 1 Profile of 14 aneurysms re-treated using a microsurgical technique

No	Age	Sex	Hunt and Hess Grade	Ruptured	Location	Size (mm)	Results of initial embolization	Interval (day)	Recurrent status	Additional treatment	Extraction of coils
1	63	F	4	Ruptured	ICA	4	Neck remnant	740	Type 3	Neck clipping	No
2	66	F	2	Ruptured	ICA	4	Neck remnant	646	Type 3	Neck clipping	No
3	42	M	2	Ruptured	ICA	5	Neck remnant	786	Type 3	Neck clipping	No
4	38	M	5	Ruptured	ACA	5	Nearly complete occlusion	499	Type 4	Partial clipping	No
5	43	M	5	Ruptured	VA	4	Partial embolization	49	Type 3	Neck clipping	No
6	48	F	4	Ruptured	ICA	6	Partial embolization	36	Type 4	Partial clipping	No
7	38	F	3	Ruptured	ICA	3	Nearly complete occlusion	57	Type 3	Neck clipping	No
8	32	M	2	Ruptured	ICA	7	Nearly complete occlusion	730	Type 3	Neck clipping	No
9	28	F	3	Ruptured	ICA	5	Neck remnant	240	Type 3	Neck clipping	No
10	68	M	0	Unruptured	ICA	7	Neck remnant	390	Type 3	Neck clipping	No
11	66	F	0	Unruptured	ICA	5	Neck remnant	340	Type 3	Neck clipping	No
12	55	M	3	Ruptured	A-com A	7	Nearly complete occlusion	311	Type 3	Neck clipping	No
13	79	F	5	Ruptured	A-com A	4	Nearly complete occlusion	22	Type 4	Bypass trapping	No
14	38	M	3	Ruptured	ICA	5	Neck remnant	96	Type 3	Neck clipping	No

ICA internal carotid artery, *A-com A* anterior communicating artery, *ACA* anterior cerebral artery, *VA* vertebral artery

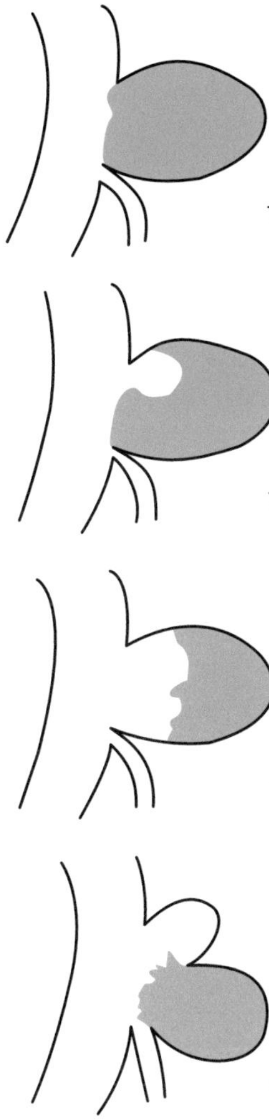

Fig. 1 Schema of recurrent status. The status was classified into four types: Type 1: The previous frames cover the aneurysms all around. Type 2: The previous frames cover the aneurysms almost around except a part of the neck. Type 3: The remnant neck is sufficiently tall. Type 4: The remnant neck is short, and the border between the thrombosed and non-thrombosed portion is distinct

Illustrated Cases

Case 14 (Fig. 2)

A 38-year-old man presented with subarachnoid hemorrhage (SAH) (Hunt and Hess Grade 3). On the onset day, the patient underwent coil embolization of a ruptured right ICA top aneurysm. The initial size of the aneurysm was 5 mm. After coil embolization a remnant neck persisted. Approximately 3 months after the initial treatment, regrowth of the remnant neck was observed. The shape of the remnant neck was irregular, but the average height was more than 2 mm and the width was 2.5 mm. The recurrence was classed as Type 3 based on our schema, and neck clipping was planned.

Via a right trans-sylvian approach, the embolized aneurysm and surrounding structures were exposed using a microsurgical technique. Under temporal occlusion of the ICA, selective clipping of the remnant neck was performed, without removal of the coils, under MEP monitoring.

The postoperative course was uneventful. The patient was discharged without any neurological complications.

Case 13 (Fig. 3)

A 79-year-old woman presented with SAH (Hunt and Hess Grade 5). On the onset day, the patient underwent coil embolization of an ACom aneurysm. The initial size of the aneurysm was 4 mm. After coiling, nearly complete occlusion was obtained in the absence of procedural complications. As severe vasospasm caused cerebral infarction in both hemispheres during the post-SAH course, the status deteriorated to modified Rankin Scale (mRS) 5. Twenty-two days after the initial treatment, re-rupture of the aneurysm occurred. Cerebral angiography revealed a rapid aneurysmal enlargement adjacent to the coil-embolized section of the aneurysm. The recurrence was classed as Type 4, and partial clipping of the non-embolized portion was planned.

Via an interhemispheric approach, the embolized part of the aneurysm and the aneurysmal enlargement adjacent to it were exposed using a microsurgical technique. As it was thought to be a pseudoaneurysmal formation and it ruptured intraoperatively, trapping with bypass was performed. In order to trap the aneurysm, ACom and the origin of the right A2 of the ACA were occluded (using two clips) after the construction of an A3-A3 bypass. Patency of the bypass was confirmed by ICG videoangiography.

Although there was no apparent evidence of new ischemic lesions after the operation and the postoperative course was uneventful, the status remained mRS 5 and the patient was transferred to a long-term care hospital.

Discussion

As a re-treatment option for recurrent aneurysms after coiling, re-coil embolization is a safe and effective strategy. There are many reports of coil embolization being adopted as the first-line option for the treatment of recurrent aneurysms [6–8]. In addition, using a stent or flow diverter has

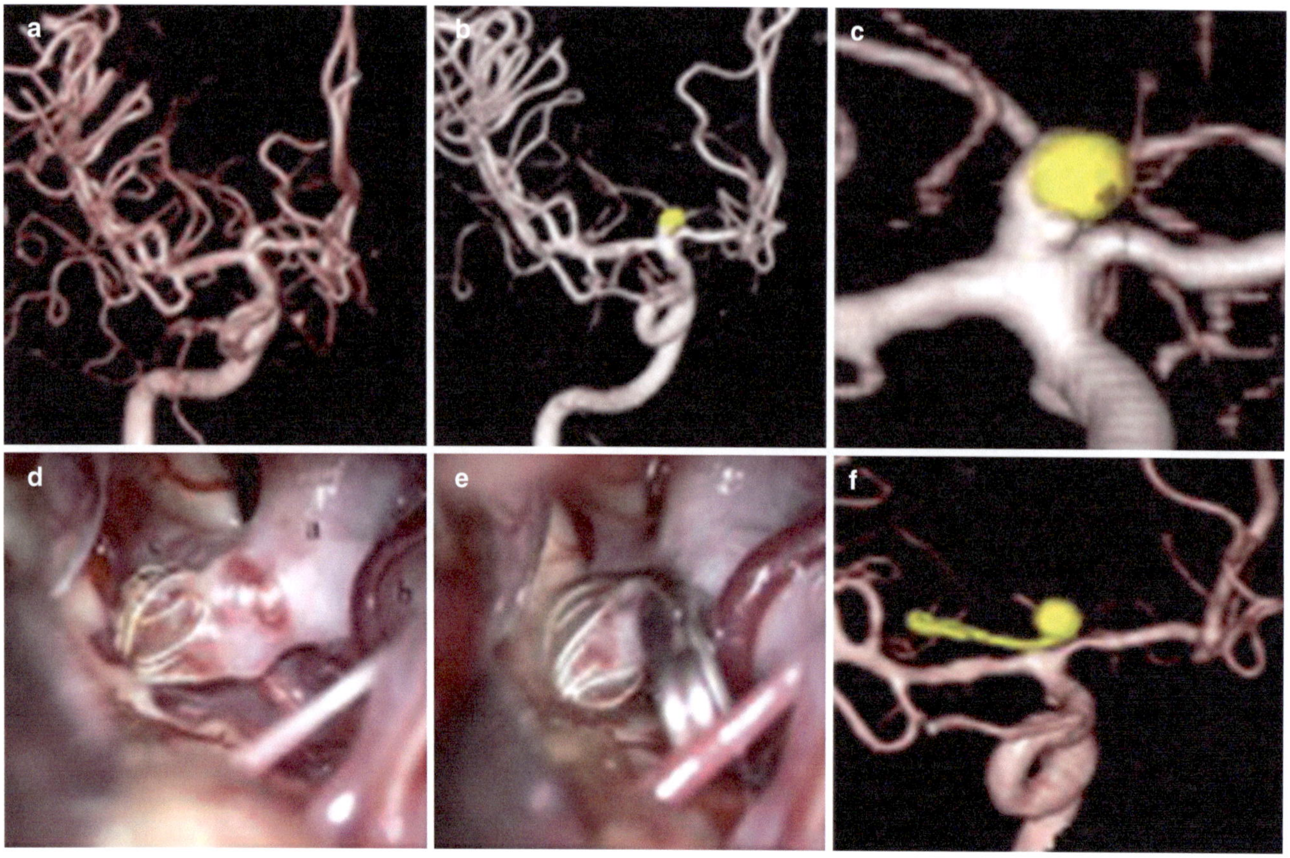

Fig. 2 Case 14: A 38-year-old man. (**a**) A ruptured right ICA top aneurysm was recognized with 3D digital subtraction angiography. (**b**) After coiling, a neck remnant was documented. (**c**) Approximately 3 months after the initial treatment, regrowth of the remnant neck was revealed. (**d**) In the operative findings, coils and regrowth of the remnant neck were observed. (**e**) Neck clipping was performed. (**f**) Neck clipping without removal of previously embolized coils. (**a**) ICA, (**b**) M1 portion of MCA, (**c**) A1 portion of ACA

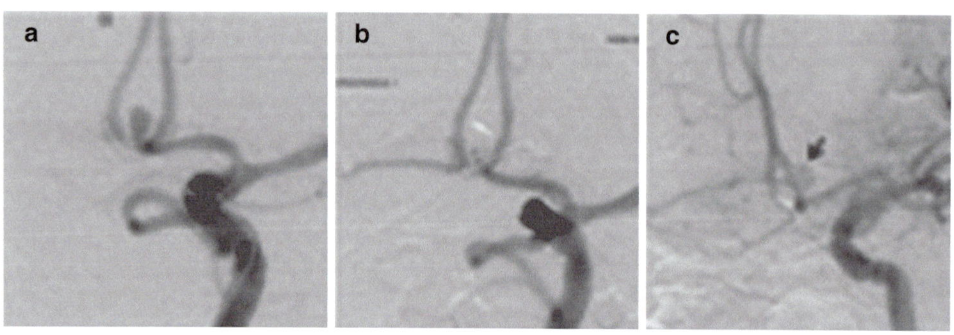

Fig. 3 Case 13: A 79-year-old woman. (**a**) A ruptured ACom aneurysm was recognized with angiography. (**b**) After coiling, nearly complete occlusion was obtained. (**c**) Twenty-two days after the initial treatment, angiography revealed a rapid aneurysmal enlargement (arrow) adjacent to the coil-embolized section. (**d**) In the operative findings, embolized coils and pseudoaneurysmal formation were observed. (**e**) A3-A3 bypass was performed before trapping of the aneurysm. (**f**) In order to trap the aneurysm, ACom and the origin of the right A2 were occluded (by means of two clips). (**g**) Trapping with bypass documented via ICG videoangiography. (**a**) The right A2 portion of the ACA, (**b**) the left A2 portion of the ACA, (**c**) pseudoaneurysmal formation, (**d**) the right A1 portion of the ACA

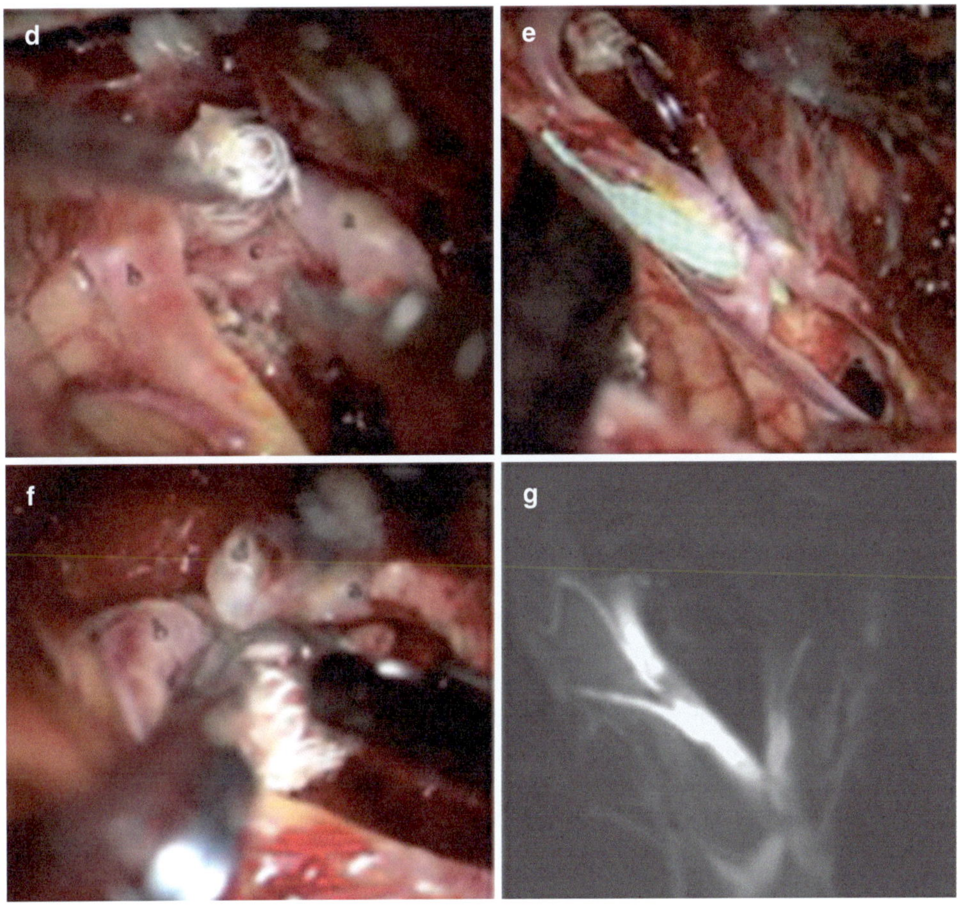

Fig. 3 (continued)

expanded the indication of endovascular surgery for retreatment, although we should consider the thromboembolic complications and the possible disadvantages of dual antiplatelet therapy [18]. However, it is well-known that not all configurations of recurrent aneurysms are suitable for endovascular treatment. In cases unsuitable for coil embolization, direct surgery can be an alternative option [9, 12, 19].

Herein we present a schema for surgical decision making for managing recurrent aneurysms after coiling (not suitable for endovascular treatment). The strategy is based on the morphology of the remnant neck. Coils are not removed. According to the schema presented above, Type 1 and Type 2 recurrent aneurysms are not ideal candidate for selective clipping of the neck without removal of the coils. Type 3 and Type 4 recurrent aneurysms are possible good candidates for selective clipping. This strategy could reduce the need for clipping procedures with associated coils removal, which may be associated with high morbidity [11, 12]. Clipping for recurrent aneurysms after coiling is performed with or without removal of the coils. Removal of the coils may help to provide enough space for clipping, but may also present disadvantages [11, 13, 19]. Dorfer et al. reported a case where opening of the aneurysm and attempting coil removal resulted in aneurysm rupture at the neck and ultimately led to the sacrifice of the parent artery [19]. Furthermore, as the extraction of the coils may require temporary occlusion of the parent artery or bypass surgery, or may cause intimal injury of the parent artery, clipping without removal of the coils may be preferable when technically feasible [12].

In two cases of Type 4, we planned and performed partial clipping of the non-thrombosed portion of the aneurysms in order to avoid complications related to the extraction of the coils. In partial clipping, it is necessary to confirm that the border between the thrombosed and non-thrombosed portions is distinct before surgery, and clips should be applied as closely as possible to the coil mass.

Predicting whether coil extraction during microsurgery may be necessary has significant implications in preoperative planning [9, 12, 13, 19–21]. For safe clipping of the aneurysm neck without coil removal, the remnant neck should be "tall enough" to provide space for neck clipping [13, 20]. Waldon et al. evaluated the ratio of coil width to compaction height (C:H ratio) at re-treatment. They suggested that aneurysms with a C:H ratio greater than 2.5 or with minimal compaction (compaction height <2 mm) were not amenable to clipping without coil removal [13]. In our opinion, the average height of the neck should be more than 2 mm: if not, neck clipping without coil removal should not be performed. For instance, in Case 14 (Type 3), we planned and accomplished selective neck clipping without coils removal because the average height of the remnant neck was more than 2 mm, and the C:H ratio was less than 2.5.

During surgical procedures, dissection all around aneurysms is not always straightforward because the coil mass cannot be reduced even if we use temporary occlusion of the parent artery [12]. The difficulties associated with microsurgical clipping of aneurysms previously treated via endovascular means were reported by several authors [9, 11–13, 19]. Tough arachnoid scarring and adhesions surrounding the coiled aneurysms can complicate dissection, and extrusion of the coil into the subarachnoid space and cerebral parenchyma is frequently observed [22]. Coiled aneurysms are relatively immobile, making dissection and visualization in the surrounding area more difficult [13, 19]. As neck clipping without removal of coils may cause a longitudinal stretch force along the neck, it is preferable to prepare a temporary occlusion of the parent artery [12]. Additionally, a donor artery, such as the superficial temporal artery, should be prepared for bypass surgery in case of temporary occlusion of the parent artery during coil extraction [11–13, 19]. In Case 13 (Type 4), A3-A3 bypass was required because ACom and the origin of the right A2 of the ACA were clipped to trap the pseudoaneurysm. Especially in the re-treatment of recurrent ACom aneurysms after coiling, the interhemispheric approach, which can provide a wide working space and A3-A3 bypass, is considered an option. During application of the aneurysm clip, it is not necessary to close and release the clips many times: this may be important to prevent thromboembolic events. All the recurrent aneurysms after coil embolization are thought to be "thrombosed aneurysms."

In this study, several limitations should be noted. First, the number of treated aneurysms was small. Second, the diameters of the aneurysms were relatively small. In large or giant aneurysms the possibility of neck clipping without removal of coils is thought to be low. As the choice of the re-treatment greatly depends on the individual microsurgery and endovascular surgery skills, it is desirable to establish objective criteria for the choice of re-treatment.

Conclusions

Surgical clipping of recurrent aneurysms after coiling can compensate for the failure of the initial endovascular treatment. For clipping without coil removal, a precise evaluation of the remnant neck is required. Bypass surgery is key to treatment in the case of aneurysm trapping.

Conflict of Interests Disclosure Nothing to report.

References

1. Molyneux A, Kerr R, Stratton I, Sandercock P, Clarke M, Shrimpton J, Holman R, International Subarachnoid Aneurysm Trial Collaborative G. International Subarachnoid Aneurysm Trial (ISAT) of neurosurgical clipping versus endovascular coiling in 2143 patients with ruptured intracranial aneurysms: a randomised trial. Lancet. 2002;360:1267–74.
2. Shigematsu T, Fujinaka T, Yoshimine T, Imamura H, Ishii A, Sakai C, Sakai N, Investigators J-N. Endovascular therapy for asymptomatic unruptured intracranial aneurysms: JR-NET and JR-NET2 findings. Stroke. 2013;44:2735–42.
3. Campi A, Ramzi N, Molyneux AJ, Summers PE, Kerr RS, Sneade M, Yarnold JA, Rischmiller J, Byrne JV. Retreatment of ruptured cerebral aneurysms in patients randomized by coiling or clipping in the International Subarachnoid Aneurysm Trial (ISAT). Stroke. 2007;38:1538–44.
4. Investigators C. Rates of delayed rebleeding from intracranial aneurysms are low after surgical and endovascular treatment. Stroke. 2006;37:1437–42.
5. Molyneux AJ, Kerr RS, Birks J, Ramzi N, Yarnold J, Sneade M, Rischmiller J, Collaborators I. Risk of recurrent subarachnoid haemorrhage, death, or dependence and standardised mortality ratios after clipping or coiling of an intracranial aneurysm in the International Subarachnoid Aneurysm Trial (ISAT): long-term follow-up. Lancet Neurol. 2009;8:427–33.
6. Kang HS, Han MH, Kwon BJ, Kwon OK, Kim SH. Repeat endovascular treatment in post-embolization recurrent intracranial aneurysms. Neurosurgery. 2006;58:60–70; discussion 60–70.
7. Slob MJ, Sluzewski M, van Rooij WJ, Roks G, Rinkel GJ. Additional coiling of previously coiled cerebral aneurysms: clinical and angiographic results. AJNR Am J Neuroradiol. 2004;25:1373–6.
8. van Rooij WJ, Sprengers ME, Sluzewski M, Beute GN. Intracranial aneurysms that repeatedly reopen over time after coiling: imaging characteristics and treatment outcome. Neuroradiology. 2007;49:343–9.

9. Izumo T, Matsuo T, Morofuji Y, Hiu T, Horie N, Hayashi K, Nagata I. Microsurgical clipping for recurrent aneurysms after initial endovascular coil embolization. World Neurosurg. 2015;83(2):211–8.
10. Kai Y, Hamada J, Morioka M, Yano S, Nakamura H, Makino K, Kuratsu J. Re-treatment of patients with embolized ruptured intracranial aneurysms. Surg Neurol. 2008;70:378–85.
11. Romani R, Lehto H, Laakso A, Horcajadas A, Kivisaari R, von und zu Fraunberg M, Niemela M, Rinne J, Hernesniemi J. Microsurgery for previously coiled aneurysms: experience with 81 patients. Neurosurgery. 2011;68:140–53; discussion 153–144.
12. Toyota S, Taki T, Wakayama A, Yoshimine T. Retreatment of recurrent internal carotid-posterior communicating artery aneurysm after coil embolization. Neurol Med Chir (Tokyo). 2015;55:838–47.
13. Waldron JS, Halbach VV, Lawton MT. Microsurgical management of incompletely coiled and recurrent aneurysms: trends, techniques, and observations on coil extrusion. Neurosurgery. 2009;64:301–15; discussion 315–317.
14. Kinouchi H, Yanagisawa T, Suzuki A, Ohta T, Hirano Y, Sugawara T, Sasajima T, Mizoi K. Simultaneous microscopic and endoscopic monitoring during surgery for internal carotid artery aneurysms. J Neurosurg. 2004;101:989–95.
15. Toyota S, Taki T, Wakayama A, Yoshimine T. Unruptured internal carotid-posterior communicating artery aneurysm splitting the oculomotor nerve: a case report and literature review. J Neurol Surg Rep. 2014;75:e180–2.
16. Raabe A, Nakaji P, Beck J, Kim LJ, Hsu FP, Kamerman JD, Seifert V, Spetzler RF. Prospective evaluation of surgical microscope-integrated intraoperative near-infrared indocyanine green videoangiography during aneurysm surgery. J Neurosurg. 2005;103:982–9.
17. Suzuki K, Kodama N, Sasaki T, Matsumoto M, Konno Y, Sakuma J, Oinuma M, Murakawa M. Intraoperative monitoring of blood flow insufficiency in the anterior choroidal artery during aneurysm surgery. J Neurosurg. 2003;98:507–14.
18. Tahtinen OI, Manninen HI, Vanninen RL, Rautio R, Haapanen A, Seppanen J, Niskakangas T, Rinne J, Keski-Nisula L. Stent-assisted embolization of recurrent or residual intracranial aneurysms. Neuroradiology. 2013;55:1221–31.
19. Dorfer C, Gruber A, Standhardt H, Bavinzski G, Knosp E. Management of residual and recurrent aneurysms after initial endovascular treatment. Neurosurgery. 2012;70:537–53; discussion 553–554.
20. Bulsara KR, Hoh B, Rosen C, Tanikawa R, Carpenter J. Preliminary observation on predicting the need for coil extraction during microsurgery: the clip-coil ratio. Acta Neurochir. 2010;152:431–4.
21. Lejeune JP, Thines L, Taschner C, Bourgeois P, Henon H, Leclerc X. Neurosurgical treatment for aneurysm remnants or recurrences after coil occlusion. Neurosurgery. 2008;63:684–91; discussion 691–692.
22. Mizoi K, Yoshimoto T, Takahashi A, Nagamine Y. A pitfall in the surgery of a recurrent aneurysm after coil embolization and its histological observation: technical case report. Neurosurgery. 1996;39:165–8; discussion 168–169.

Complex Aneurysm: The Unpredictable Pathological Entity

L. Pescatori, M.P. Tropeano, and A. Santoro

Abstract *Background.* Surgical treatment of complex aneurysms often requires the execution of a revascularization procedure. Even if avoiding the concomitant trapping of the aneurysm during the bypass procedure (waiting for the subsequent endovascular or spontaneous closure) permits one to verify the graft's patency and patient's adaptation to increased flow, the hemodynamic changes induced by the bypass may cause the aneurysmal rupture. Whether or not to perform the concomitant trapping of the aneurysm still remains a dilemma. Here we illustrate our management protocol through the critical analysis of some illustrative cases of our series.

Materials and methods. Between 1990 and 2016, 48 of 157 patients affected by complex aneurysms underwent a revascularization procedure. In 19 cases (1990–1997) only a bypass procedure was performed. Spontaneous or endovascular closure was obtained within the first postoperative week once the graft patency had been verified (staged revascularization strategy). In the remaining 29 cases (1997–2016) the revascularization procedure and the closure of the aneurysm were performed simultaneously during the same surgical procedure (single-stage strategy).

Results. In the staged revascularization era, one patient died because of the rupture of the aneurysm before its closure.

In the single-stage era no further cases of rebleeding were observed. Neurologic status of this group was unvaried or improved.

Conclusions. Given the unpredictable response of complex aneurysms to the hemodynamic changes induced by the revascularization, in our opinion it is always preferable to perform complete or at least incomplete trapping of the aneurysm during the bypass procedure.

L. Pescatori (✉) · M. P. Tropeano · A. Santoro
Department of Neurosurgery, Sapienza University of Rome, Rome, Italy

Keywords Bypass · Complex aneurysm · Hemodynamic · Trapping

Introduction

Complex aneurysms are a particular subtype of aneurysm in which the dimensions, the localization, the presence of collateral flows, specific wall characteristics, and previous endovascular or surgical treatment often preclude the possibility of a sole endovascular closure [1, 2]. This category of aneurysms often requires surgical therapy, including cerebral revascularization procedures [1–3]. Such procedures require the execution of an extra-intracranial bypass alone or in combination with incomplete or complete trapping of the aneurysm. In the case of bypass alone, the closure is expected to take place at a variable time in the postoperative course (through thrombosis or endovascularly) [1–6]. During this period the aneurysm is at potential risk of rupture [3, 7–9]. In the case of partial trapping, induced aneurysmal thrombosis may take place directly after trapping or during the postoperative course. During this period the aneurysm remains at risk of rupture. In the case of complete trapping, the aneurysm is excluded from the intracranial circle in the same surgical procedure simultaneously with the bypass and the risk of rupture is no longer present [1–3].

In choosing one of these two surgical alternatives, neurosurgeons must bear in mind that the natural history of complex aneurysms, as well as their response to similar surgical strategies, is extremely heterogeneous and unpredictable and that unpleasant events may characterize each phase of the therapeutic course.

Through the description of some illustrative cases extrapolated from our series, we demonstrate how variable the behavior of such pathological entities could be and what rationale lies behind the surgical strategy we decided to adopt at our Institution.

G. Esposito et al. (eds.), *Trends in the Management of Cerebrovascular Diseases*, Acta Neurochirurgica Supplement, Vol. 129,
https://doi.org/10.1007/978-3-319-73739-3_9, © Springer International Publishing AG, part of Springer Nature 2018

Materials and Methods

Between 1990 and 2016, 157 complex aneurysms were treated at our institution (Department of Neurosurgery, Sapienza University of Rome). Among these, 119 required surgical treatment. In 48 cases a cerebral revascularization procedure was performed. In all but one of the other cases, surgical treatment involved direct clipping of the aneurysm. Hunterian ligation of the internal carotid artery (ICA) was performed only in one case. In the first part of our experience (1990–1997, 19 patients) revascularization was performed according to the so-called staged revascularization strategy. This consisted of four different Phases:

- Preoperative balloon occlusion test (BOT) to verify patient's toleration to the occlusion of the ICA and to select ICA/external carotid artery (ECA) as donor vessel
- Bypass
- Postoperative angiography and BOT to verify the patency of the graft and the patient's adaptation to the improved flow
- Endovascular or spontaneous closure of the aneurysm

In the second part of this series (1997–2016, 29 patients) the strategy was shifted to the "single stage revascularization strategy." In this technique, BOT, EC-IC bypass, and closure of the parent vessel were all performed during the surgical procedure.

The results of our series are briefly summarized and four emblematic illustrative cases (two cases treated in the "staged" era and two other cases in the "single stage" era) are presented.

Results

Of the 48 aneurysms treated by revascularization procedures, 15 (32%) were localized in the paraclinoid region whereas the other 33 were intracavernous aneurysms with subarachnoidal extension.

Among the 19 patients treated in the "staged" revascularization strategy era, 15 presented with an intracavernous aneurysm with subarachnoidal extension, whereas in 4 cases the aneurysm was in the paraclinoidal region.

Among the 29 patients treated in the "single" stage revascularization strategy era, 18 were affected by an intracavernous aneurysm with subarachnoidal extension, whereas the other 11 aneurysms were localized in the paraclinoidal region.

Among the 19 patients treated by the staged strategy, at 6 months follow-up 17 patients experienced an improvement of the neurological status or at least did not deteriorate. Two patients died in the immediate postoperative course. In one case death was caused by a widespread middle cerebral artery (MCA) ischemia, probably related to the distal spread of intra-aneurysmal thrombus. The cause of the death of the second patient was an intraparenchymal hematoma with subarachnoidal hemorrhage determined by the rupture of the aneurysm in the postoperative course while awaiting its spontaneous thrombosis.

At 6 months follow-up, neurological examination of the 29 patients treated in the single stage era showed no variation or was improved. During the second part of our experience we did not experience further cases of re-bleeding.

Illustrative Cases

Case 1

This 22-year-old man presented with sudden onset of severe headache in April 1994. Cerebral computed tomography revealed subarachnoid hemorrhage, and the patient therefore underwent angiography, which detected an aneurysm of the right internal carotid artery (ICA) (Fig. 1a). Surgical clipping

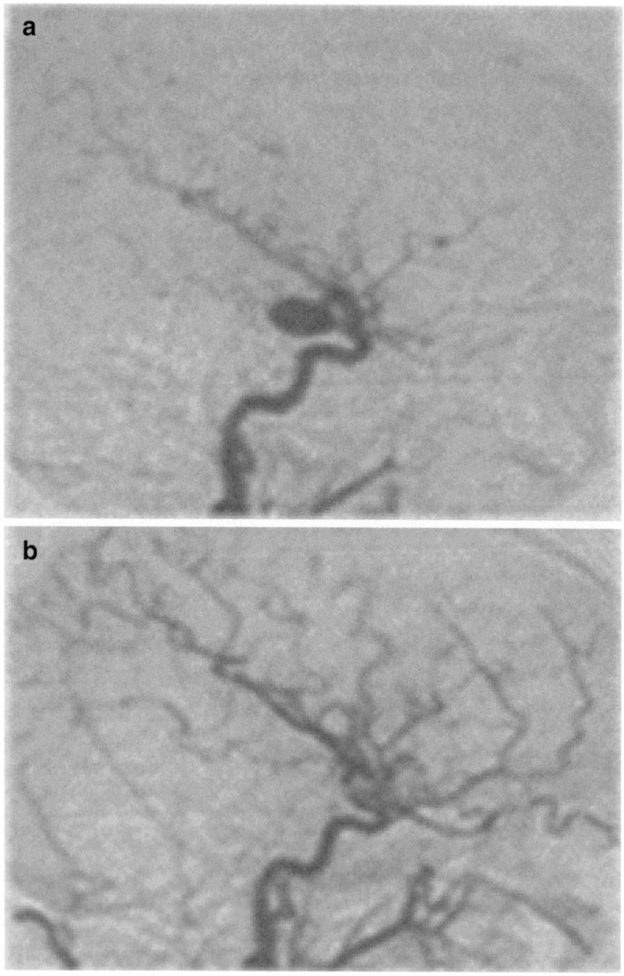

Fig. 1 (**a**) Angiography documenting a right ICA aneurysm. (**b**) Postoperative angiography after the clipping of the aneurysm

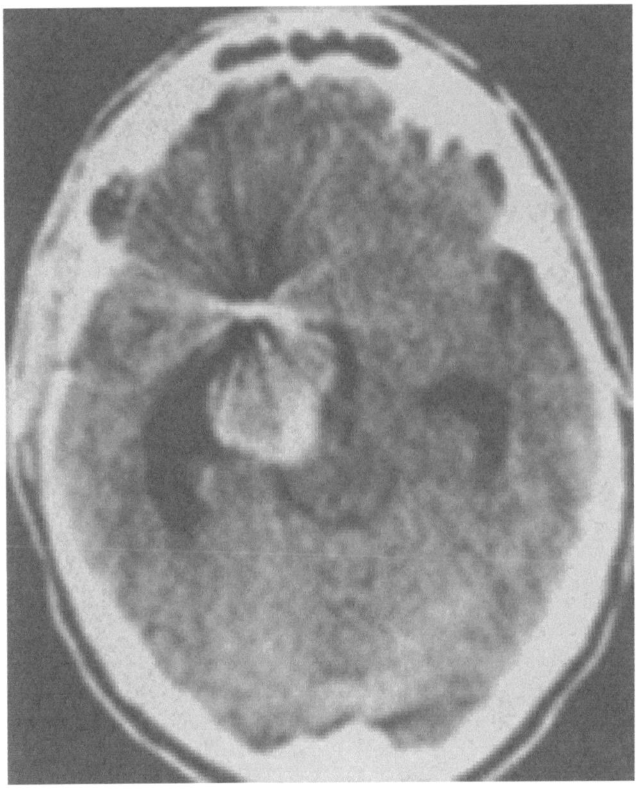

Fig. 2 Computed tomography enhanced with contrast medium, detecting a large area of hyperdensity in the area surrounding the clips previously positioned

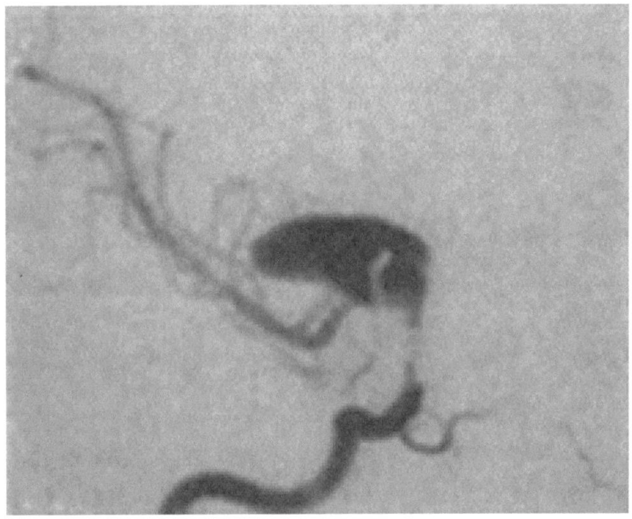

Fig. 3 A further angiographic study revealed a large, partly thrombosed aneurysm situated in the supraclinoidal segment of the right ICA, the formation of which was probably caused by sliding of the clips

of the aneurysm, the results of which are illustrated in the postoperative angiograms (Fig. 1b), was performed elsewhere. The postoperative period was uneventful, and the patient was discharged on Day 7 in good neurological condition. After a period of well-being lasting 4 months, the patient started again to complain of headache, followed by left hemiparesis. Computed tomography with contrast medium showed a large area of hyperdensity around the clips (Fig. 2). A further angiographic study revealed a large, partly thrombosed aneurysm situated in the supraclinoidal segment of the right ICA, the formation of which was probably caused by sliding of the clips (Fig. 3). The patient was operated on again, but it was impossible to exclude the aneurysm because no clear neck could be identified. Angiography was therefore repeated, this time with a balloon occlusion test (BOT); the balloon was deflated because it accentuated the left hemiparesis. Consequently, we decided to construct an extra-intracranial bypass with a saphenous vein graft between the ECA and the temporal branch of the MCA and then to proceed with endovascular occlusion of the aneurysm.

Five days later, control angiograms (Fig. 4) confirmed the patency of the venous graft, good intracranial perfusion, exclusion of the aneurysm from the arterial circulation, and

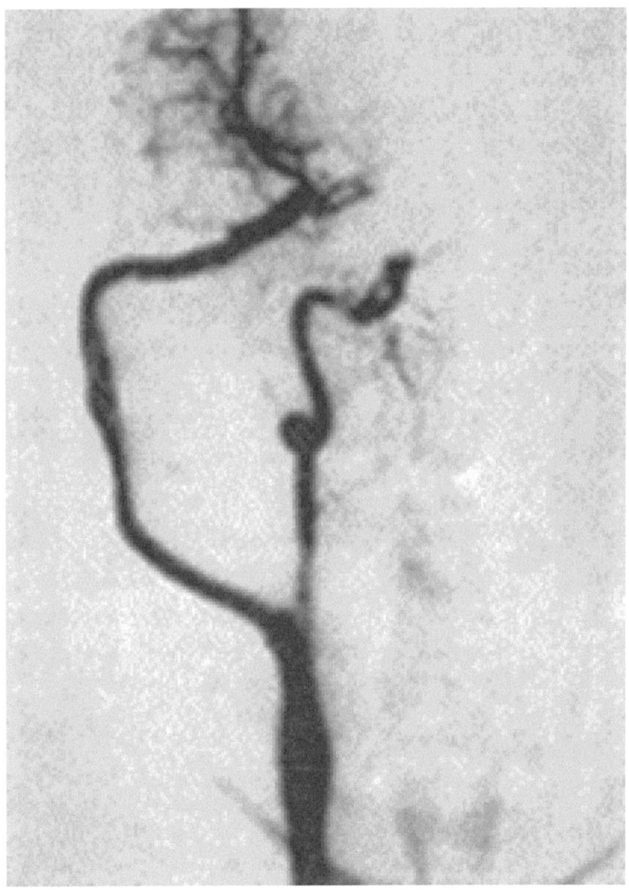

Fig. 4 Control angiograms confirming patency of the venous graft, good intracranial perfusion, exclusion of the aneurysm from the arterial circulation, and occlusion of the ICA just after the origin of the ophthalmic artery

occlusion of the ICA just after the origin of the ophthalmic artery. The patient was discharged on Day 10 in good neurological condition. At the 6-month clinical and radiological follow-up examinations, the hemiparesis had completely regressed and magnetic resonance (MR) imaging confirmed complete thrombosis of the aneurysm.

Case 2

This 45-year-old woman came to our attention because of the progressive onset of left visual disturbances. A brain CT scan with contrast documented the presence of a supraclinoidal aneurysm of the left ICA (Fig. 5). Angiography confirmed the presence of the aneurysm (Fig. 6). Electroencephalographic (EEG) modification during BOT induced us to deflate the balloon and to plan a revascularization surgical procedure consisting of extra-intracranial bypass with saphenous vein graft between the left ECA and the temporal branch of the middle cerebral artery. Given the result of the preoperative BOT, we decided to postpone the closure of the ICA once the patency of the bypass was confirmed by the postoperative angiography. An EC-IC bypass was successfully created. Intraoperative ultrasonography confirmed the patency of the graft. Three days later a control angiography was performed. It demonstrated the patency of the graft and the progressive thrombosis of the aneurysm (Fig. 7). Three days later the patient became comatose, unresponsive, and mydriatic bilaterally. A brain CT scan was then performed. It demonstrated the presence of a voluminous left frontal intraparenchymal hemorrhage (Fig. 8). Given the neurological assessment, the patient was not operated on. She died 2 days later.

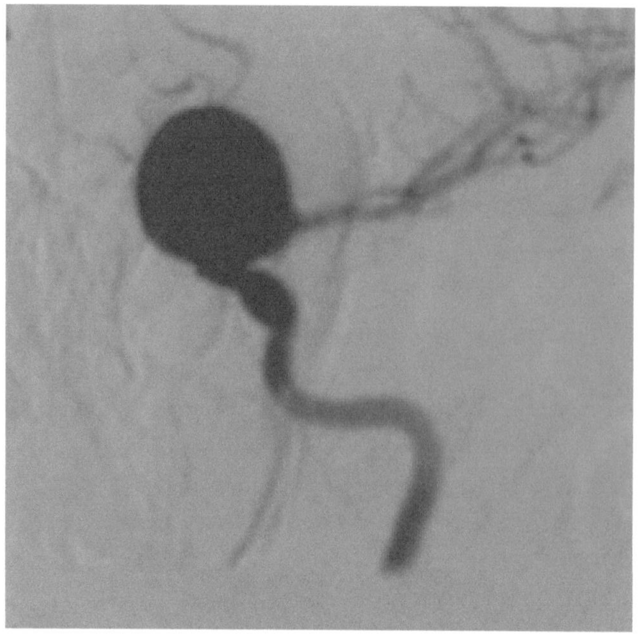

Fig. 6 Angiography confirming the presence of a paraclinoidal-supraclinoidal aneurysm of the left ICA

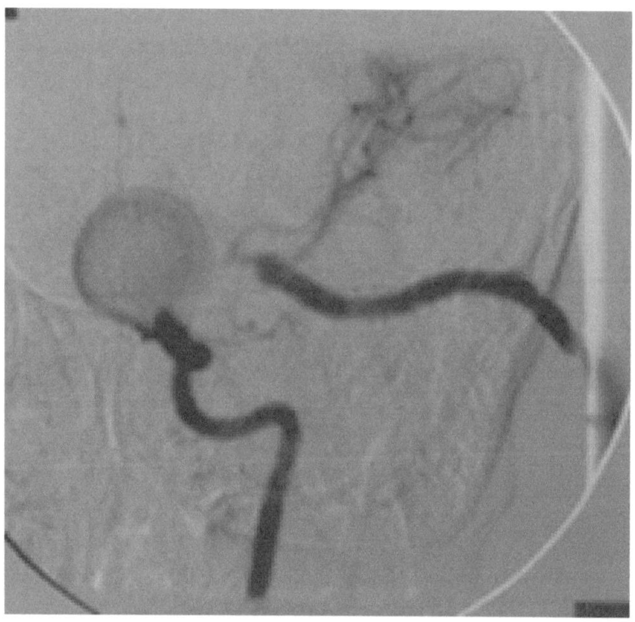

Fig. 7 Postoperative angiography. After the EC-IC bypass procedure the aneurysm partially thrombosed.

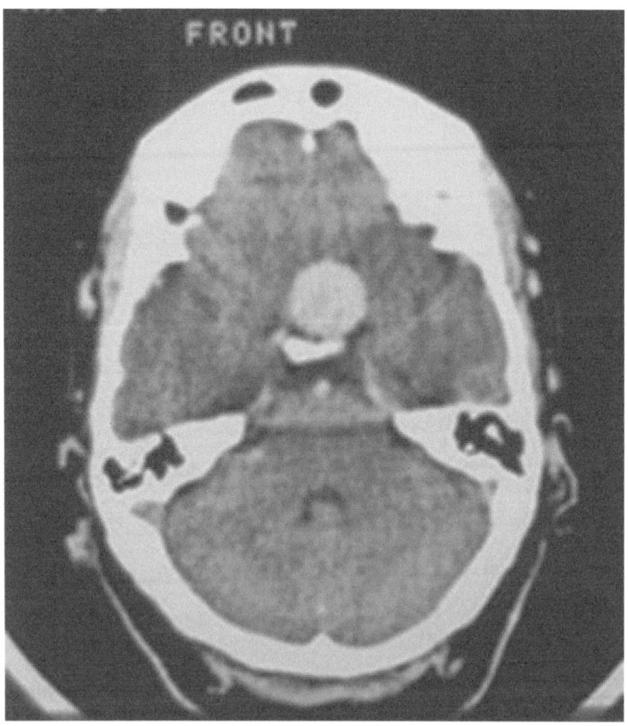

Fig. 5 Brain CT scan with contrast documenting the presence of a supraclinoidal aneurysm of the left ICA

Case 3

This 50-year-old male came to our attention because of persistent drug-resistant headache and progressive onset of mild right hemiparesis. A brain MRI was performed. It demonstrated the presence of a left giant partially thrombosed MCA aneurysm (Fig. 9). Cerebral angiography confirmed the presence of the aneurysm (Fig. 10). The patient was scheduled for a surgical procedure of cerebral revascularization through an EC-IC bypass and concomitant trapping of the aneurysm.

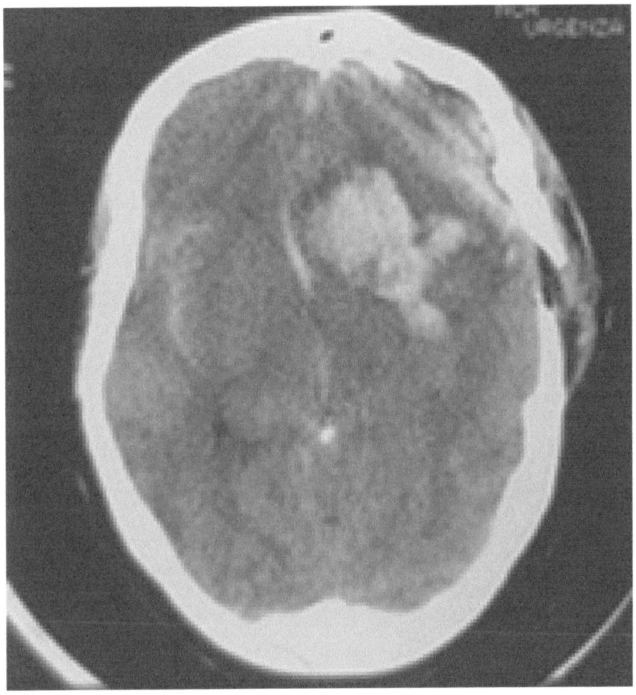

Fig. 8 Three days after the surgical procedure the patient became comatose, unresponsive, and mydriatic bilaterally. A brain CT scan was then performed. It demonstrated the presence of a voluminous left frontal intraparenchymal hemorrhage

Intraoperative closure of the ICA was tolerated by the patient. An EC-IC bypass through a saphenous graft connecting the ICA with the temporal branch of the MCA was executed. Intraoperative ultrasonography confirmed the presence of flow within the graft. After the bypass procedure, the MCA was closed with a clip as close as possible to the bifurcation, thereby obtaining an incomplete trapping of the aneurysm. A clip distal to the aneurysm (to obtain complete trapping) was not placed because of the localization of the aneurysm. The postoperative course was regular in the absence of the new neurological deficit. CT-angiography demonstrated the patency of the bypass (Fig. 11). Ten days after the surgical procedure a cerebral angiography was performed. It confirmed the patency of the graft, the occlusion of the aneurysm, and retrograde flow through the perforating arteries of M1 (Fig. 12a). Another angiography performed at 30 days confirmed the patency of the graft, the complete occlusion of the aneurysm, and improved flow within the perforating vessels (Fig. 12b). Neurological examination at 2 months follow-up documented improvement of the right hemiparesis. The headache disappeared.

Case 4

This 49-year-old woman came to our attention because of a sudden onset of headache with vomiting. A brain CT scan demonstrated the presence of a subarachnoid hemorrhage mainly localized within the left Sylvian fissure (Fig. 13a). A CT-angiography scan documented the presence of a left ICA aneurysm extending from the supraclinoidal segment to the

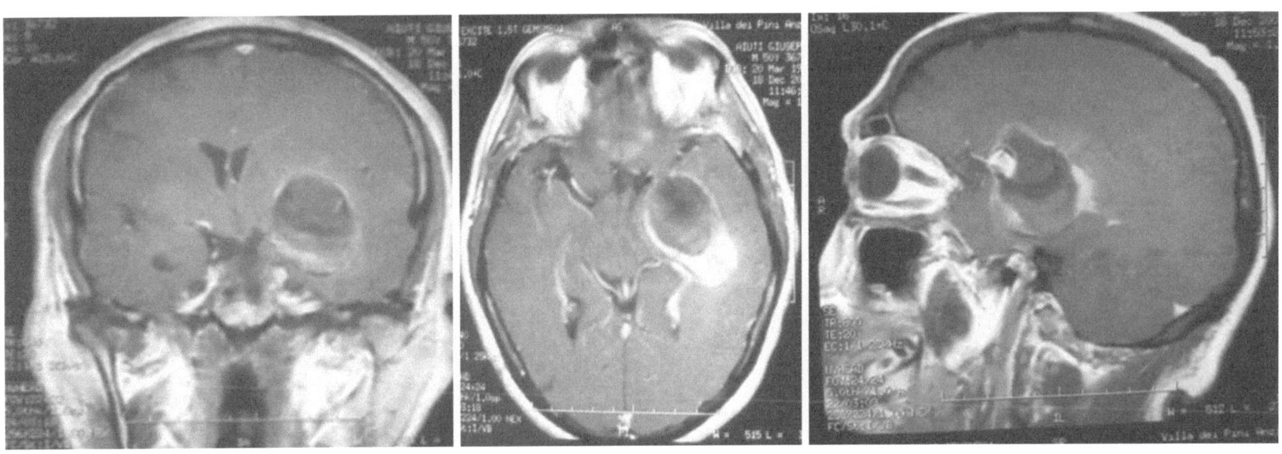

Fig. 9 Preoperative MRI, coronal, axial, and sagittal projection. It demonstrated the presence of a left giant partially thrombosed MCA aneurysm localized at the bifurcation

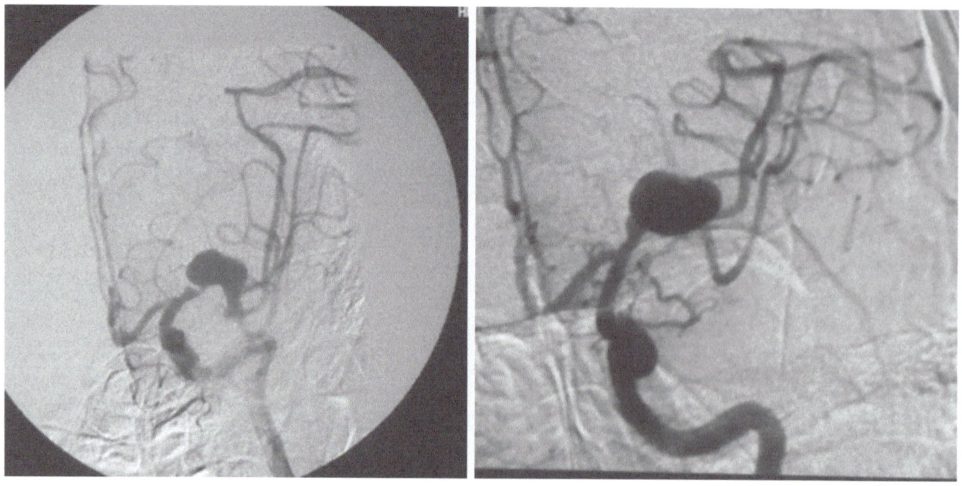

Fig. 10 Angiographic study confirming the presence of the partially thrombosed left MCA aneurysm

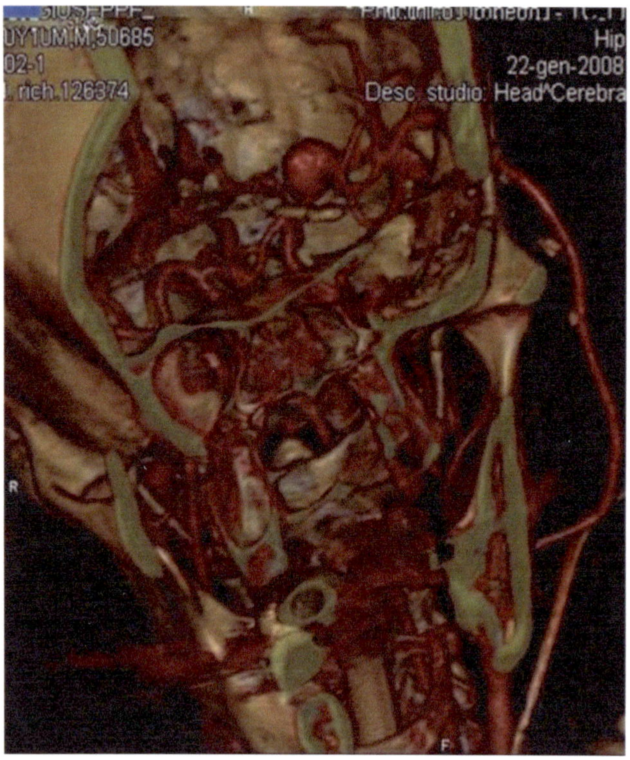

Fig. 11 Early postoperative CT scan showing patency of the EC-IC bypass

ICA bifurcation (Fig. 13b). The aneurysm was embolized (Fig. 13c). A follow-up cerebral angiography 2 years later showed the regrowth of the aneurysm (Fig. 14). A cerebral revascularization procedure was then planned. Intraoperative closure of the ICA was tolerated. An EC-IC bypass with saphenous graft connecting the ICA with the temporal branch of the MCA was constructed. Intraoperative ultrasonography confirmed the presence of flow within the graft. Incomplete trapping through the closure of the ICA was also performed. Control angiography showed the patency of the graft and the exclusion of the aneurysm (Fig. 15). The postoperative course was uneventful.

At 1 year follow-up, angiography showed a new recanalization of the aneurysm (Fig. 16). This time, in awake surgery, we closed the MCA and the ipsilateral A1 segment as close as possible to the aneurysm. Motor and speech functions were monitored for 40 min after the closure of the artery. During this period the patient did not experience any neurological deficits. Postoperative angiography documented the exclusion of the aneurysm and the presence of flow within the MCA supplied by the previous graft distally to the point of closure (Fig. 17). The postoperative course was uneventful.

Discussion

Giant and complex intracranial aneurysms are among the most challenging pathologies encountered in neurosurgical practice [1–3]. Although complex aneurysms are often assimilated to giant ones, many other characteristics contribute to define the complexity of an aneurysm. They include the localization, previous endovascular or surgical treatment, the presence or absence of collateral circulation, intraluminal thrombus, and calcification of the aneurysmal wall [1–3].

The treatment of complex aneurysms requires a multidisciplinary approach that includes both surgical and endovascular expertise [1]. It often requires revascularization procedures (cerebral bypass) [1–4, 8, 10–12].

Intra-aneurysmal hemodynamics is one the most accepted factors contributing to aneurysmal formation, growth, rupture, and thrombosis [4–7, 10, 13–15]. As a consequence, the hemodynamic changes induced by the revascularization procedures represent an important element for managing complex aneurysms. Since hemodynamic characteristics differs from patient to patient, both the natural history and the response of complex aneurysms to a similar surgical strategy

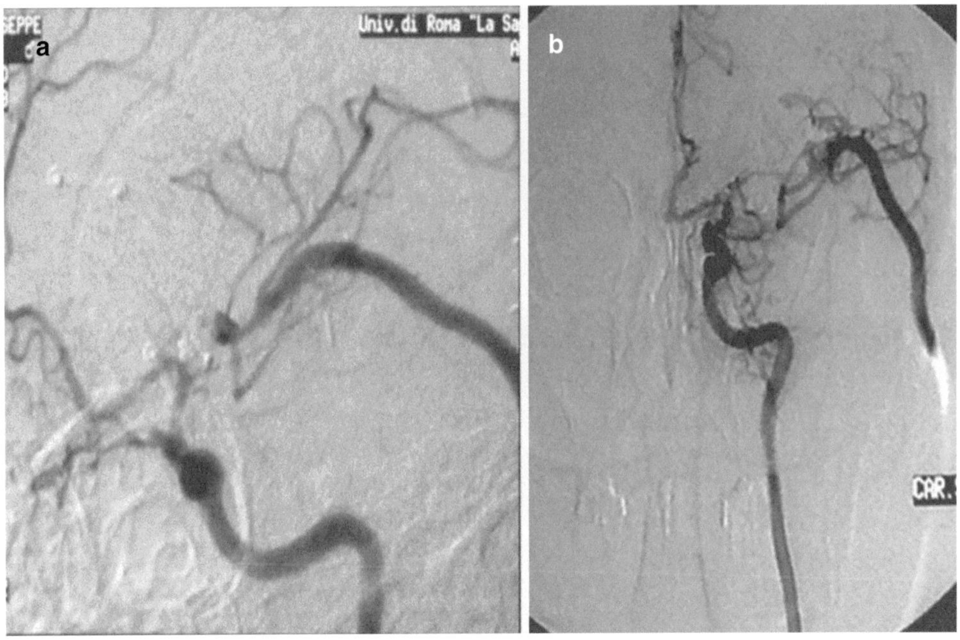

Fig. 12 (**a**) Angiographic study performed 10 days after the surgical procedure. It shows the patency of the graft, the exclusion of the aneurysm, and the presence of flow proximally and distally to the site of the clip used placed for the incomplete trapping. (**b**) Thirty days later the angiography demonstrates an even better flow within the MCA

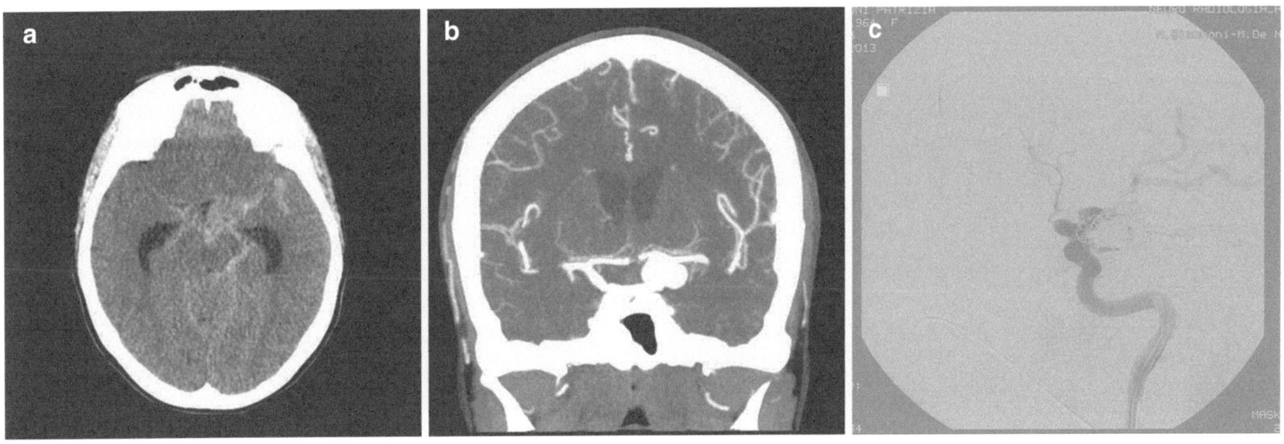

Fig. 13 (**a**) Brain CT scan demonstrating the presence of subarachnoid hemorrhage mainly localized within the left Sylvian fissure. (**b**) Angio-CT scan documents the presence of a left ICA aneurysm extended from the supraclinoidal segment to the ICA bifurcation. (**c**) Cerebral angiography and embolization of the aneurysm

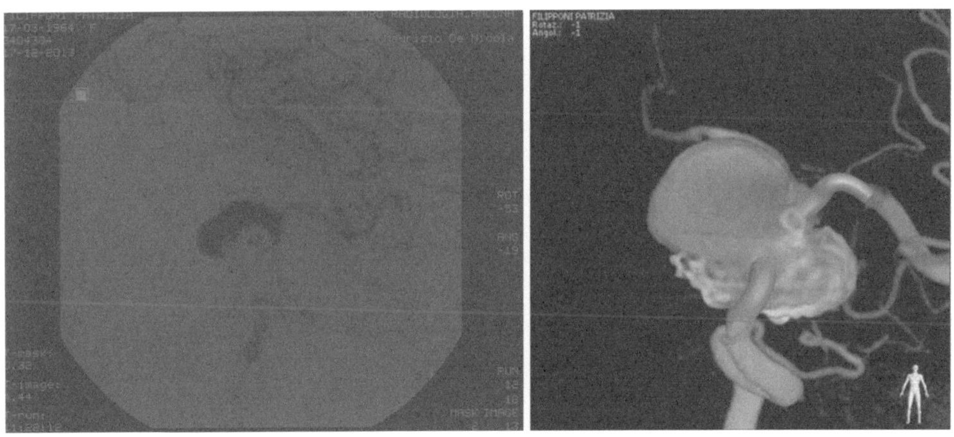

Fig. 14 Follow-up angiography demonstrating the progressive recanalization of the aneurysm

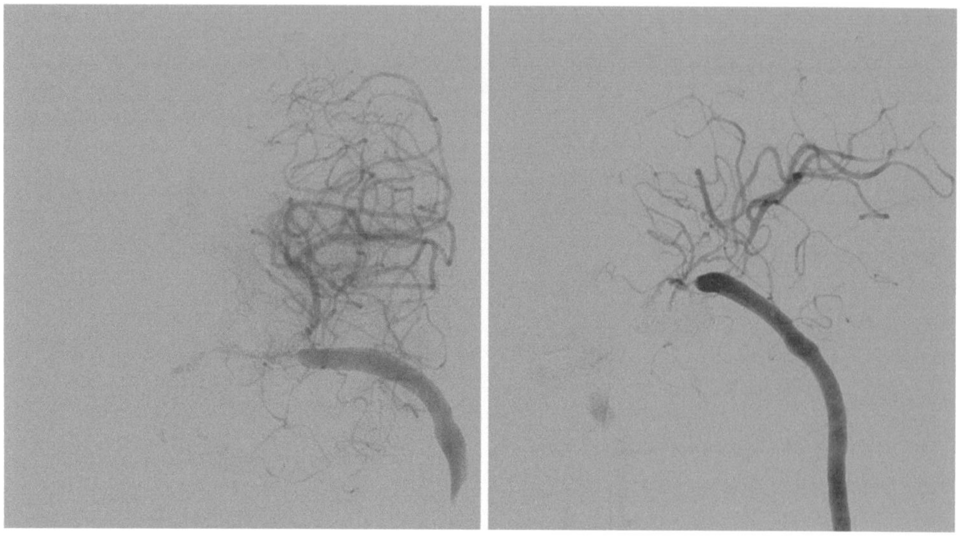

Fig. 15 Angiography performed after the procedure of EC-IC bypass and closure of the ICA. The graft is patent and ensures an adequate distal flow. After closure of the ICA the aneurysm cannot be visualized

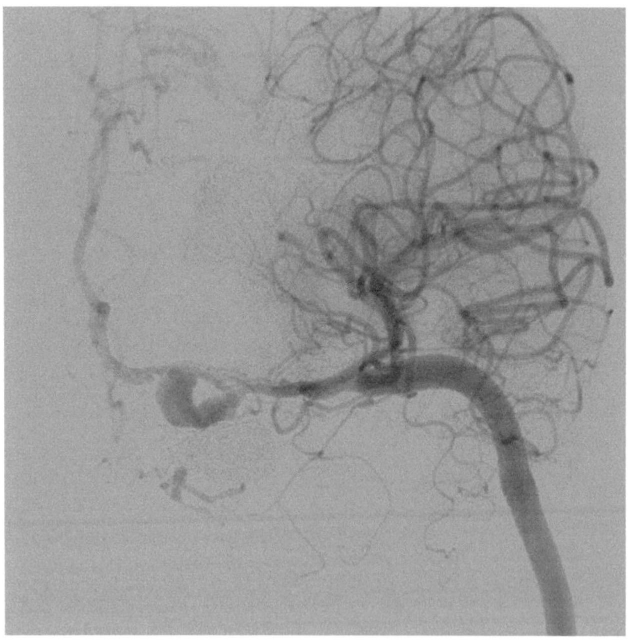

Fig. 16 Follow-up angiography shows further recanalization of the aneurysm

is absolutely variable and unpredictable [4–10]. The awareness of this heterogeneity must inevitably influence the choice of the most suitable and safe revascularization strategy.

The experience gained during two decades dedicated to the improvement of revascularization techniques induced us to substantially modify our therapeutic strategy and protocol [10].

In the first part of our experience we used the so-called "staged revascularization strategy" [10]. With this technique the occlusion of the aneurysm was obtained through a "multi-step" process. After the initial angiography and BOT performed in order to verify the patient's toleration to the occlusion of the ICA, the revascularization procedure was performed through the creation of an EC-IC bypass between the ICA/ECA (selected depending on the result of the preoperative BOT) and the MCA. Considering the well-known limitations regarding the predictive value of the BOT [1, 15], we did not choose to close the parent vessel intraoperatively but preferred to postpone the trapping procedure after the patency of the graft and the patient's adaptation to the improved flow had been verified during the first postoperative week. Closure of the vessel could be obtained endovascularly or through the spontaneous thrombosis of the aneurysm caused by local hemodynamic changes induced by the bypass [5, 10]. The first case presented in this work is illustrative. Thrombosis of the aneurysm was obtained spontaneously 5 days after the EC-IC bypass procedure. The role of hemodynamic modification in this case is evident. Alteration of flow, establishment of balanced flow, and flow inversion could have redirected blood away from the unstable inflow zone of the aneurysm. The final outcome of this hemodynamic modification is the decrease of flow within the aneurysm and subsequent thrombosis. In addition, there may have also been a decrease or balance in anterograde flow from the ipsilateral carotid artery or MCA due to the opposing flow of the bypass graft [6].

Unfortunately the hemodynamic changes induced by the bypass could also determine the onset of turbulent flow and redirect the flow vectors within the aneurysm toward weakened areas of its wall, exceeding the rupture threshold and causing bleeding of the aneurysm [3, 8, 9, 13, 14]. This is what probably happened in the second case described. The progressive thrombosis documented on postoperative angiography was linked to the counterbalance of the retrograde flow coming from the graft with the anterograde one coming

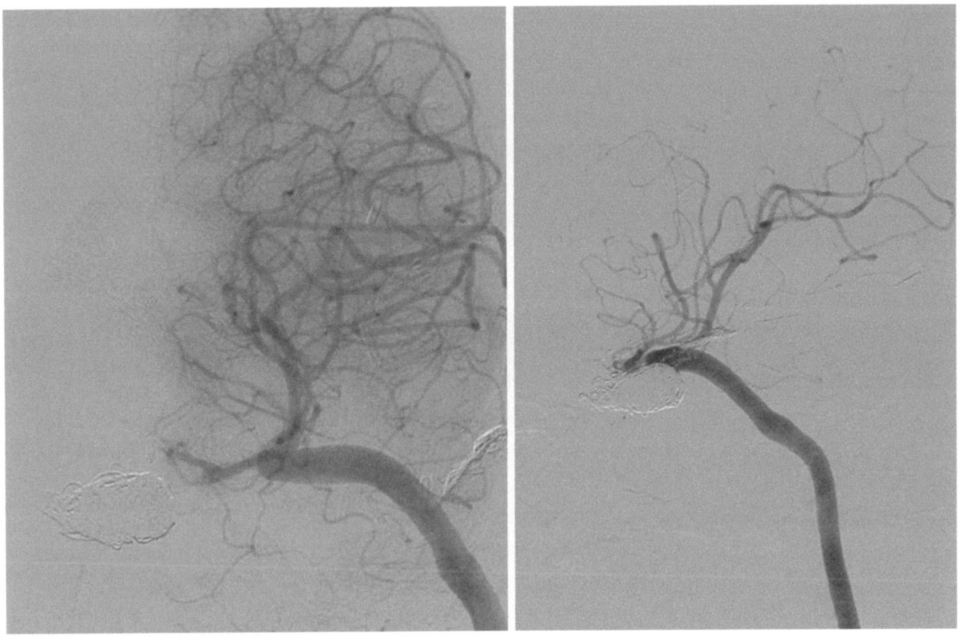

Fig. 17 Angiographic study after closure of the MCA (in awake surgery). The aneurysm has been definitively excluded

from the ICA. At the same time, these opposite forces determined the onset of turbulent flows that exceeded the rupture threshold of the aneurysmal wall determining the devastating bleeding showed on the CT scan.

This significant variability in the results obtained in the treatment of complex aneurysms with the "staged revascularization strategy" convinced us that the hemodynamic changes induced by the bypass, including the redistribution of the vectors flows, as well as the rupture threshold of the aneurysmal wall, were too variable and unpredictable to take the risk of waiting for the spontaneous or endovascular closure of the aneurysm to evaluate the patency of the graft and the adaptation of the patient to the new hemodynamic setting [10].

Our intuition has been confirmed by the modern studies of computational fluid dynamics, showing that we are far from finding a unifying theory regarding the hemodynamic modifications induced by the bypass and their role in the process of thrombosis or rupture of aneurysms [9, 11, 13, 15].

Given these considerations, our surgical strategy was muted radically. We shifted from the "staged revascularization strategy" to the so-called single stage revascularization strategy [10]. Using this procedure we eliminated preoperative and postoperative BOT and performed the closure of the ICA immediately after the creation of the bypass during the same surgical procedure [10].

Since this technique did not give us the possibility to verify postoperatively the patency of the graft and the patient's adaptation to the new hemodynamic setting, we have been obliged to develop new methods to test the correct functionality of the bypass during the surgical procedure [10]. The measurement of the flow within the graft through flowmetry techniques gave us important information regarding the likelihood of the patency of the graft. Flow values greater than 40 mL/min were correlated to an increased probability of good results [10].

Using this technique we did not experience further cases of aneurysm rebleeding and graft closure [10].

In the third case presented, as documented by the postoperative angiography, it is possible to appreciate how the intraoperative closure of the ICA after the creation of the bypass resulted in the immediate occlusion of the aneurysm. Although the blood flow through the graft could theoretically determine a retrograde filling of the aneurysm, it is highly probable that the proximal increase of resistance determined by the closure of the ICA directed the flow mainly distally toward the M2 segment, reducing the retrograde component and so determining the consequent thrombosis of the aneurysm.

However, the extent of the retrograde flow through the bypass and toward the aneurysm does not depend only on the values of resistance induced by the closure of the parent vessel. Other factors probably influence this phenomenon. They include the systemic blood pressure, the anatomic peculiarities of the intracranial circulation, the patency and dimension of anterior and posterior communicating arteries, the presence of collateral flows, the characteristics of aneurysmal wall, and so on [1–15].

Considering all these variables, not even incomplete trapping could be considered completely safe regarding the capacity to determine the definitive occlusion of the aneurysm. The fourth case presented is paradigmatic from this point of view. Despite the aggressive treatment consisting in the creation of an EC-IC bypass accompanied by the closure of the parent vessel, the retrograde flow from the graft was still strong enough to determine the recanalization of the aneurysm. Because of this, we needed to trap the aneurysm completely. The procedure was performed in awake surgery in order to verify the neurological integrity of motor and speech functions.

Conclusion

Complex aneurysms represent one of the most challenging pathologies neurosurgeons have to face. On the basis of our experience, we can state that the only common feature characterizing these lesions is their complete unpredictability. The cases presented demonstrate how, at least nowadays, it is still impossible to foresee the natural history as well as the response of this subcategory of aneurysm to similar therapeutic strategies. This heterogeneous behavior reflects the complexity of the hemodynamic changes induced by the creation of an EC-IC bypass. Until new technologies are able to predict the peculiar response of each aneurysm to a specific treatment, we believe that the creation of the bypass should be always accompanied by complete or at least incomplete trapping of the aneurysm. In our opinion the single-stage revascularization strategy currently represents the safest and most efficient therapy available for the successful treatment of complex aneurysms not amenable to endovascular therapies or selective clipping reconstruction.

References

1. Hanel RA, Spetzler RF. Surgical treatment of complex intracranial aneurysms. Neurosurgery. 2008;62(6 suppl 3):1289–97.
2. Mohit AA, Sekhar LN, Natarajan SK, Britz GW, Ghodke B. High-flow bypass grafts in the management of complex intracranial aneurysms. Neurosurgery. 2007;60(2 Suppl 1):ONS105–22.
3. Scott RM, Liu HC, Yuan R, Adelman L. Rupture of a previously unruptured giant middle cerebral artery aneurysm after extracranial-intracranial bypass surgery. Neurosurgery. 1982;10(5):600–3.
4. Benashvili GM, Alexander LF, Zubkov YN. Thrombosis of a giant aneurysm after extracranial-intracranial bypass. Neurosurgery. 1992;31(2):360–4.
5. Cantore G, Santoro A, Da Pian R. Spontaneous occlusion of supraclinoid aneurysms after the creation of extra-intracranial by passes using long grafts: report of two cases. Neurosurgery. 1999;44(1):216–9.
6. Haque R, Kellner C, Solomon RA. Spontaneous thrombosis of a giant fusiform aneurysm following extracranial-intracranial bypasssurgery. J Neurosurg. 2009;110(3):469–674.
7. Anson JA, Stone JL, Crowell RM. Rupture of a giant carotid aneurysm after extracranial-to-intracranial bypass surgery. Neurosurgery. 1991;28(1):142–7.
8. Heros RC, Ameri AM. Rupture of a giant basilar aneurysm after saphenous vein interposition graft to the posterior cerebral artery. Case report. J Neurosurg. 1984;61(2):387–90.
9. Hopkins LN, Grand W. Extracranial-intracranial arterial bypass in the treatment of aneurysms of the carotid and middle cerebralarteries. Neurosurgery. 1979;5(1 Pt 1):21–31.
10. Cantore G, Santoro A, Guidetti G, Delfinis CP, Colonnese C, Passacantilli E. Surgical treatment of giant intracranial aneurysms: current viewpoint. Neurosurgery. 2008;63(4 Suppl 2):279–89.
11. Kawaguchi T, Nishimura S, Kanamori M, Takazawa H, Omodaka S, Sato K, Maeda N, Yokoyama Y, Midorikawa H, Sasaki T, Nishijima M. Distinctive flow pattern of wall shear stress and oscillatory shear index: similarity and dissimilarity in ruptured and unruptured cerebral aneurysm blebs. J Neurosurg. 2012;117(4):774–80.
12. Yeh H, Tomsick TA. Obliteration of a giant carotid aneurysm after extracranial-to-intracranial bypass surgery: case report. Surg Neurol. 1997;48(5):473–6.
13. Meng H, Tutino VM, Xiang J, Siddiqui A. High WSS or low WSS? Complex interactions of hemodynamics with intracranial aneurysm initiation, growth, and rupture: toward a unifying hypothesis. AJNR Am J Neuroradiol. 2014;35(7):1254–62.
14. Omodaka S, Sugiyama S, Inoue T, Funamoto K, Fujimura M, Shimizu H, Hayase T, Takahashi A, Tominaga T. Local hemodynamics at the rupture point of cerebral aneurysms determined by computational fluiddynamics analysis. Cerebrovasc Dis. 2012;34(2):121–9.
15. Russin J, Babiker H, Ryan J, Rangel-Castilla L, Frakes D, Nakaji P. Computational fluid dynamics to evaluate the management of a giant internal carotid artery aneurysm. World Neurosurg. 2015;83(6):1057–65.

Part II

Cerebral Revascularization

Cerebral Bypass Surgery: Level of Evidence and Grade of Recommendation

Giuseppe Esposito, Martina Sebök, Sepideh Amin-Hanjani, and Luca Regli

Abstract *Background and aims.* Cerebral bypasses are categorized according to function (flow augmentation or flow preservation) and to characteristics: direct, indirect or combined bypass, extra-to-intracranial or intra-to-intracranial bypass, and high-, moderate- or low-capacity bypass. We critically summarize the current state of evidence and grades of recommendation for cerebral bypass surgery.

Methods. The current indications for cerebral bypass are discussed depending on the function of the bypass (flow preservation or augmentation) and analyzed according to level of evidence criteria.

Results. Flow-preservation bypass plays an important role in managing complex intracranial aneurysms (level of evidence 4; grade of recommendation C). Flow-preservation bypass is currently only very rarely indicated in the treatment of cerebral tumors involving major cerebral arteries (level of evidence 5; grade of recommendation D). The trend has evolved in favor of partial resection and radiotherapy. To preserve the flow, the bypass is always a direct bypass.

Flow-augmentation bypass is currently recommended for Moyamoya patients with ischemic symptoms and compromised hemodynamics (level of evidence 4; grade of recommendation C) and patients with hemorrhagic onset (level of evidence 1B; grade of recommendation A). Flow-augmentation bypass is currently not recommended for patients with recently symptomatic carotid artery occlusion, even in the setting of compromised cerebral hemodynamics (level of evidence 1A; grade of recommendation A), but may be considered in patients with hemodynamic failure and recurrent medically refractory symptoms as a final resort (level of evidence 5; grade of recommendation D).

Conclusions. The results of recent randomized clinical trials narrow the indication for cerebral bypass in the setting of ischemic cerebrovascular disease. However, cerebral bypass is still very useful for managing complex intracranial aneurysms (not amenable to selective clipping or endovascular therapies) and is the only treatment option for managing symptomatic patients with Moyamoya vasculopathy and impaired brain hemodynamics.

Keywords Cerebral bypass · Cerebral revascularization · Evidence-based medicine · Grades of recommendation · Indications · Level of evidence

G. Esposito, M.D., Ph.D. (✉) · M. Sebök · L. Regli
Department of Neurosurgery, University Hospital Zurich, University of Zurich, Zürich, Switzerland
e-mail: giuseppe.esposito@usz.ch

S. Amin-Hanjani
Department of Neurosurgery, University of Illinois at Chicago, Neuropsychiatric Institute, Chicago, IL, USA

Background

In current neurosurgical practice, different types of bypasses can be distinguished. According to their function, cerebral bypasses can be classified into "flow-augmentation" and "flow-preservation" [1, 2] (Table 1).

The aim of a flow-augmentation bypass is to restore blood flow to a hypoperfused brain territory in order to avoid strokes in patients with symptomatic steno-occlusive diseases of major cerebral arteries [2, 3].

The aim of a flow-preservation bypass is to replace blood flow to a brain territory previously perfused via a major vessel, the sacrifice of which is necessary to treat an underlying disease (such as an aneurysm) [2, 4, 5].

Bypass surgery is categorized into direct, indirect, and combined procedures. A direct bypass consists of a direct microvascular anastomosis between a donor artery (for instance the superficial temporal artery [STA]) and an intracranial recipient artery, and instantly delivers blood flow to the brain [2–4, 6, 7]. Depending on the choice of the donor artery, direct bypass is classified as extra-to-intracranial (EC-IC) or intra-to-intracranial (IC-IC). Furthermore, the donor and the recipient artery can be anastomosed with or without graft interposition, depending on the interposition or not of a

G. Esposito et al. (eds.), *Trends in the Management of Cerebrovascular Diseases*, Acta Neurochirurgica Supplement, Vol. 129, https://doi.org/10.1007/978-3-319-73739-3_10, © Springer International Publishing AG, part of Springer Nature 2018

Table 1 Bypass types

Function of bypass	*Flow-augmentation*		
	Flow-preservation		
Type of revascularization	*Direct bypass*	EC-IC bypass	No graft interposition
			Graft interposition
		IC-IC bypass	No graft interposition
			Graft Interposition
	Indirect bypass	EMS	
		EDMS	
		EAS	
		EMAS	
		EDAMS	
		EDAS	
		EDPS	
		Multiple burr-holes	
		Omental transplantation	
	Combined bypass	Direct + indirect bypass procedures	
Characteristics of the anastomosis	*Type*	Occlusive (conventional)	
		Non-occlusive (ELANA)	
	Anatomy	End-to-side	
		End-to-end	
		Side-to-side	
Capacity	*Low* (<50 mL/min)		
	Intermediate (50–100 mL/min)		
	High (>100 mL/min)		

EAS encephalo-arterio-synangiosis, *EC-IC* extra-to-intracranial, *EDAMS* encephalo-duro-arterio-myo-synangiosis, *EDAS* encephalo-duro-arterio-synangiosis, *EDMS* encephalo-duro-myo-synangiosis, *EDPS* encephalo-duro-periosteal-synangiosis, *ELANA* excimer laser assisted non-occlusive anastomosis, *EMAS* encephalo-myo-arterio-synangiosis, *EMS* encephalo-myo-synangiosis, *IC-IC* intra-to-intracranial

vascular graft (arterial or venous) [2]. The bypass is traditionally named according to the donor and the recipient vessels (e.g., STA to middle cerebral artery [MCA] bypass) [2, 4, 8]. Direct bypass procedures can be further categorized according to the amount of flow (capacity) provided: low (<50 mL/min), intermediate (50–100 mL/min) or high (>100 mL/min) capacity (see Table 1) [2, 5]. It is important to match the flow to demand, that is, the bypass must supply adequate flow for the needs of the vascular territory that is revascularized.

Indirect bypasses rely on the overlay of vascularized tissue (e.g., muscle, dura, pericranium, omentum) onto the cerebral cortex. The aim is to promote neoangiogenesis over time and achieve delayed revascularization [2, 7, 9, 10].

Combined bypass consists of the "combination" of direct and indirect bypass in the same surgical session [2, 3].

To *preserve* flow, the bypass must be a direct bypass and needs to be performed before permanent occlusion of the vessel. To *augment* flow, direct, indirect, and combined techniques can be applied.

Herein we summarize the current state of evidence and discuss the grades of recommendation for cerebral bypass surgery, using the "Oxford Centre for Evidence-Based Medicine (OCEBM) Levels of Evidence" for grading levels of evidence and recommendations (http://www.cebm.net).

Flow-Preservation Bypass

Bypass surgery plays an important role in managing complex intracranial aneurysms not amenable to endovascular therapy or selective clip reconstruction [4]. The treatment of such lesions may in fact require vessel occlusion or "trapping," which involves sacrifice of the artery bearing the aneurysm and/or efferent arteries [2, 4, 11]. The goal of any aneurysm treatment is, however, both aneurysm exclusion and preservation of blood flow to the brain. Therefore, bypass is essential to replace the flow provided by the sacrificed artery [4, 11]. In flow-preservation bypass surgery, a key point is that the bypass has to match the flow of the sacrificed artery: intraoperative quantitative flow measurements allow confirmation of flow matching [2, 4, 12].

The type of bypass performed in this setting is always a direct bypass in order to deliver the flow instantly to the involved territory. By varying the bypass construct (i.e., end-to-side, end-to-end, or side-to-side anastomosis or single or double bypass), the bypass can be customized to the intracranial angioanatomy [2, 4, 5, 11, 13, 14]. Complex aneurysms are rare lesions and their variety and heterogeneity do not lend themselves to randomized clinical trials (RCTs) [2]. The utility of the bypass for managing complex intracranial aneurysms has been demonstrated primarily by many case series (level of evidence 4; grade of recommendation C—see Table 2) [4, 5, 14, 15].

Radical removal of cerebral tumors involving the proximal brain vasculature may be impossible without sacrificing a major artery and replacing it with a bypass [2, 16]. The risk-benefit ratio for complete tumor resection combined with a bypass or partial resection has evolved toward partial resection and adjuvant therapy (radiotherapy or chemotherapy) [2, 16, 17]. The flow-preservation bypass for tumors has substantially declined in frequency during the past few decades. Bypass surgery can be considered only in very select cases, and has to be balanced against whether the benefit of radical

Table 2 Current indications for cerebral bypass: level of evidence

Bypass role	Indication	Bypass indicated	Level of evidence	Grade of recommendation	RCT
Flow-preservation	Complex Aneurysms[a]	Yes	4	C	N.A.
	Tumors	Rarely	5	D	N.A.
Flow–augmentation	Moya ischemic	Yes	4	C	/
	Moya hemorrhagic	Yes	1B	A	Yes
	Symptomatic cerebrovascular atherosclerotic steno-occlusive disease	No[b]	1A	A	Yes

The "Oxford Centre for Evidence-Based Medicine (OCEBM) Levels of Evidence" has been used for grading levels of evidence and recommendations (http://www.cebm.net)
N.A. not applicable
[a]Complex aneurysms not amenable to direct clipping or definitive endovascular therapy
[b]May be indicated in select cases presenting with ongoing hemodynamic symptoms (postural or with blood pressure variations) despite maximal medical management or patients having acute stroke with evidence of persistent oligemic brain tissue at risk of infarction (penumbra)

resection plus arterial sacrifice and bypass outweighs the risks in terms of improving survival with good quality of life. Cerebral tumors involving the proximal brain vasculature (e.g., skull base tumors) are also rare: the variety and heterogeneity of these lesions preclude RCTs. Only a few case series and expert opinions are available (level of evidence 5; grade of recommendation D—see Table 2) [2, 15, 18, 19].

Flow-Augmentation Bypass

Bypass surgery is the only effective treatment for managing patients with symptomatic Moyamoya vasculopathy and impaired brain hemodynamics. Bypass surgery has been shown to decrease both ischemic and hemorrhagic stroke rates [2, 3, 10, 20].

Direct, indirect, and combined bypass procedures are used for treating Moyamoya [10, 21]. There is no definitive consensus on which procedure is superior [9, 10]. Traditionally, direct or combined bypass is used in adults, while indirect or combined bypass is applied in children [2, 10, 21].

The most common direct bypass is the STA-MCA bypass [2, 3, 21]. Among the indirect techniques, the following can be considered: encephalo-myo-synangiosis (EMS) [2, 3], encephalo-duro-myo-synangiosis (EDMS) [3], encephalo-arterio-synangiosis (EAS) [22], encephalo-myo-arterio-synangiosis (EMAS) [23], encephalo-duro-arterio-myo-synangiosis (EDAMS) [24], encephalo-duro-arterio-synangiosis (EDAS) [25], encephalo-duro-periosteal-synangiosis (EDPS) [3], multiple burr-holes [26], and omental transplantation [27].

Combined bypass offers the advantages of direct and indirect methods. However, the procedures are somewhat more complex and time-consuming [2, 3, 10].

There are no RCTs on the value of bypass surgery for prevention of ischemic stroke and cognitive deterioration in Moyamoya patients. However, there are a number of observational studies which strongly indicate that bypass benefits these patients [10, 28, 29] compared to natural history; there is an unfavorable annual ischemic stroke rate in untreated patients (up to 13.3%) [30] and a high rate of disease progression with subsequent symptom occurrence in non-surgically treated hemispheres [2, 31]. In light of existing data, an RCT to test bypass surgery efficacy for prevention of ischemic stroke recurrence and cognitive deterioration in symptomatic Moyamoya patients is unlikely be performed [2, 10, 28, 29] because of a lack of equipoise. Based on existing observational studies, surgery is routinely recommended for children and adults with ischemic symptoms and compromised hemodynamics (level of evidence 4; grade of recommendation C—see Table 2) [2, 3, 10, 15, 28, 29, 32].

As for hemorrhagic Moyamoya disease (MMD), bypass surgery has RCT evidence demonstrating its efficacy in preventing recurrence of hemorrhagic stroke in patients with MMDs [20]. Although statistically marginal, the Japanese Adult Moyamoya Trial showed that direct (or combined) bypass surgery for adult patients with hemorrhagic MMD reduces the rebleeding rate and improves patient prognosis during the 5 years following enrollment (level of evidence 1B; grade of recommendation A – see Table 2) [15, 20]. Bypass is thought to improve cerebral hemodynamics, and reduce the hemodynamic stress on, the rupture-prone fragile Moyamoya collateral vessels [20].

The topic of flow-augmentation bypass in patients with symptomatic cerebrovascular atherosclerotic occlusion of extracranial or intracranial major arteries has been extensively debated in the past [33–35]. The main question has been whether STA-MCA bypass (plus medical therapy) benefits patients with symptomatic cerebrovascular atherosclerotic occlusion in comparison to medical therapy.

To answer this question, RCTs have been conducted. The "*EC-IC Bypass Trial*" [33], the first prospective RCT in this field, published in 1985, showed no significant advantage of bypass surgery in reducing the incidence of fatal and nonfatal ischemic strokes [33, 36]. This study was hotly debated [37]: among the various criticisms, the most important related to the lack of hemodynamic criteria used to identify and select high-risk patients who might benefit from a bypass [2].

A Cochrane review [38], published in 2010, reported the results of 21 trials (2 randomized and 19 non-randomized studies) for patients with symptomatic carotid occlusion. Bypass was shown to be neither superior nor inferior to medical care alone [2, 38].

The "*Carotid Occlusion Surgery Study* (*COSS*)" [35] is an RCT whose results were published in 2011. In this study, patients were selected based on very strict hemodynamic criteria, to identify those high-risk patients who might benefit most from bypass [36, 39, 40]. However, STA-MCA bypass (plus medical therapy) was shown to provide no clinical benefit over medical therapy alone [2, 35].

An ancillary study to COSS, the "*Randomized Evaluation of Carotid Occlusion and Neurocognition*" *(RECON) Trial* [41] tested neurocognition at 2 years in COSS patients and was unable to identify a benefit of bypass when compared to medical therapy alone [41].

Both EC-IC Bypass Trial and COSS have generated level I evidence indicating no benefit of bypass for patients with recently symptomatic carotid artery occlusion (in comparison to medical therapy alone) [33, 35, 36]. Bypass failed to show benefit both because medical therapy performed better than in the past and because of the relatively high complication rate in the perioperative period (most of which was non-bypass related) potentially due to the fragility of these flow-compromised patients [2]. Bypass is therefore currently not indicated for these patients (level of evidence 1A; grade of recommendation A) [2, 15, 35, 41].

However, there are subcategories of patients not included in these RCTs (EC-IC Bypass trial and COSS) for whom flow-augmentation bypass could still be of benefit and may be used as a last resort to avoid disabling strokes despite optimal medical and interventional management [2, 42]: (1) patients presenting with ongoing hemodynamic symptoms (postural or with blood pressure variations) and (2) patients having acute stroke with evidence of persistent oligemic brain tissue at risk of infarction (penumbra).

Currently, two other studies are underway. One, "*Carotid and Middle Cerebral Artery Occlusion Surgery Study*" *(CMOSS)* in China (ClinicalTrials.gov NCT01758614), and the other, "*EDAS (Surgical) Revascularization in patients with Symptomatic Intracranial Arterial Stenosis (ERSIAS)*" in the USA. Both may give new insights into the role of direct and indirect bypass, respectively (ClinicalTrials.gov NCT01819597).

Conclusion

Cerebral bypass still represents an important treatment option for managing specific cerebrovascular conditions.

Flow-preservation bypass plays an important role for managing complex intracranial aneurysms (level of evidence 4; grade of recommendation C). Flow-preservation bypass is only very rarely indicated in the treatment of cerebral tumors involving major arteries (level of evidence 5; grade of recommendation D), where the trend has evolved in favor of partial resection and radiotherapy. To preserve flow, the bypass is always a direct bypass.

Flow-augmentation bypass is currently recommended for Moyamoya patients with ischemic symptoms and compromised hemodynamics (level of evidence 4; grade of recommendation C) and Moyamoya patients with hemorrhagic onset (level of evidence 1B; grade of recommendation A). Flow-augmentation bypass is currently not recommended for patients with recently symptomatic carotid artery occlusion failure of cerebral hemodynamics (level of evidence 1A; grade of recommendation A), but may be considered in select patients with refractory hemodynamic symptoms (level of evidence 5; grade of recommendation D).

Disclosures The authors report no conflicts.

References

1. Charbel FT, Guppy KH, Ausman JI. Cerebral revascularization: superficial temporal middle cerebral artery anastomosis. In: Sekhar LN, Fessler RG, editors. Atlas of neurosurgical techniques. New York: Thieme; 2006.
2. Esposito G, Amin-Hanjani S, Regli L. Role of and indications for bypass surgery after carotid occlusion surgery study (COSS)? Stroke. 2016;47:282–90.
3. Esposito G, Kronenburg A, Fierstra J, Braun KP, Klijn CJ, van der Zwan A, Regli L. "STA-MCA bypass with encephalo-duro-myo-synangiosis combined with bifrontal encephalo-duro-periosteal-synangiosis" as a one-staged revascularization strategy for pediatric moyamoya vasculopathy. Childs Nerv Syst. 2015;31:765–72.
4. Esposito G, Durand A, Van Doormaal T, Regli L. Selective-targeted extra-intracranial bypass surgery in complex middle cerebral artery aneurysms: correctly identifying the recipient artery using indocyanine green videoangiography. Neurosurgery. 2012;71:ons274–84; discussion ons284–275.
5. Sekhar LN, Natarajan SK, Ellenbogen RG, Ghodke B. Cerebral revascularization for ischemia, aneurysms, and cranial base tumors. Neurosurgery. 2008;62:1373–408; discussion 1408–1310.
6. Burkhardt JK, Esposito G, Fierstra J, Bozinov O, Regli L. Emergency non-occlusive high capacity bypass surgery for ruptured giant internal carotid artery aneurysms. Acta Neurochir Suppl. 2016;123:77–81.
7. Kronenburg A, Esposito G, Fierstra J, Braun KP, Regli L. Combined bypass technique for contemporary revascularization of unilateral mca and bilateral frontal territories in moyamoya vasculopathy. Acta Neurochir Suppl. 2014;119:65–70.

8. Charbel FT, Meglio G, Amin-Hanjani S. Superficial temporal artery-to-middle cerebral artery bypass. Neurosurgery. 2005;56:186–90; discussion 186–190.
9. Esposito G, Fierstra J, Kronenburg A, Regli L. A comment on "contralateral cerebral hemodynamic changes after unilateral direct revascularization in patients with moyamoya disease". Neurosurg Rev. 2012;35:141–3; author reply 143.
10. Kronenburg A, Braun KP, van der Zwan A, Klijn CJ. Recent advances in moyamoya disease: pathophysiology and treatment. Curr Neurol Neurosci Rep. 2014;14:423.
11. Esposito G, Regli L. Surgical decision-making for managing complex intracranial aneurysms. Acta Neurochir Suppl. 2014;119:3–11.
12. Amin-Hanjani S, Alaraj A, Charbel FT. Flow replacement bypass for aneurysms: decision-making using intraoperative blood flow measurements. Acta Neurochir. 2010;152:1021–32; discussion 1032.
13. Esposito G, Albanese A, Sabatino G, Scerrati A, Sturiale C, Pedicelli A, Pilato F, Maira G, Di Lazzaro V. Large middle cerebral artery dissecting aneurysm mimicking hemorrhagic stroke. Clin Neurol Neurosurg. 2011;113:901–3.
14. Kivipelto L, Niemela M, Meling T, Lehecka M, Lehto H, Hernesniemi J. Bypass surgery for complex middle cerebral artery aneurysms: impact of the exact location in the MCA tree. J Neurosurg. 2014;120:398–408.
15. Burns PB, Rohrich RJ, Chung KC. The levels of evidence and their role in evidence-based medicine. Plast Reconstr Surg. 2011;128:305–10.
16. Berg-Johnsen J, Helseth E, Langmoen IA. Cerebral revascularization for skull base tumors. World Neurosurg. 2014;82:575–6.
17. Kalani MY, Kalb S, Martirosyan NL, Lettieri SC, Spetzler RF, Porter RW, Feiz-Erfan I. Cerebral revascularization and carotid artery resection at the skull base for treatment of advanced head and neck malignancies. J Neurosurg. 2013;118:637–42.
18. Kalavakonda C, Sekhar LN. Cerebral revascularization in cranial base tumors. Neurosurg Clin N Am. 2001;12:557–74, viii–ix.
19. Yang T, Tariq F, Chabot J, Madhok R, Sekhar LN. Cerebral revascularization for difficult skull base tumors: a contemporary series of 18 patients. World Neurosurg. 2014;82:660–71.
20. Miyamoto S, Yoshimoto T, Hashimoto N, Okada Y, Tsuji I, Tominaga T, Nakagawara J, Takahashi JC, Investigators JAMT. Effects of extracranial-intracranial bypass for patients with hemorrhagic moyamoya disease: results of the Japan Adult Moyamoya Trial. Stroke. 2014;45:1415–21.
21. Scott RM, Smith ER. Moyamoya disease and moyamoya syndrome. N Engl J Med. 2009;360:1226–37.
22. Khan N, Schuknecht B, Boltshauser E, Capone A, Buck A, Imhof HG, Yonekawa Y. Moyamoya disease and Moyamoya syndrome: experience in Europe; choice of revascularisation procedures. Acta Neurochir. 2003;145:1061–71; discussion 1071.
23. Matsushima T, Inoue T, Katsuta T, Natori Y, Suzuki S, Ikezaki K, Fukui M. An indirect revascularization method in the surgical treatment of moyamoya disease—various kinds of indirect procedures and a multiple combined indirect procedure. Neurol Med Chir (Tokyo). 1998;38(Suppl):297–302.
24. Kim DS, Kye DK, Cho KS, Song JU, Kang JK. Combined direct and indirect reconstructive vascular surgery on the fronto-parieto-occipital region in moyamoya disease. Clin Neurol Neurosurg. 1997;99(Suppl 2):S137–41.
25. Tenjin H, Ueda S. Multiple EDAS (encephalo-duro-arterio-synangiosis). Additional EDAS using the frontal branch of the superficial temporal artery (STA) and the occipital artery for pediatric moyamoya patients in whom EDAS using the parietal branch of STA was insufficient. Childs Nerv Syst. 1997;13:220–4.
26. Kawaguchi T, Fujita S, Hosoda K, Shose Y, Hamano S, Iwakura M, Tamaki N. Multiple burr-hole operation for adult moyamoya disease. J Neurosurg. 1996;84:468–76.
27. Yoshioka N, Tominaga S, Suzuki Y, Yamazato K, Hirano S, Nonaka K, Inui T, Matuoka N. Cerebral revascularization using omentum and muscle free flap for ischemic cerebrovascular disease. Surg Neurol. 1998;49:58–65; discussion 65–66.
28. Roach ES, Golomb MR, Adams R, Biller J, Daniels S, Deveber G, Ferriero D, Jones BV, Kirkham FJ, Scott RM, Smith ER, American Heart Association Stroke C, Council on Cardiovascular Disease in the Y. Management of stroke in infants and children: a scientific statement from a Special Writing Group of the American Heart Association Stroke Council and the Council on Cardiovascular Disease in the Young. Stroke. 2008;39:2644–91.
29. Smith ER, Scott RM. Spontaneous occlusion of the circle of Willis in children: pediatric moyamoya summary with proposed evidence-based practice guidelines. A review. J Neurosurg Pediatr. 2012;9:353–60.
30. Gross BA, Du R. The natural history of moyamoya in a North American adult cohort. J Clin Neurosci. 2013;20:44–8.
31. Kuroda S, Ishikawa T, Houkin K, Nanba R, Hokari M, Iwasaki Y. Incidence and clinical features of disease progression in adult moyamoya disease. Stroke. 2005;36:2148–53.
32. Research Committee on the P, Treatment of Spontaneous Occlusion of the Circle of W, Health Labour Sciences Research Grant for Research on Measures for Infractable D. Guidelines for diagnosis and treatment of moyamoya disease (spontaneous occlusion of the circle of Willis). Neurol Med Chir (Tokyo). 2012;52:245–66.
33. The EC/IC Bypass Study Group. Failure of extracranial-intracranial arterial bypass to reduce the risk of ischemic stroke. Results of an international randomized trial. N Engl J Med. 1985;313:1191–200.
34. Esposito G, Della Pepa GM, Sabatino G, Gaudino S, Puca A, Maira G, Marchese E, Albanese A. Bilateral flow changes after extracranial-intracranial bypass surgery in a complex setting of multiple brain-feeding arteries occlusion: the role of perfusion studies. Br J Neurosurg. 2015;29:1–3.
35. Powers WJ, Clarke WR, Grubb RL Jr, Videen TO, Adams HP Jr, Derdeyn CP, Investigators C. Extracranial-intracranial bypass surgery for stroke prevention in hemodynamic cerebral ischemia: the carotid occlusion surgery study randomized trial. JAMA. 2011;306:1983–92.
36. Reynolds MR, Derdeyn CP, Grubb RL Jr, Powers WJ, Zipfel GJ. Extracranial-intracranial bypass for ischemic cerebrovascular disease: what have we learned from the carotid occlusion surgery study? Neurosurg Focus. 2014;36:E9.
37. Amin-Hanjani S, Barker FG II, Charbel FT, Connolly ES Jr, Morcos JJ, Thompson BG, Cerebrovascular Section of the American Association of Neurological S, Congress of Neurological S. Extracranial-intracranial bypass for stroke-is this the end of the line or a bump in the road? Neurosurgery. 2012;71:557–61.
38. Fluri F, Engelter S, Lyrer P. Extracranial-intracranial arterial bypass surgery for occlusive carotid artery disease. Cochrane Database Syst Rev. 2010;2010:CD005953. https://doi.org/10.1002/14651858.CD005953.pub2.
39. Derdeyn CP, Gage BF, Grubb RL Jr, Powers WJ. Cost-effectiveness analysis of therapy for symptomatic carotid occlusion: PET screening before selective extracranial-to-intracranial bypass versus medical treatment. J Nucl Med. 2000;41:800–7.
40. Grubb RL Jr, Powers WJ, Derdeyn CP, Adams HP Jr, Clarke WR. The carotid occlusion surgery study. Neurosurg Focus. 2003;14:e9.
41. Marshall RS, Festa JR, Cheung YK, Pavol MA, Derdeyn CP, Clarke WR, Videen TO, Grubb RL, Slane K, Powers WJ, Lazar RM, Investigators R. Randomized evaluation of carotid occlusion and neurocognition (RECON) trial: main results. Neurology. 2014;82:744–51.
42. Albanese A, Esposito G, Puca A, Tuttolomondo A, Tirpakova B, Di Giuda D, Maira G, Di Lazzaro V. Positional brain ischemia with MCA occlusion successfully treated with extra-intracranial bypass. Cerebrovasc Dis. 2010;29:408–9.

STA-MCA Bypass Under Local Anesthesia

Yasuhiko Kaku, Tetsuya Yamada, Kiyomitsu Kanou, Naoki Oka, Kentarou Yamashita, and Jouji Kokuzawa

Abstract *Background and aims.* The superficial temporal artery to middle cerebral artery (STA-MCA) bypass procedure has continually evolved and new strategies have been advocated to reduce anesthetic or surgical mortality and morbidity. Further simplifying and decreasing the invasiveness of STA-MCA bypass by performing this operation without endotracheal general anesthesia was deemed feasible in certain subsets of patients.

Methods. We performed STA-MCA bypass using local anesthesia using a sedative in 45 patients with hemodynamically compromised cerebrovascular occlusive disease as well as multiple comorbidities in the period between February 2010 and April 2016. The technique is based on preoperative identification of the point at which the donor and recipient vessels are in closest proximity. The preoperative use of computed tomography angiography allowed us to identify the target point precisely and use a minimally invasive procedure. All patients received dexmedetomidine as the sole sedative agent, together with scalp block local anesthesia with an unsecured airway.

Results. Successful STA-MCA bypass surgeries were achieved via a preselected minimally invasive approach in all cases. There was good hemodynamic stability throughout surgery. No airway/ventilation complications occurred and no patient was converted to general anesthesia. The patients subjectively tolerated this technique well with a high rate of satisfaction. Postoperative magnetic resonance angiography confirmed patent bypass in 44 of 45 patients (patency rate of 97.8%). There were two postoperative hyper-perfusion syndromes and one cerebral ischemia with transient neurological symptoms (postoperative complication rate of 6.3%). No recurrence of ipsilateral cerebral ischemia was observed during the follow-up periods. There was one contralateral cardiogenic cerebral embolism during the follow-up period. The overall stroke rate was calculated as 1%/patient/year.

Conclusions. Our initial experience confirms the feasibility of performing STA-MCA bypass under local anesthesia without endotracheal general anesthesia.

Keywords Local anesthesia · Minimally invasive technique · STA-MCA bypass

Y. Kaku, M.D. (✉) · T. Yamada, M.D. · K. Kanou, M.D.
N. Oka, M.D. · K. Yamashita, M.D. · J. Kokuzawa, M.D.
Department of Neurosurgery, Asahi University Murakami Memorial Hospital, Gifu, Japan
e-mail: kaku@murakami.asahi-u.ac.jp

Introduction

The superficial temporal artery to middle cerebral artery (STA-MCA) bypass is an established cerebral revascularization procedure. It has continually evolved, and new strategies have been advocated to reduce anesthetic or surgical mortality and morbidity [1–4]. Further simplifying and decreasing the invasiveness of STA-MCA bypass by performing this operation without endotracheal general anesthesia was deemed feasible in certain subsets of patients [5]. Since 2010 we have conducted STA-MCA bypass with mini-targeted craniotomy under local anesthesia.

Methods

Patient Selection

The patient selection criteria included (1) non-Moyamoya adult patients (≥ 20 years of age) who had ischemic neurological symptoms (transient ischemic attack or minor completed stroke); (2) patients who had hemodynamically significant cerebrovascular occlusive disease in the middle cerebral artery territory (resting regional cerebral blood flow <90% of the normal value and cerebrovascular reserve capacity <15% upon diamox challenge ^{123}I-iodoamphetamine

G. Esposito et al. (eds.), *Trends in the Management of Cerebrovascular Diseases*, Acta Neurochirurgica Supplement, Vol. 129,
https://doi.org/10.1007/978-3-319-73739-3_11,

single-photon emission computed tomography (IMP-SPECT); (3) patients who had no cognitive deficits and were cooperative; and (4) patients who had pulmonary dysfunction, such as chronic obstructive pulmonary disease (COPD) or other multiple systemic comorbidities.

A total of 45 patients, including 6 with impending stroke were enrolled in this study and underwent an STA-MCA bypass using local anesthesia and a sedative in the period between February 2010 and April 2016. All patients were symptomatic, and had a mean age of 74.3 years, including 14 cases over 80 years. Forty patients had multiple systemic comorbidities, including 10 with COPD and 15 with coronary heart disease.

Preoperative Examinations

We selected patients as candidates for STA-MCA bypass using MRI/A, 3D CT angiography (3D CTA) and SPECT with acetazolamide challenge. Conventional angiography is not routinely used for preoperative evaluation.

A 3D CTA used for preoperative planning of a craniotomy was obtained with a 256-channel multi-detector row spiral CT scanner (Revolution: GE medical systems, Milwaukee, WI, USA) and a slice thickness of 0.6 mm to target recipient and donor arteries. On the original images of 3D CTA, the closest point of the appropriate donor branch of the STA and the most suitable recipient M4 having a diameter of approximately 1 mm could be identified within the scalp and on the brain surface, respectively (Fig. 1). This segment provided both the donor (Fig. 1, arrow) and recipient arteries (Fig. 1, arrowhead) for STA-MCA bypass. The afore-mentioned segment could be considered as the center of a mini-craniotomy, and the distance between the afore-mentioned segment of the donor artery and the rostral attachment of the ear was calculated (Fig. 2).

Sedation, Local Anesthesia, and Monitoring

All patients received dexmedetomidine as the sole sedative agent, together with scalp block local anesthesia and intravenous bolus administration of buprenorphine (0.4 mg) as the analgesic. Dexmedetomidine was started with an initial dose of 1 μg/kg in 10 min and followed by infusions of 0.2–0.7 μg/kg/h, which were continued throughout the procedures. Spontaneous ventilation was preserved, and no endotracheal tube or laryngeal mask airway was used. Oxygen (50%) was administered via a facial mask at 4–5 L/min. The ECG, heart rate (HR), systolic and diastolic blood pressure (BP), respiratory rate, pulse oximetry (SpO2), and end-tidal CO2 were monitored. Systolic and diastolic BP, HR, SpO2, and end-tidal CO2 were recorded every 5 min. No pin fixation was applied, but the head of the patient was fixed with an adjustable pillow for the shape of the individual patient's head (Fig. 2a). All patients received local anesthetic infiltration immediately after induction of the sedative before surgery, first to a superficial layer of the preselected scalp incision line on the superficial temporal artery (STA), then as a circular scalp block around the scalp incision line throughout the entire thickness of the scalp, and finally to the temporal muscle, using approximately 35–40 mL of a combined solution of 2% lidocaine and 0.25% bupivacaine (Fig. 3b).

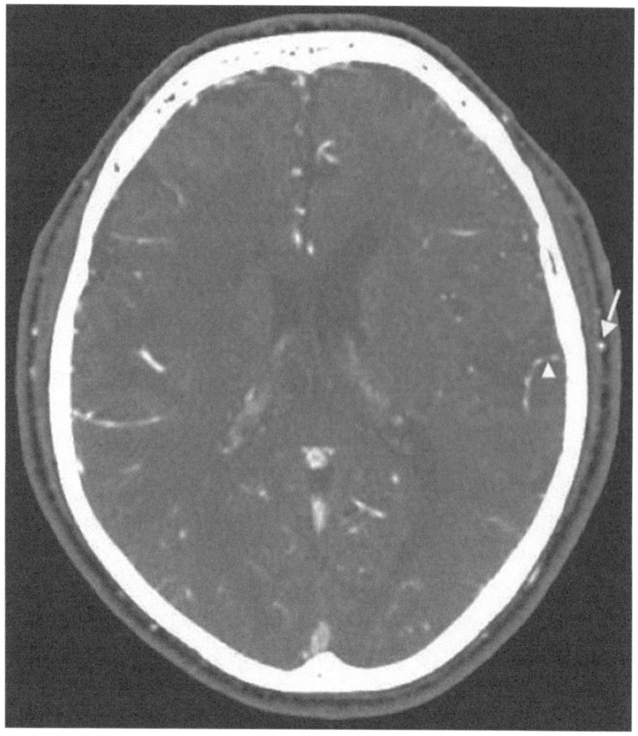

Fig. 1 The original image of a 3D CTA demonstrates a parietal branch of the STA within the scalp and a cortical artery on the brain surface. The most suitable segments of both the artery provided as the donor (arrow) and the recipient arteries (arrowhead) for EC-IC bypass are demonstrated. The distance between the above-mentioned segment of the donor artery and the superior border of the helix can be calculated

Surgical Technique

The surgical technique used was as follows: a 5-cm linear skin incision on the preselected segment of the parietal or frontal branch of the STA (Fig. 3a, c), the center of which was the point measured on preoperative 3D CTA, was made. The temporal muscle was divided in the same fashion, and a 2.5- to 3-cm small craniotomy was made. The dura was

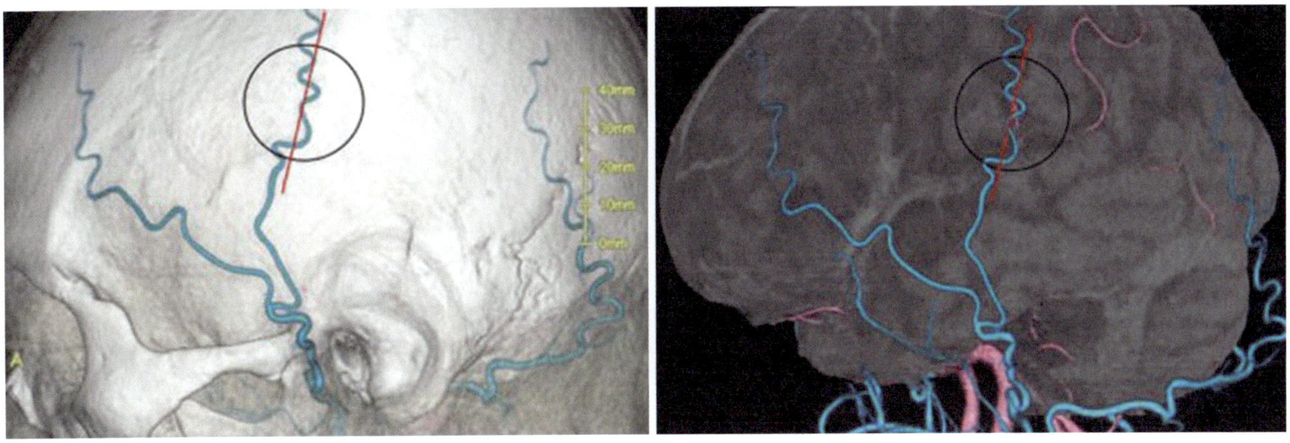

Fig. 2 The image of the craniotomy superimposed on the skull and the brain surface images of the preoperative 3D CTA. The red line indicates the scalp incision and the black circle indicates the bone window

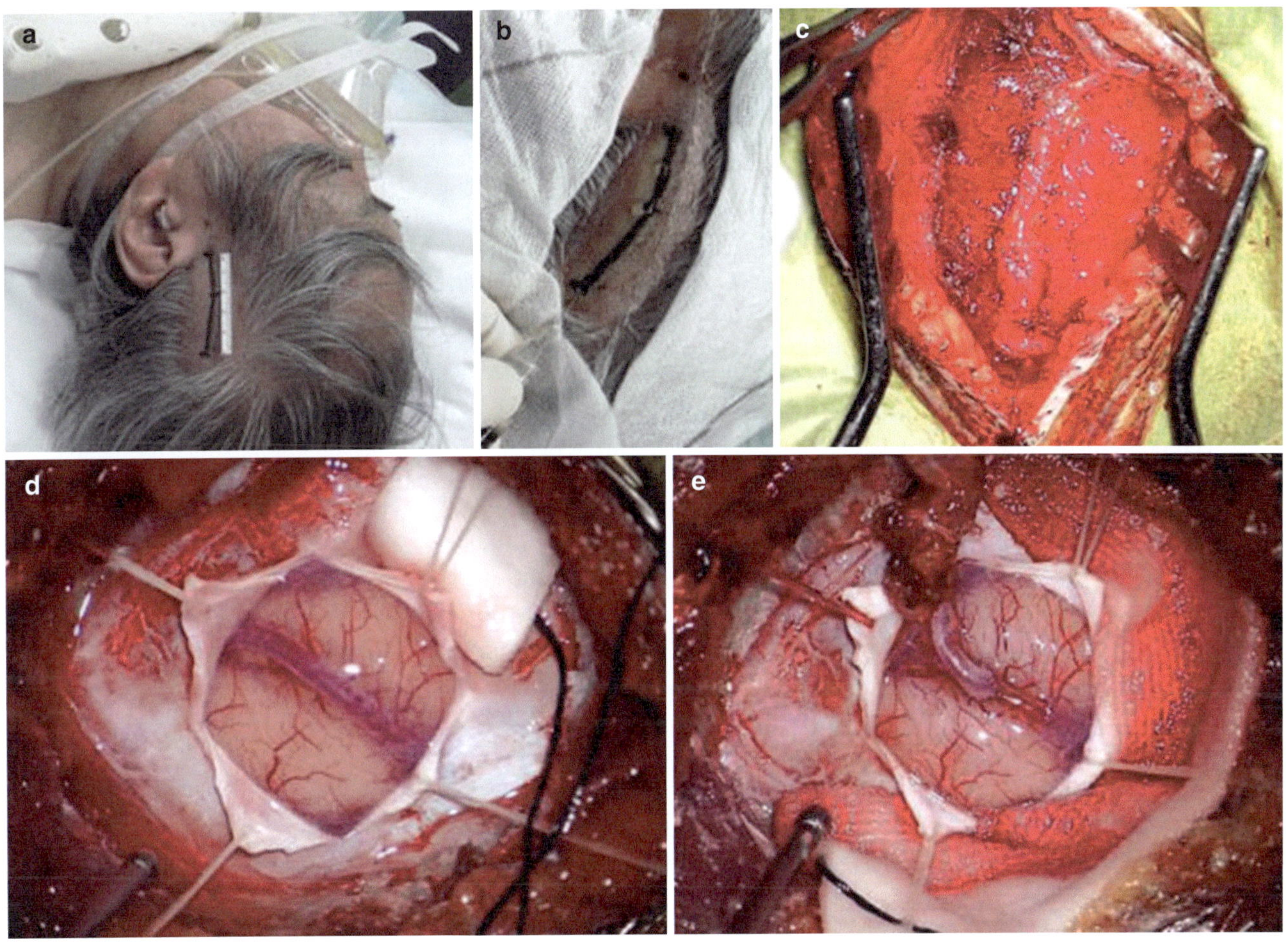

Fig. 3 (**a**) The head of the patient is fixed with an adjustable pillow for the shape of the individual patient's head with an unsecured airway. (**b**) A sufficient amount of local anesthesia infiltrates to superficial layer of the preselected scalp incision line on the superficial temporal artery and around the scalp incision line throughout the entire thickness of the scalp, and finally to the temporal muscle. (**c**) The donor artery (parietal branch of the STA) is dissected. (**d**) The recipient artery can be identified at the center of the craniotomy. (**e**) The end-to-side anastomosis is completed

opened in a cruciate fashion in the center of the craniotomy. The recipient artery could be identified on the center of the craniotomy (Fig. 3d). End-to-side anastomosis was performed in the usual fashion. Two anchoring sutures at the apices of the incision and an additional 10 interrupted sutures were placed with 10–0 nylon sutures (Fig. 3e).

Results

Successful STA-MCA bypass surgeries were achieved via a preselected minimally invasive approach in all 45 patients. Subsequent enlargement of the craniotomy was not necessary. All operations were performed by the same surgeon (Y.K.). The patients tolerated this procedure well. There were good hemodynamic stabilities throughout the surgery. The patients' BP and HR were maintained within 20% of the initial values. There were no episodes of bradycardia (defined as less than 40 bpm) or hypotension (defined as systolic arterial pressure of less than 80 mmHg). No airway/ventilation complication occurred and no patient was converted to general anesthesia. Oxygen saturation levels were maintained between 99 and 100% in all patients throughout the procedure. The ETCO2 was maintained within 25% of the initial value, although a mild accumulation of carbon dioxide was noted. The duration of the whole procedure ranged from 87 to 151 min (mean 126 min) with minimal blood loss. The lack of endotracheal general anesthesia and muscle paralysis did not compromise the quality of the anastomoses.

Postoperative MRA confirmed patent bypass in 44 of 45 patients (patency rate of 97.8%). There were two postoperative hyper-perfusion syndromes and one cerebral ischemia due to low cardiac output with transient neurological symptoms (periprocedural complication rate of 6.3%). All of the patients had no permanent neurological deterioration. No recurrence of ipsilateral cerebral ischemia was observed during the follow-up period. There was one contralateral cardiogenic cerebral embolism during the follow-up period. The overall stroke rate was calculated as 1%/patient/year.

Illustrative Case

This 80-year-old male patient had esophageal cancer. During radiation and chemotherapy he had a minor completed stroke. MRA revealed occlusion of the left internal carotid artery (Fig. 4) and SPECT demonstrated misery perfusion in the territory of left MCA (Fig. 5). According to his strong request we decided to perform STA-MCA bypass under local anesthesia. STA-MCA bypass was performed through a target mini-craniotomy using the afore-mentioned technique. He tolerated the bypass surgery well, but the day after the operation he became confused. IMP-SPECT demonstrated 118% of hyper-perfusion in the territory of the left MCA (Fig. 6) and MRA demonstrated the widely patent bypass (Fig. 7). A strict control of blood pressure was initiated. He recovered in the following 2 weeks and there were no ischemic episodes thereafter. He maintained or somewhat gained preoperative activity.

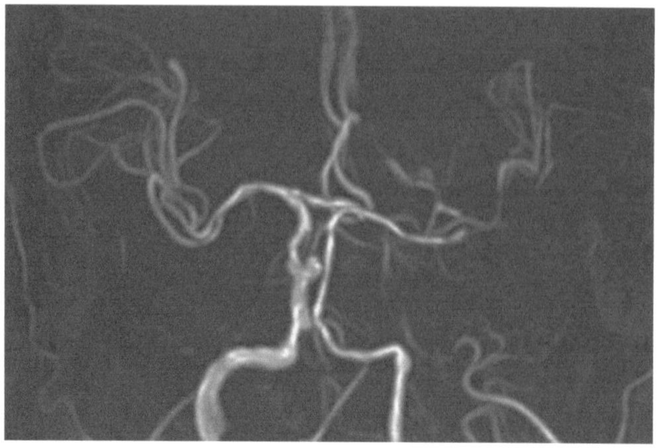

Fig. 4 Preoperative MRA demonstrating an occlusion of the left internal carotid artery

Discussion

STA-MCA bypass has continually evolved and new strategies have been advocated for reducing anesthetic or surgical mortality and morbidity [1–4]. Although STA-MCA bypass is an established cerebral revascularization procedure, Carotid occlusion surgery study (COSS) study demonstrated that it was not superior to medical treatment in a 2-year follow-up [6]. Those unfavorable results depend on the perioperative complications. After the perioperative period, bypass surgery might have a preventive effect for cerebral ischemia. Therefore, if we could reduce the perioperative complications, STA-MCA bypass might be meaningful for stroke prevention.

The conventional STA-MCA bypass technique, however, cannot solve the problems associated with general anesthesia and positive pressure ventilation. Patients with severe systemic diseases such as pulmonary dysfunction are predicted to be at high risk of postoperative complications associated with general anesthesia and positive pressure ventilation. For these high-risk cases, avoiding general anesthesia and mechanical ventilation seems to be another way to decrease the invasiveness and risk of the STA-MCA bypass [5].

It has been suggested that performing the operation under local anesthesia, rather than general anesthesia, may be safer [7]. The potential benefits of local anesthesia in a wider range of surgical procedures are supported by an overview of randomized trials of spinal and epidural anesthesia vs general anesthesia [8, 9]. The overall mortality was reduced by about one-third in the patients allocated to a neuraxial blockade. Furthermore, neuraxial blockade reduced the odds of deep vein thrombosis by 44%, pulmonary embolism by 55%, pneumonia by 39%, and respiratory depression by 59% (all $P < 0.001$). There was also reduction in myocardial

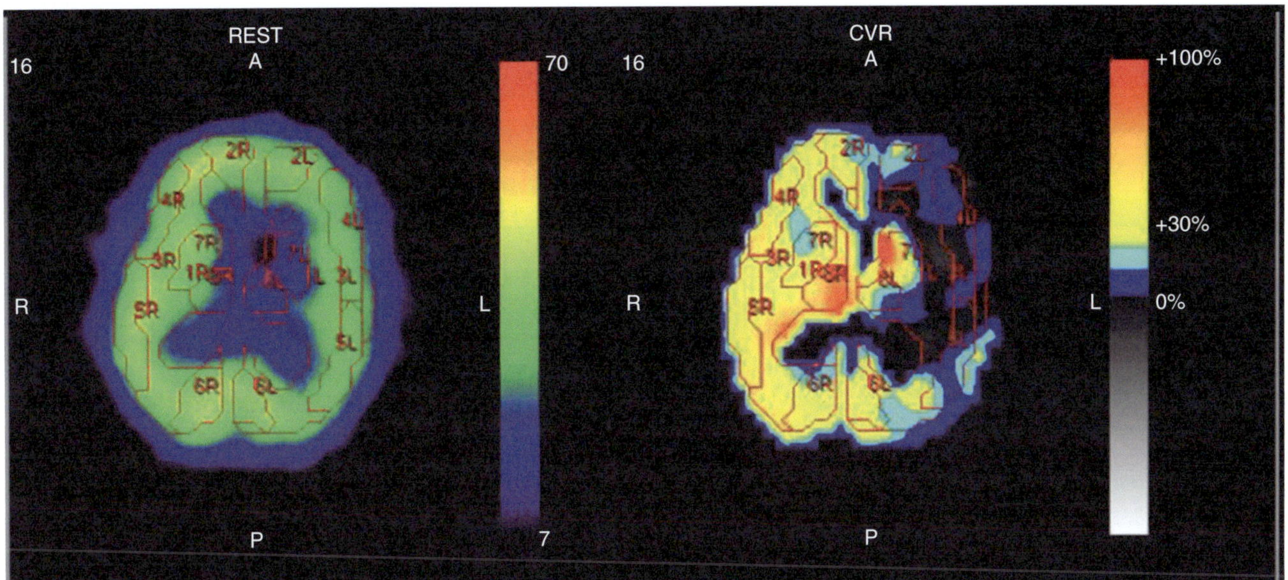

#	Territory	Right	Left	L/R
1	hemisphere	33.14	28.33	0.85
2	ACA	35.61	35.01	0.98
3	MCA	35.73	30.17	0.84
4	(M2ant)	34.81	29.60	0.85
5	(M2post)	36.77	30.97	0.84
6	PCA	37.75	36.11	0.96
7	B.G.	31.33	19.71	0.63

#	Territory	Right	Left
1	hemisphere	35.46	9.39
2	ACA	26.45	7.71
3	MCA	36.19	3.94
4	(M2ant)	33.78	0.41
5	(M2post)	37.45	8.14
6	PCA	27.95	30.24
7	B.G.	31.57	20.80

Fig. 5 Preoperative IMP-SPECT demonstrating a resting CBF decreased to 85% of the normal value (Left) and a decreased cerebrovascular reserve capacity (CVR) to less than10% in the left MCA territory (Right)

infarction and renal failure. The benefits seen for local anesthesia may be conferred by multifactorial mechanisms, including an improved ability to breath, altered coagulation, increased blood flow, and a reduction in surgical stress responses.

We performed our minimally invasive STA-MCA bypass under local anesthesia for patients with hemodynamically compromised cerebrovascular occlusive disease as well as multiple comorbidities. The procedure was performed using a local anesthetic agent in combination with a sedative. Spontaneous respiration was preserved, no endotracheal tube or laryngeal mask airway was used, and no skull fixation was adopted. The patients received dexmedetomidine as the sole sedative agent, together with the scalp block. Dexmedetomidine is a lipophilic imidazole derivative which acts as an α-2 agonist. It can induce anesthesia via its effect on the α-2a receptor subtype and has analgesic properties as well. Dexmedetomidine has little to no effect on respiration at clinically relevant doses, and allows arousal from a state mimicking sleep. It has been used in a wide variety of clinical situations including the provision of sedation in awake craniotomies [10, 11]. Other beneficial qualities of dexmedetomidine were the effect on hemodynamic stability and its anxiolytic effect. As dexmedetomidine provides sedation which resembles natural sleep and a certain extent of analgesia without respiratory depression, this sedative may be a suitable agent for STA-MCA bypass under local anesthesia.

In our initial clinical experience, there was good hemodynamic stability throughout surgery, and no airway/ventilation complications developed in any of our patients. The patients subjectively tolerated this technique well, with a high rate of satisfaction. This procedure did not compromise the quality of the anastomoses. Our initial experience confirms the feasibility of performing STA-MCA bypass under local anesthesia with a sedative, thereby representing an alternative to the procedure under endotracheal general anesthesia. These results might also encourage the wider application of this technique to include patients without significant comorbidities.

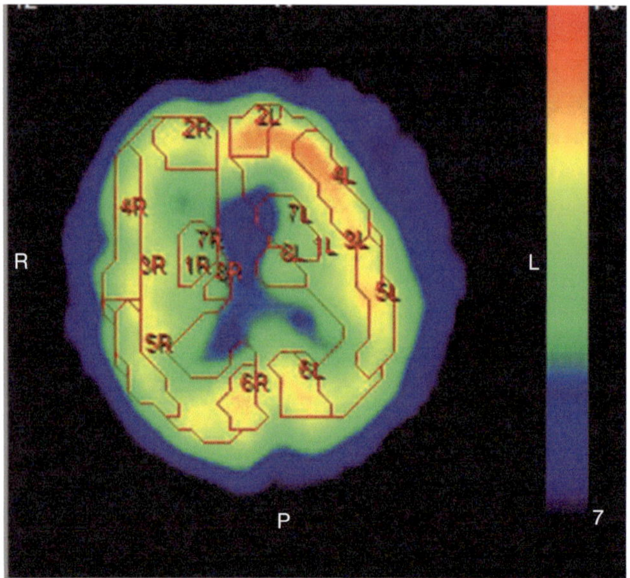

#	Territory	Right	Left	L/R
1	hemisphere	40.84	43.71	1.07
2	ACA	45.11	50.54	1.12
3	MCA	42.79	48.27	1.13
4	(M2ant)	43.15	50.79	1.18
5	(M2post)	42.54	46.15	1.08
6	PCA	48.39	47.32	0.98
7	B.G.	35.64	34.00	0.95
8	Thalamus	28.57	33.69	1.18

Fig. 6 Post-operative IMP-SPECT demonstrating 118% of hyperperfusion in the territory of the left MCA

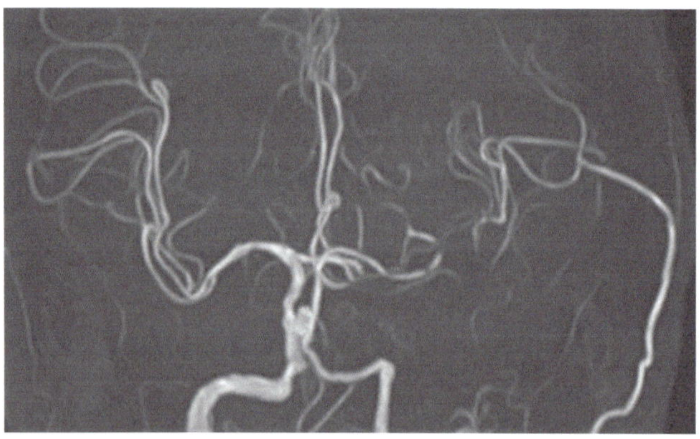

Fig. 7 Post-operative MRA demonstrating the widely patent bypass

Conclusions

Avoiding general anesthesia and mechanical ventilation seems to be another way to decrease the invasiveness and risk of the STA-MCA bypass.

There was good hemodynamic stability throughout surgery, and no airway/ventilation complications developed in any of our patients. The patients tolerated this technique well, with a high rate of satisfaction. This method could be recommended, especially for patients with systemic comorbidities such as COPD.

Conflict of Interest The authors declare that they have no conflict of interest.

References

1. Coppens JR, Cantando DO, Abdulrauf SI. Mininimally invasive superficial temporal artery to middle cerebral artery bypass through an enlarged bur hole: the use of computed tomography angiography neuronavigation in surgical planning. J Neurosurg. 2008;109:553–8.
2. Fischer G, Stadie A, Schwandt E, Gawehn J, Boor S, Marx J, Oertel J. Minimally invasive superficial temporal artery to middle cerebral artery bypass through a minicraniotomy: benefit of three-demensional virtual reality planning using magnetic resonance angiography. Neurosurg Focus. 2009;26(5):E20.
3. Kaku Y, Watarai H, Kokuzawa J, Tanaka T, Andoh T. Less invasive technique for EC-IC bypass. Acta Neurochir. 2008;103(suppl):83–6.
4. Kikuta K, Takagi Y, Fushimi Y, Ishizu K, Okada T, Hanakawa T, Miki Y, Fukuyama H, Nozaki K, Hashimoto N. "Target Bypass": a method for preoperative targeting of a recipient artery in superficial temporal artery-to-middle cerebral artery anastomoses. Operative Neurosurgery. 2006;4:320–7.
5. Kaku Y, Yamashita K, Kokuzawa J, Kanou K, Tsujimoto M. Superficial temporal artery-middle cerebral artery bypass using local anesthesia and a sedative without endotracheal general anesthesia. J Neurosurg. 2012;117:288–94.
6. Powers WJ, Clarke WR, Grubb RL Jr, Videen TO, Adams HP Jr, Derdeyn CP, COSS Investigators. Extracranial-intracranial bypass surgery for stroke prevention in hemodynamic cerebral ischemia: the Carotid Occlusion Surgery Study randomized trial. JAMA. 2011;306:1983–92.
7. Abou-Chebl A, Lin R, Hussain MS, Jovin TG, Levy EI, Liebeskind DS, Yoo AJ, Hsu DP, Rymer MM, Tayal AH, Zaidat OO, Natarajan SK, Nogueira RG, Nanda A, Tian M, Hao Q, Kalia JS, Nguyen TN, Chen M, Gupta R. Consious sedation versus general anesthesia during endovascular therapy for acute anterior circulation stroke. Stroke. 2010;41:1175–9.
8. Gough MJ, Bodenham A, Horrocks M, Colam B, Lewis SC, Rothwell PM, Banning AP, Torgerson D, Gough M, Dellagrammaticas D, Leigh-Brown A, Liapis C, Warlow C. GALA: an international multicentre randomized trial comparing general anaesthesia versus local anaesthesia for carotid surgery. Trials. 2008;9:28.
9. Rodgers A, Walker N, Schug S, McKee A, Kehlet H, van Zundert A, Sage D, Futter M, Saville G, Clark T, MacMahon S. Reduction of postoperative mortality and morbidity with epidural or spinal anaesthesia: results from overview of randomized trials. BMJ. 2000;321(7275):1493.
10. Souter MJ, Rozet I, Ojemann JG, Souter KJ, Holmes MD, Lee L, Lam AM. Dexmedetomidine sedation during awake craniotomy for seizure resection: effects on electrocorticography. J Neurosurg Anesthesiol. 2007;19:38–44.
11. Triltsch AE, Welte M, von Homeyer P, Große J, Genähr A, Moshirzadeh M, Sidiropoulos A, Konertz W, Kox WJ, Spies CD. Bispectral index-guided sedation with dexmedetomidine in intensive care: a prospective, randomized, double blind, placebo-controlled phase II study. Crit Care Med. 2002;30:1007–14.

Role of Indocyanine Green Videoangiography in Identification of Donor and Recipient Arteries in Cerebral Bypass Surgery

Giuseppe Esposito, Sandra Dias, Jan-Karl Burkhardt, Oliver Bozinov, and Luca Regli

Abstract The identification and preparation of a very good quality donor artery is a crucial step in every superficial temporal artery to middle cerebral artery (STA-MCA) bypass.

For flow-preservation bypass performed for trapping of complex MCA aneurysms, the key element is the correct target of the recipient artery. When a cortical recipient artery (M4 segment of the MCA) is selected, this vessel must be a terminal branch of the artery whose sacrifice is necessary for definitive aneurysmal treatment.

In this chapter we report on two techniques for (1) intraoperative mapping and preparation of good quality STA branch as the donor artery for STA-MCA bypass (mostly in the case the frontal branch of the STA needs to be used) and (2) selective identification of the correct superficial (M4 cortical) "recipient" artery in flow-preservation STA-MCA bypass performed for managing complex MCA aneurysms.

Both techniques are based on the use of microscope-integrated indocyanine green videoangiography (ICG-VA), an intraoperative tool allowing observation and real-time assessment of blood flow in large and small vessels, with distinct evaluation of arterial, capillary, and venous phases.

The two techniques contribute, respectively, to (1) reduce the risk of erroneous identification or injury of the donor artery in STA-MCA bypass procedures and (2) eliminate the risk of erroneous revascularization of a non-involved arterial territory in flow-preservation bypass surgery for managing complex MCA aneurysms.

Keywords Cerebral bypass · Donor artery · Extra-intracranial bypass · Flow-preservation bypass · Indocyanine green videoangiography—ICGVA · Neurosurgery · Recipient artery · Selective revascularization

G. Esposito, M.D., Ph.D. (✉) · S. Dias · J-K. Burkhardt
O. Bozinov · L. Regli
Department of Neurosurgery, University Hospital Zurich, University of Zurich, Zurich, Switzerland
e-mail: giuseppe.esposito@usz.ch

Abbreviations

DSA	Digital subtraction angiography
EC-IC	Extracranial to intracranial
ICGVA	Indocyanine green videoangiography
MCA	Middle cerebral artery
STA	Superficial temporal artery
STA-MCA	Superficial temporal artery to middle cerebral artery

Introduction

A crucial step in every STA-MCA bypass procedure (both flow-preservation and flow-augmentation) is the reliable identification and safe dissection of the donor artery, namely the superficial temporal artery (STA) [1].

For flow-preservation bypass performed to trap complex aneurysms of the middle cerebral artery (MCA), a key element is the correct target of the recipient artery [2–8]. The bypass must supply adequate blood flow to the brain perfused by the trapped vessel [2–4, 6, 7, 9–11]. When a cortical recipient artery (M4 segment of the MCA) is selected, this vessel must be a terminal branch of the artery whose sacrifice is necessary for definitive aneurysm treatment [3, 6].

Microscope-integrated indocyanine green videoangiography (ICGVA) allows intraoperative and real-time assessment of blood flow in large and small vessels, with distinct evaluation of arterial, capillary, and venous phases [12, 13].

With this work, we present the way we use ICGVA to (1) intraoperatively map and prepare good-quality STA branch as the donor artery for STA-MCA bypass (mostly in cases when the frontal branch of the STA needs to be used) and (2) selectively identify the correct superficial (M4 cortical) "recipient" artery in flow-preservation STA-MCA bypass performed to manage complex MCA aneurysms. These two techniques have been separately reported by us in the past few years [1, 3].

G. Esposito et al. (eds.), *Trends in the Management of Cerebrovascular Diseases*, Acta Neurochirurgica Supplement, Vol. 129,
https://doi.org/10.1007/978-3-319-73739-3_12,

ICGVA-Assisted Identification of Bypass Donor Artery

The STA divides into two branches: an anterior frontal branch and a posterior parietal branch [14]. If only the parietal branch needs to be prepared, a linear incision above this parietal branch allows its dissection under the microscope [1]. In the case the frontal branch of the STA has to be used (for instance, in the case of an absent/hypoplasic parietal branch as well as for double-barrel STA-MCA bypass), the surgeon usually dissects the frontal branch from the underside of a fronto-temporal scalp flap [1]. This dissection can, however, be difficult because of the additional skin retraction required to expose the artery and dissection through the fat plane, as well as variability in the anatomy of the STA branches [1].

The ICGVA-assisted technique described here allows intraoperative mapping and preparation of a good quality STA branch as the donor artery for STA-MCA bypass: the technique is useful mostly in the case where the frontal branch of the STA needs to be dissected [1].

This technique is based on the analysis of the difference in time of filling of scalp vessels illuminated via ICG-VA from the underside of a scalp flap [1].

ICG-VA is performed using a commercially available surgical microscope (OPMI® Pentero™, The Carl Zeiss Co, Oberkochen, Germany). A standard dose of 25 mg ICG is dissolved in 5 mL of water and injected into a central vein as a bolus. The underside of the fronto-temporal scalp flap is illuminated with near-infrared light and the anatomy of the visualized vasculature studied. ICG-VA videos are analyzed on a video screen and recorded for further analysis [1].

ICG-VA allows one to visualize the whole pattern of the STA at once before preparation (Fig. 1a), differentiate the STA-branches running parallel (Fig. 1a), map precisely the donor in the case of serpiginous STA (Fig. 1b), localize the bifurcation-points of the STA branches (Fig. 1a), and precisely define the location of all the branching points in the late arterial phase (Fig. 1a, b).

This technique is very effective for mapping and preparing a very good quality donor artery [1]. It may reduce the risk of erroneous identification or injury of the donor artery, mainly in the case of anatomical variations of the STA, such as changes in main bifurcation site (over or below the zygomatic arch), absence of bifurcation, hypoplasia or absence of one of the branches, double parietal branches, further bifurcation along the branches, and a serpiginous course [1]. The technique presented is not intended to substitute for the use of intraoperative Doppler for identification of the STA branches, but rather as an alternative/complementary tool [1].

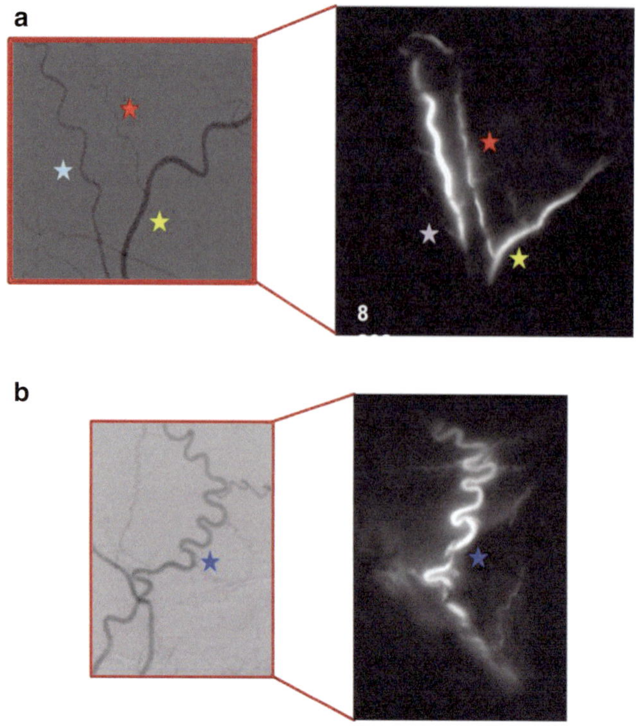

Fig. 1 (**a**) Left: Preoperative DSA with selective injection of the left external carotid artery showing the frontal and parietal branches of the left STA. Right: ICG-VA demonstrating the course of the frontal (yellow star) and parietal (light blue star) branches of the STA from the underside of the left fronto-temporal scalp flap. ICG-VA differentiates the STA branches running parallel (light blue and red stars) and shows (in the late arterial phase of the angiography, 8 s) all the branching points of the STA. The red star indicates a subbranch of the frontal STA. (**b**) Left: Preoperative DSA with selective injection of the left external carotid artery demonstrating a serpiginous course of the frontal branch of the STA (blue star). Right: ICGVA shows the frontal branch has a serpiginous course and all the branching points of the STA (*Modified from Esposito* et al., *Acta Neurochir, 2016*) [1]

ICGVA-Assisted Identification of Bypass Recipient Artery

For flow-preservation bypass performed for trapping complex MCA aneurysms, the selection of the correct recipient artery is an essential step. When microsurgical dissection of the Sylvian fissure and of the aneurysmal angioanatomy is safe, the selection of an M2-M3 segment of MCA as recipient is a valid choice. When microsurgical dissection is considered more risky or when avoiding a deep site for the anastomosis is preferred, a cortical recipient artery (M4 segment of MCA) can be selected [3, 6]. It is essential that this recipient artery indeed represents a distal branch of the artery whose sacrifice is needed to treat the aneurysms (by aneurysmal trapping). Because each M2 segment feeds several cortical (M4) arteries, there is the risk of revascularization into a wrong territory despite the use of anatomical landmarks,

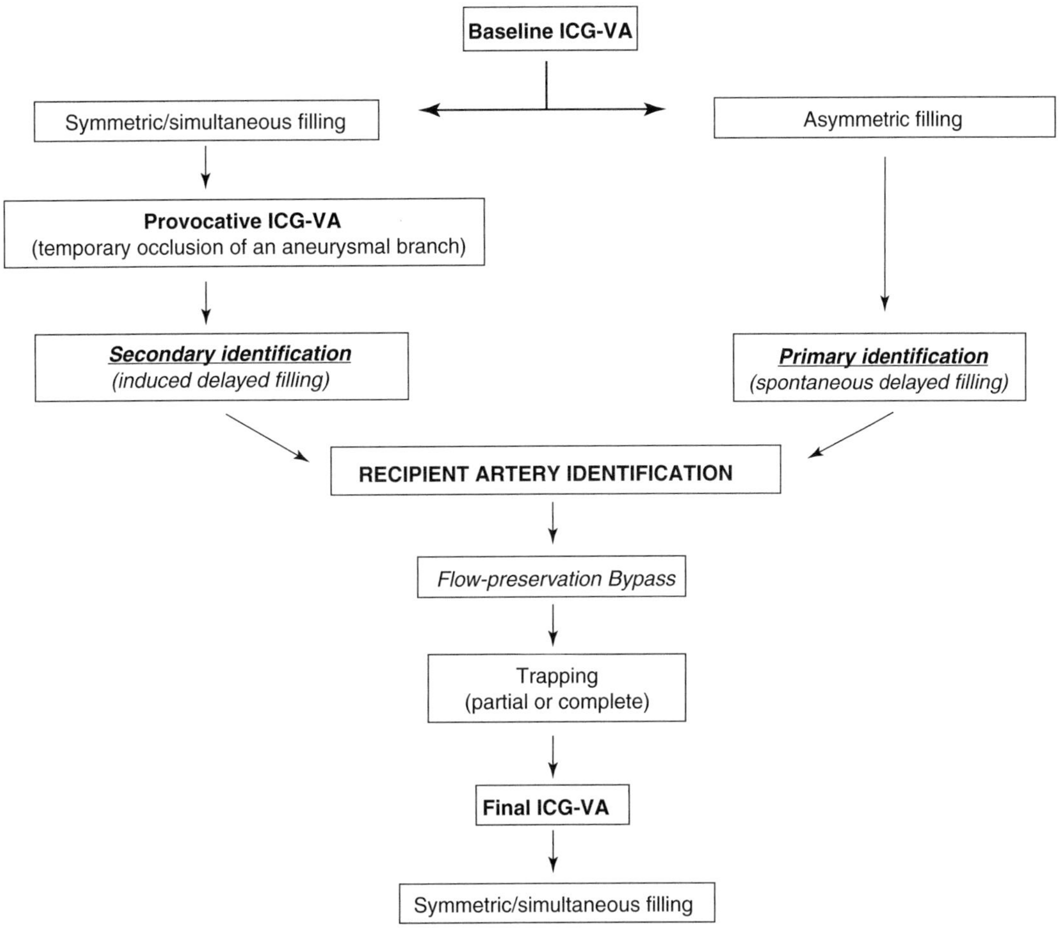

Fig. 2 Flowchart illustrating the strategy in serial ICG-VAs performed for selective-targeted identification of the cortical recipient artery in flow-preservation EC-IC bypass surgery (*Modified from: Esposito* et al., *Neurosurgery, 2012*) [3]

preoperative neuroimaging, neuronavigation, and stereotactic techniques) [3, 6].

The ICGVA-assisted technique presented allows selective identification of the correct superficial (M4 cortical) "recipient" artery in flow-preservation STA-MCA bypass performed to manage complex MCA aneurysms by using trapping strategies. In this way it eliminates the risk of erroneous revascularization of a non-involved arterial territory.

The possibility of selecting a superficial recipient (M4) artery makes the bypass easier and less invasive. Furthermore, tolerance to ischemia is better during temporary occlusion of a cortical M4 artery as compared to occlusion of a more proximal M2 or M3 branch [3, 6].

ICG-VA is performed as described above. This time, however, the cortex around the Sylvian fissure is illuminated with near-infrared light: the difference in the direction and in the time of filling of M4 cortical arteries is analyzed [3]. In fact, ICGVA allows one to assess a delayed or reversed arterial filling, as well as delayed capillary/venous filling [3, 6, 13].

As schematized in the flowchart in Fig. 2, a delay in cortical M4 arteries filling may be seen in two different circumstances. The first is *primarily* on a baseline ICG-VA without any temporary occlusion of arteries. Such a delay can be caused by any increased resistance to flow (e.g., stenosis/occlusion of an aneurysmal branch, intra-aneurysmatic turbulent flow, serpiginous aneurysm). We define this as *primary* identification (Fig. 2) [3]. The second circumstance is the detection of delayed flow *secondarily,* after provocative temporary occlusion of an artery. This implies temporary test-occlusion (via application of a temporary clip) of any MCA branch that may need to be occluded for final aneurysm treatment. We define this as *secondary* identification [3] (Figs. 2 and 3). These two conditions are defined as *primary identification* and *secondary identification*, respectively (Fig. 2) [3].

Any *primary* or *secondary* delayed fluorescence of M4 branches (fluorescence is visualized during the capillary/venous phases of ICG-VA) defines a cortical area around the Sylvian fissure with delayed vascular filling. The most suitable cortical artery within this cortical area can be targeted as bypass recipient artery (Figs. 2 and 3) [3].

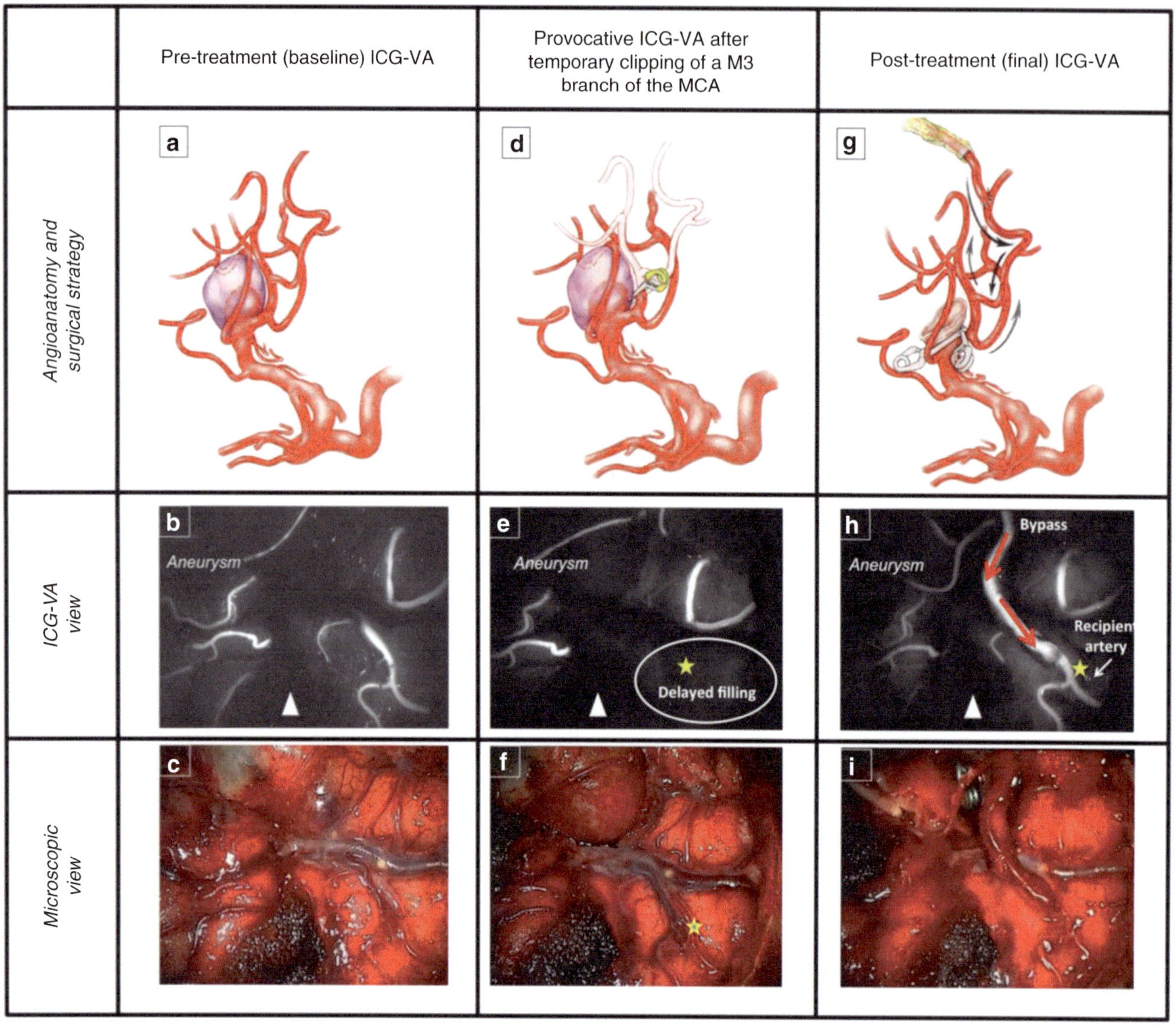

Fig. 3 (Patient 2)—secondary identification. (**a**) Drawing: partially thrombosed aneurysm of the right M1 bifurcation. (**b**) Baseline ICG-VA: simultaneous filling of all the exposed cortical (M4) arteries. (**c**) Intraoperative microscopic view of the ICG-VA field shown in (**b**). (**d**) Drawing: a temporary clip on the M3 segment of the MCA is placed to perform a provocative ICG-VA. (**e**) Provocative ICG-VA: an area presenting a delayed filling is evident. A suitable artery in this territory is then selected as recipient (yellow asterisk). (**f**) Intraoperative microscopic view of the ICG-VA field shown in (**e**) (yellow asterisk represents the recipient artery). (**g**) Drawing: final aneurysm treatment: trapping + flow-preservation bypass. (**h**) Final (post-bypass) ICG-VA: the bypass is patent and the cortex takes fluorescence simultaneously. (**i**) Intraoperative microscopic view of the ICG-VA field shown in (**h**). (*Asterisk*) White triangles indicate surgery-related decreased fluorescence on ICG-VA. DSA: digital subtraction angiography; ICG-VA: indocyanine green videoangiography (*Modified from: Esposito* et al., *Neurosurgery, 2012 and Esposito* et al., *Neurosurgery, 2014*)

ICG-VA can be repeated as many times as needed; it is important to remain within the daily dose limit of ICG (5 mg/kg) and to wait at least 10 min between two consecutive intravenous ICG injections (to allow washout of the previously administered ICG).

The possibility of repeating ICGVA enabled us to study the cortical filling before (*baseline ICG-VA*), as well as during temporary occlusion of MCA branches (*provocative ICG-VA*), and after bypass construction and aneurysm treatment (*final ICG-VA*) (Fig. 2) [3].

Conclusions

The two reported ICGVA-assisted techniques allow (1) mapping and preparation of very good quality donor vessel in STA-MCA bypass (mostly if the frontal branch of the STA has to be used) and (2) reliable and accurate identification of the cortical recipient artery and elimination of the risk of erroneous revascularization of a non-involved arterial territory in flow-preservation bypass surgery performed to manage complex MCA aneurysms.

Disclosure The authors report no conflicts.

References

1. Esposito G, Burkhardt JK, Bozinov O, Regli L. Indocyanine green videoangiography for the identification of superficial temporal artery branches in EC-IC bypass surgery. Acta Neurochir. 2016;158:565–70.
2. Esposito G, Amin-Hanjani S, Regli L. Role of and indications for bypass surgery after carotid occlusion surgery study (COSS)? Stroke. 2016;47:282–90.
3. Esposito G, Durand A, Van Doormaal T, Regli L. Selective-targeted extra-intracranial bypass surgery in complex middle cerebral artery aneurysms: correctly identifying the recipient artery using indocyanine green videoangiography. Neurosurgery. 2012;71:ons274–84; discussion ons284–285.
4. Esposito G, Fierstra J, Regli L. Distal outflow occlusion with bypass revascularization: last resort measure in managing complex MCA and PICA aneurysms. Acta Neurochir. 2016;158:1523–31.
5. Esposito G, Fierstra J, Regli L. Partial trapping strategies for managing complex intracranial aneurysms. Acta Neurochir Suppl. 2016;123:73–5.
6. Esposito G, Regli L. Selective targeted cerebral revascularization via microscope integrated indocyanine green videoangiography technology. Acta Neurochir Suppl. 2014;119:59–64.
7. Esposito G, Regli L. Surgical decision-making for managing complex intracranial aneurysms. Acta Neurochir Suppl. 2014; 119:3–11.
8. Kronenburg A, Esposito G, Fierstra J, Braun KP, Regli L. Combined bypass technique for contemporary revascularization of unilateral MCA and bilateral frontal territories in moyamoya vasculopathy. Acta Neurochir Suppl. 2014;119:65–70.
9. Burkhardt JK, Esposito G, Fierstra J, Bozinov O, Regli L. Emergency non-occlusive high capacity bypass surgery for ruptured giant internal carotid artery aneurysms. Acta Neurochir Suppl. 2016;123:77–81.
10. Jafar JJ, Russell SM, Woo HH. Treatment of giant intracranial aneurysms with saphenous vein extracranial-to-intracranial bypass grafting: indications, operative technique, and results in 29 patients. Neurosurgery. 2002;51:138–44; discussion 144–146.
11. Sekhar LN, Natarajan SK, Ellenbogen RG, Ghodke B. Cerebral revascularization for ischemia, aneurysms, and cranial base tumors. Neurosurgery. 2008;62:1373–408; discussion 1408–1410.
12. Raabe A, Beck J, Gerlach R, Zimmermann M, Seifert V. Near-infrared indocyanine green video angiography: a new method for intraoperative assessment of vascular flow. Neurosurgery. 2003;52:132–9; discussion 139.
13. Scerrati A, Della Pepa GM, Conforti G, Sabatino G, Puca A, Albanese A, Maira G, Marchese E, Esposito G. Indocyanine green video-angiography in neurosurgery: a glance beyond vascular applications. Clin Neurol Neurosurg. 2014;124:106–13.
14. Pinar YA, Govsa F. Anatomy of the superficial temporal artery and its branches: its importance for surgery. Surg Radiol Anat. 2006;28:248–53.

Incidence of Moyamoya Disease in Denmark: A Population-Based Register Study

Peter Birkeland and Jens Lauritsen

Abstract In this first population-based study of moyamoya disease (MMD) in Europe, the authors identified 56 patients with MMD in Denmark during the period 1994–2015 using nationwide registers. The overall incidence was 0.047 per 100,000 person-years, which is about one-tenth that reported in Japan. Otherwise the epidemiological features were comparable: there was a bimodal age distribution with peaks in the age groups 0–9 years and 30–39 years, with twice as many females as males.

Keywords Moyamoya disease · Epidemiology · Stroke · Cerebrovascular · 1994–2015 · Scandinavian

Introduction

Moyamoya disease (MMD) is an idiopathic cerebrovascular disease characterized by progressive stenosis of the internal carotid arteries and their proximal branches. Reduced blood flow to the anterior circulation of the brain leads to the development of compensatory collaterals at the base of the brain. The disease predisposes affected patients to stroke [1]. When the characteristic vasculopathy is seen with recognized associated conditions such as neurofibromatosis type 1, Down syndrome, and sickle cell disease [1, 2], patients are classified as having moyamoya syndrome (MMS). First described in Japan and originally considered to affect mainly persons of Asian heritage, MMD is now recognized as an unusual cause of stroke in people of many ethnic backgrounds around the world, including in Denmark [3, 4]. The incidence in Japan is in the range 0.34–0.94 per 100,000 person-years, with peaks in two age groups: 5–9 years and 45–49 years, and it is about twice as common in females as in males [5–7]. A case series [8] and a recent review [9] indicate that MMD in Europe may have distinct characteristics, although population-based data are scarce [10]. By taking advantage of Danish nationwide registers, this study investigated the epidemiology of MMD in a European population.

P. Birkeland, M.D. (✉)
Department of Neurosurgery, Aalborg University Hospital, Aalborg, Denmark
e-mail: Peter@Birkeland.dk

J. Lauritsen, M.D., Ph.D.
Department of Orthopaedic Surgery, Odense University Hospital, Odense, Denmark

Institute of Clinical Research, University of Southern Denmark, Odense, Denmark

Materials and Methods

This study was based on data from three nationwide registers: the Danish National Patient Register, the Danish Central Person Register, and the Danish Mortality Register. Information on essentially all discharges from Danish hospitals has been recorded in the Danish National Patient Register since 1977, and information on outpatient clinic visits has also been included since 1994. Recorded data include the patient's unique civil registration number, the dates of admission and discharge, discharge diagnoses, hospital and department codes, and any surgical or diagnostic (from 1999) procedure(s) performed [11]. For this study the civil registration numbers were encrypted. MMD first appeared as a diagnostic code in Denmark in the International Classification of Diseases 10th Revision (ICD-10) in 1994 (diagnoses had previously been coded according to ICD-8), although ICD-10 does not distinguish between MMD and MMS. Thus, patients with other diagnostic codes suggesting an underlying condition (such as MMS) were excluded from further analysis.

We identified patients with a diagnosis of MMD (ICD-10 code I675) in the Danish National Patient Register from 1

G. Esposito et al. (eds.), *Trends in the Management of Cerebrovascular Diseases*, Acta Neurochirurgica Supplement, Vol. 129, https://doi.org/10.1007/978-3-319-73739-3_13,

January 1994 to 31 December 2015 and retrieved data on all hospitalizations or clinic visits registered with a diagnosis of MMD. An incident case was defined as the first registered admission or clinic visit to a hospital with a diagnosis of MMD. For the calculation of incidence, person-years were approximated by the number of persons on 1 January in any given calendar year. These data are accessible on Statistics Denmark (www.statistikbanken.dk). We also looked at whether the diagnosis had been made in a specialist department and what diagnostic procedures had been performed in the workup.

From the Central Person Register we obtained information on date of birth, sex, residency, date of immigration or emigration, and date of death (if applicable) for identified cases. For each individual the civil registration numbers of the parents are also recorded, allowing us to identify familial cases (adopted children are recorded under their adoptive parents). From the Mortality Register we collected data on cause of death.

Analyses were performed using STATA (version 14, College Station, TX, USA) and the OpenEpi software (www.openepi.com). For statistics we used the Fisher exact test with significance level $P < 0.05$. The study was approved by The Danish Data Protection Agency.

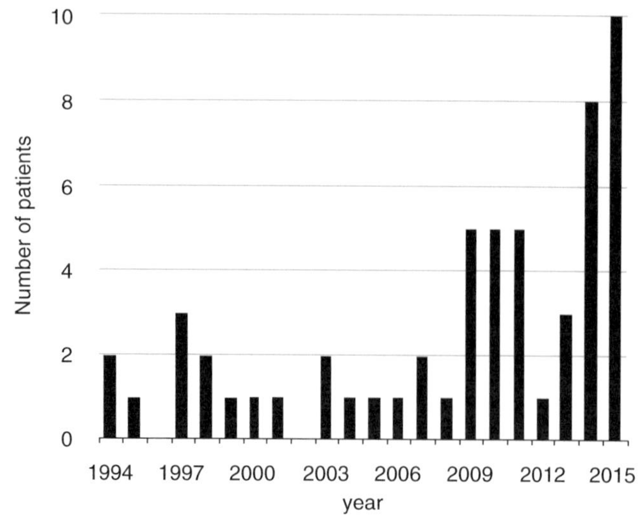

Fig. 1 Annual number of incident cases of moyamoya disease

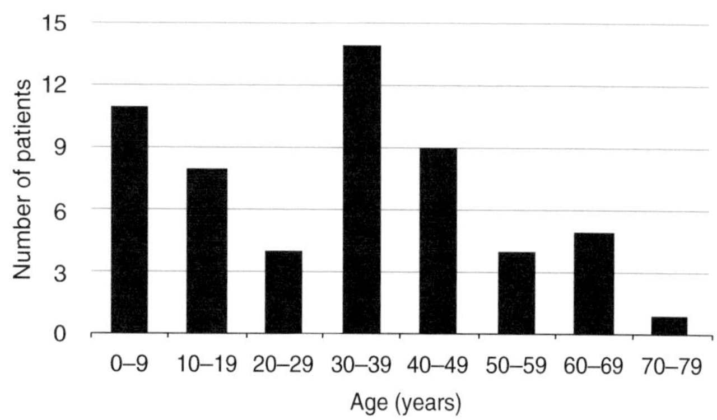

Fig. 2 Onset age distribution of moyamoya disease

Results

Overall, 64 patients were identified with the ICD-10 diagnostic code for MMD between 1994 and 2015. Digital subtraction angiography (DSA) and/or magnetic resonance imaging and angiography (MRI/MRA) were recorded in the register for 31 patients (48%). All but one diagnosis was made in specialist departments (pediatrics, neurology, and/or neurosurgery). The one patient diagnosed outside this setting was admitted to a medical ward in a hospital with a neurological service. Four patients died during the study period, three being females. In one case the cause of death was neurovascular disease, namely intracerebral hemorrhage.

A further eight patients had other diagnostic codes, suggesting an underlying disease: four had neurofibromatosis, two congenital heart disease, one thalassaemia minor, and one Down's syndrome, leaving 56 patients for further analysis.

Thirty eight of the 56 patients were females. Thus, the female:male ratio was 2.1. The overall incidence was 0.047 per 100,000 person-years (95% confidence interval, 0.035–0.061 per 100,000 person-years). Of note, from 1994 until 2008, 1 or 2 cases were diagnosed most years, and this number rose to 5–10 cases from 2009 (see Fig. 1). There was a bimodal age distribution at presentation with peaks in the age groups 0–10 years and 30–39 years (Fig. 2). There were four cases of familial MMD (7.1%): siblings and a parent and child.

Discussion

In this Danish register study we found an incidence of MMD that was about one tenth of that reported in Japan, but the sex and age distribution at presentation and proportion of familial cases were comparable. Thus, our preliminary data do not indicate that MMD has distinct epidemiological characteristics in Scandinavia.

When comparing incidence data with that of other populations, part of the discrepancy may be attributable to different case finding methods, as has been discussed previously [10]. Using hospital discharge databases and a somewhat similar approach to ours, an incidence of 0.086 per 100,000 person-years has been reported in the U.S. [12]. The authors of a survey from French neuropediatric centers found an incidence of 0.065 per 100,000 person-years in children [13]. Both studies included both MMS and MMD in their analyses and this may account for the higher incidences reported. For research purposes it would be useful if future disease classification distinguished between MMD and MMS.

By assuming that the first hospitalization/clinic visit in the study period was the incident event, we may have missed earlier events. This could lead to a higher number of incident cases during the first years of analysis. However, incidence has risen during the study period. The register data do not provide us with an explanation for this trend. Rather than a true increase, it may reflect a higher detection rate because of an increased index of suspicion for this disease and increased availability of magnetic resonance angiography. Our data show that in Europe MMD should be considered in the differential diagnosis of stroke in children and in adults, particularly females in the age group 30–49 years.

It should be noted that DSA and/or MRI with MRA were only recorded in the register for about half of the patients. These are investigations that are considered essential in MMD diagnosis [14]. However, more patients may have been investigated than those recorded, particularly in the first years of the study period. In 2000, register data became the basis of hospital reimbursement in Denmark and the registration is assumed to be complete only after that date [11]. Interestingly, in the U.S. study a similar proportion of the patients had appropriate investigation recorded [12].

The strength of the study is that it provides the first population-based data on MMD from a European country. However, this study has limitations. First, the sensitivity and specificity of the ICD-10 diagnostic code to identify MMD are unknown. It was not possible to validate the diagnosis according to the definition of MMD [14] because of the anonymity of the data. Similar studies of other neurological disorders may reveal the extent of this problem. For example, in a study of Parkinson's disease, a primary diagnosis of Parkinson's disease in the Danish National Patient Register could be confirmed in 82% of patients based on established criteria [15]. Second, the registers do not contain data on race and ethnicity and one should bear in mind that some of the cases may not be Caucasians. Denmark's population is diverse and. for example, also comprises Asians (e.g., adopted children) and Inuits. Third, the data do not provide information on the clinical and radiological presentation of MMD. To gain more insight on MMD in Denmark and address the shortcomings of this preliminary study, we have requested access to individual patient charts.

Ethics and Conflict of Interest

Ethical Approval For this type of study formal consent is not required.

Conflict of Interest The authors declare that they have no conflict of interest.

Funding This study was supported by a grant from Ingeniør K.A. Rohde of Hustrus Legat.

References

1. Scott RM, Smith ER. Moyamoya disease and moyamoya syndrome. N Engl J Med. 2009;360:1226–37.
2. Birkeland P, Gardner K, Kesse-Adu R, Davies J, Lauritsen J, Rom Poulsen F, Tolias CM, Thein SL. Intracranial aneurysms in sickle-cell disease are associated with the hemoglobin SS genotype but not with moyamoya syndrome. Stroke. 2016;47:1710–3.
3. Hansen RN, Andersen G, Longin E. Moyamoya. Ugeskr Laeger. 2011;173:281–2.
4. Kondziella D. Diagnosis and treatment of rare causes of ischaemic stroke. Ugeskr Laeger. 2016;178:V02160101.
5. Baba T, Houkin K, Kuroda S. Novel epidemiological features of moyamoya disease. J Neurol Neurosurg Psychiatry. 2008;79:900–4.
6. Hoshino H, Izawa Y, Suzuki N. Epidemiological features of moyamoya disease in Japan. Neurol Med Chir (Tokyo). 2012;52: 295–8.
7. Wakai K, Tamakoshi A, Ikezaki K, Fukui M, Kawamura T, Aoki R, Kojima M, Lin Y, Ohno Y. Epidemiological features of moyamoya disease in Japan: findings from a nationwide survey. Clin Neurol Neurosurg. 1997;99(Suppl 2):S1–5.
8. Acker G, Goerdes S, Schneider UC, Schmiedek P, Czabanka M, Vajkoczy P. Distinct clinical and radiographic characteristics of moyamoya disease amongst European Caucasians. Eur J Neurol. 2015;22:1012–7.
9. Hever P, Alamri A, Tolias C. Moyamoya angiopathy—is there a Western phenotype? Br J Neurosurg. 2015;29:765–71.
10. Kleinloog R, Regli L, Rinkel GJ, Klijn CJ. Regional differences in incidence and patient characteristics of moyamoya disease: a systematic review. J Neurol Neurosurg Psychiatry. 2012;83:531–6.
11. Lynge E, Sandegaard JL, Rebolj M. The Danish national patient register. Scand J Public Health. 2011;39:30–3.
12. Uchino K, Johnston SC, Becker KJ, Tirschwell DL. Moyamoya disease in Washington State and California. Neurology. 2005;65:956–8.
13. Kossorotoff M, Herve D, Toulgoat F, Renaud C, Presles E, Chabriat H, Chabrier S. Paediatric moyamoya in mainland France: a comprehensive survey of academic neuropaediatric centres. Cerebrovasc Dis. 2012;33:76–9.
14. Research Committee on the Pathology and Treatment of Spontaneous. Occlusion of the Circle of Willis, Health Labour Sciences Research Grant for Research on Measure for Infractable Diseases. Guidelines for diagnosis and treatment of moyamoya disease (spontaneous occlusion of the circle of Willis). Neurol Med Chir (Tokyo). 2012;52:245–66.
15. Wermuth L, Lassen CF, Himmerslev L, Olsen J, Ritz B. Validation of hospital register-based diagnosis of Parkinson's disease. Dan Med J. 2012;59:A4391.

Carotid Endarterectomy and Carotid Artery Stenting in the Light of ICSS and CREST Studies

V. Benes and O. Bradac

Abstract *Objective.* We analyzed the results of internal carotid artery (ICA) stenosis treatment at our institution according to the treatment modality—carotid endarterectomy (CEA) vs. carotid artery stenting (CAS).

Methods. During 2003–2015, a total of 1894 procedures were performed for ICA stenosis. CEA was done in 1064 cases and CAS in 830 cases.

The primary outcome was disabling stroke (mRS > 2) or myocardial infarction within 30 days of treatment. Secondary outcomes were transitory ischemic attacks (TIAs), minor strokes (stroke without impaired activities of daily living), and any other significant complications.

Results. Major mortality and morbidity were divided according to their treatment groups; this reached 0.9% in the CEA and 2.5% in the CAS group ($p = 0.007$). Minor stroke was recorded at 1.5% and 2.7% in the CEA and CAS groups ($p = 0.077$), TIAs in 1.0% (CEA) and 4.0% (CAS) ($p < 0.001$), and any complication in 12.4% (CEA) and 13.0% (CAS) ($p = 0.694$).

Conclusions. CEA is a safe procedure in patients who meet the correct treatment indications. In all subgroup analyses CEA proved to be equal to or better than CAS. This study supports the idea of CEA being the preferred treatment and CAS being reserved for selected cases only.

Keywords Carotid artery stenting (CAS) · Carotid endarterectomy (CEA) · Complication · Outcome · Stroke

V. Benes, M.D., Ph.D. · O. Bradac, M.D., M.Sc., Ph.D. (✉)
Department of Neurosurgery, First Medical Faculty,
Military University Hospital and Charles University,
Prague, Czech Republic
e-mail: ondrej.bradac@uvn.cz

Introduction

Internal carotid artery (ICA) stenosis is one of the most thoroughly studied cerebrovascular diseases [1]. The effectiveness of carotid endarterectomy (CEA) in preventing stroke has been seen in many studies. Modern indications for CEA in symptomatic and asymptomatic patients were shown in the NASCET [2–5], ECST [6–9], ACAS [10, 11], and ACST [12, 13] studies. Following the publication of these studies, the indications altered slightly compared with those seen in the American Heart Association guidelines. During the 1990s, carotid artery stenting (CAS) came into routine practice and is nowadays used very frequently. The indications for CAS developed to be basically the same as those for CEA, although this move occurred for no specific reason. Some randomized studies showed noninferiority of CAS against CEA [14–21]. After recent publication of long-term results from ICSS [22] and CREST [23], the question of preferred treatment modality arose again. We decided to evaluate our results of ICA stenosis treatment and compare the results of each of the treatment modalities.

Materials and Methods

During 2003–2015, a total of 1894 internal carotid stenosis procedures were performed. Of these, 1064 were CEA and 830 were CAS. Patients were prospectively followed by neurologists not performing treatment procedures, and data were retrospectively evaluated. Baseline characteristics of all the patients was divided according to treatment method and the proportion of patients with two or more vascular risk factors (hypertension, ischemic heart disease, hyperlipidemia, diabetes mellitus, tobacco smoking), and are detailed in Table 1. Initial symptoms of patients divided according to treatment

G. Esposito et al. (eds.), *Trends in the Management of Cerebrovascular Diseases*, Acta Neurochirurgica Supplement, Vol. 129,
https://doi.org/10.1007/978-3-319-73739-3_14, © Springer International Publishing AG, part of Springer Nature 2018

Table 1 Baseline characteristics of patient population

	CEA	CAS	*p* value
No. of procedures	1064 (100%)	830 (100%)	
Male	740 (70%)	606 (73%)	0.099
Age	67 ± 9	70 ± 10	**<0.001**
2+ Risk factors	666 (63%)	713 (86%)	**<0.001**

Bold values are significant with *p* below 0.05

Table 2 Presenting symptoms according to treatment groups

	CEA	CAS	*p* value
Symptomtic patients	843 (100%)	605 (100%)	
TIA	182 (21.6%)	59 (9.8%)	**<0.001**
Repeated TIA	149 (17.6%)	112 (18.5%)	0.683
Minor stroke	276 (32.7%)	293 (48.4%)	**<0.001**
Major stroke	58 (6.8%)	49 (8.1%)	0.382
Diffuse + other symptoms	178 (21.1.7%)	92 (15.2%)	**0.004**

Bold values are significant with *p* below 0.05

Table 3 Number of CEA vs. CAS procedures per year of study

Year	CEA	CAS	Total
2003	80	63	143
2004	87	64	151
2005	72	99	171
2006	99	80	179
2007	100	96	196
2008	69	56	125
2009	73	57	130
2010	74	50	124
2011	71	43	114
2012	89	48	137
2013	75	57	132
2014	92	38	130
2015	83	79	162
Overall	1064	830	1894

modalities are shown in Table 2. Number and ratio of CEA vs. CAS procedures per year of the study are depicted in Table 3.

All CEA procedures were carried out on patients taking antiplatelet monotherapy (Aspirin or Clopidogrel) under general anesthesia with SSEPs and EEG monitoring. Shunting was used selectively and was performed in 28 (2.6%) procedures. All CAS procedures were performed under local anesthesia on patients taking dual antiplatelet therapy (Aspirin + Clopidogrel in the vast majority of cases), and subsequently dual antiplatelet therapy was administered for 30 days, all done using a distal protection device.

Treatment results of CEA and CAS in the whole group were compared and subgroup analyses were performed on the following patient subgroups: those with contralateral ICA stenosis/occlusion, those with symptomatic/asymptomatic ICA stenosis, and those aged 75 years or above.

Primary Outcomes

Major morbidity and mortality were defined as a new severe neurological deficit, increasing modified Rankin scale (mRS) score above 2 or MI within 30 days after the procedure.

Secondary Outcomes

These were TIAs, minor strokes (without consequence as impaired ADL) within 30 days of the intervention, and any marked complication during the early posttreatment period (cranial nerve deficits, wound hematomas, groin hematomas, wound swelling, hyper-perfusion syndrome, seizures, a prolonged length of stay—defined as more than 2 days in CAS or more than 4 days in CEA patients—for any medical reason).

Statistical Processing

All statistical computations were performed using STATISTICA 10 software (StatSoft, Tulsa, OK, USA, distributed by StatSoft CR s.r.o., Prague, Czech Republic). Categorial variables were assessed using chi-square or Fisher exact test as appropriate. Continuous variables were compared using a two-sided t-test. As a level of statistical significance, a *p*-value of 0.05 was used.

Results

Severe morbidity and mortality, divided by treatment group, reached 0.9% (10 patients, one of them experienced severe MI after treatment) in CEA group and 2.5% (21 patients, two of them experienced severe MI after treatment) in CAS group, $p = 0.007$. Minor stroke was recorded in 1.5% (16 patients) after CEA and 2.7% (22 patients) after CAS, $p = 0.077$. TIAs occurred in 1.0% (11 patients) after CEA and 4.0% (33 patients) after CAS, $p < 0.001$. Other complications were encountered in 12.4% (132 patients) after CEA and 13.0% (108 patients) after CAS, $p = 0.694$. The results divided by treatment group, together with the results of the subgroup analyses, are shown in Table 4.

Overall results (CEA and CAS counted together) showed a major morbidity and mortality was recorded in 31 patients (1.6%), minor stroke in 38 procedures (2.0%), TIA after 44 (2.3%), and any other complication after 240 (12.7%) procedures.

Table 4 Whole cohort results and subgroup results according to treatment modality

	CEA	CAS	*p* value
No. of procedures	1064 (100%)	830 (100%)	
Whole cohort			
Major M/M	10 (0.9%)	21 (2.5%)	**0.007**
Minor stroke	16 (1.5%)	22 (2.7%)	0.077
TIA	11 (1.0%)	33 (4.0%)	**<0.001**
Any complication	132 (12.4%)	108 (13.0%)	0.694
Contralateral stenosis	379 (35.6%)	99 (11.9%)	**<0.001**
Major M/M	3 (0.8%)	3 (3.0%)	0.075
Minor stroke	7 (1.9%)	3 (3.0%)	0.464
TIA	1 (0.3%)	4 (4.0%)	**0.001**
Any complication	48 (12.7%)	18 (18.2%)	0.157
Contralateral occlusion	92 (8.6%)	87 (10.4%)	0.178
Major M/M	0 (0.0%)	2 (2.3%)	0.144
Minor stroke	0 (0.0%)	1 (1.2%)	0.302
TIA	1 (1.1%)	4 (4.6%)	0.154
Any complication	6 (6.5%)	8 (9.2%)	0.506
Symptomatic vessel	513 (48.2%)	419 (50.5%)	0.327
Major M/M	6 (1.2%)	13 (3.1%)	**0.038**
Minor stroke	13 (2.5%)	14 (3.3%)	0.465
TIA	9 (1.8%)	20 (4.8%)	**0.008**
Any complication	77 (15.0%)	61 (14.6%)	0.847
Asymptomatic vessel	551 (51.8%)	411 (49.5%)	0.327
Major M/M	4 (0.7%)	8 (2.0%)	0.092
Minor stroke	4 (0.7%)	8 (2.0%)	0.092
TIA	1 (0.2%)	13 (3.2%)	**<0.001**
Any complication	55 (10.0%)	47 (11.4%)	0.469
Elderly patients (≥75 years)	220 (20.7%)	324 (39.0%)	**<0.001**
Major M/M	3 (1.4%)	6 (1.9%)	0.661
Minor stroke	2 (0.9%)	10 (3.1%)	0.090
TIA	2 (0.9%)	16 (4.9%)	**0.001**
Any complication	26 (11.8%)	50 (15.4%)	0.233
2+ Risk factors	666 (62.6%)	713 (85.9%)	**<0.001**
Major M/M	8 (1.2%)	18 (2.5%)	0.071
Minor stroke	12 (1.8%)	19 (2.66%)	0.280
TIA	5 (0.8%)	30 (4.2%)	**<0.001**
Any complication	90 (13.5%)	98 (13.7%)	0.900

Bold values are significant with *p* below 0.05

Discussion

Recently published results of the long-term follow-up of CREST [23] and ICSS [22] studies also concluded that the long-term functional outcome is similar for patients undergoing CEA and CAS. This interpretation could lead us to conclude that CEA and CAS are interchangeable procedures, but this would be an inappropriate conclusion as there were definite differences between CEA and CAS subgroups in both studies.

The ICSS study was based in 50 centers worldwide randomizing a total of 1713 patients with symptomatic ICA stenosis; 855 underwent CAS and 858 CEA. The median follow-up was 4.2 years. The number of disabling strokes was similar in both branches (52 vs. 49 in CAS and CEA subgroups). However, the number of patients suffering from any type of stroke was significantly higher in the CAS group (119 vs. 72 in CEA group). The majority of these events happened in the periprocedural period. In the further follow-up, the frequency of any type of stroke was similar in both studies.

The CREST study was performed in 117 centers in the United States and Canada, where a total of 2502 patients with symptomatic or asymptomatic ICA stenosis were randomized. The authors found a significantly higher frequency of periprocedural strokes—4.1% in the CAS group compared to 2.3% in the CEA group. This difference was outweighed by the higher frequency of myocardial infarctions in the CEA group (2.3% in CEA vs. 1.1% in the CAS group), which produced a similar rate of primary endpoints (stroke + MI + death)—5.2% in CAS vs. 4.5% in the CEA group in the periprocedural period and 11.8% in CAS vs. 9.9% in the CEA group when periprocedural period is counted together with 10 years follow-up. Again, the frequency of strokes during the follow-up period was almost identical in both groups. However, the initial difference in periprocedural stroke frequency resulted in borderline significance ($p = 0.07$) in the Kaplan–Meier analysis of CEA vs. CAS regarding stroke occurrence.

The ICSS study authors published a subanalysis of 1036 patients concerning MR findings of white-matter brain lesions before the procedure [24]. They conclude that patients presenting with more extensive white-matter lesions had a three times higher risk of periprocedural stroke during stenting than patients with less extensive white-matter changes. Similar dependence was not observed in patients undergoing endarterectomy.

Kuliha et al. [25] studied silent infarction frequency in 150 patients after CEA and CAS in a prospective randomized setting. New infarctions were found significantly more frequently after CAS (49%) than CEA procedures (25%). The lesion volumes were significantly greater after CAS than CEA. However, no significant differences were found between groups with regard to cognitive testing results.

Our institutional results agree well with published data regarding periprocedural morbidity and mortality. Furthermore, our results suggest that the traditional risk factors for CEA such as contralateral stenosis or occlusion are in fact negligible when adequate measures, such as intraoperative neuromonitoring, are performed. Similarly, CEA seems to be safer than CAS even in the elderly, who are deemed to be high-risk patients in terms of vascular events.

It is obvious that CAS carries higher risk of ischemic periprocedural complications (either silent or manifested stroke) compared to CEA, suggesting CEA as the method of choice for the treatment of carotid stenosis, although during long-term follow-up, stenting was proven to be stable and effective.

Randomized trials and subsequent recommendations are necessary for the recent philosophy of evidence-based medicine. However, it must be appreciated that all the recommendations are nothing better than maps or traffic signs. They have general implications, are internationally understood, allow the individual results to be compared to them, and give general directions. However, they can never be applied blindly to individual patients, who always have specific and local particularities and individual features. Under local conditions, it is the art of medicine to follow the rules but accept the exceptions. On the other hand, individual results should always be compared to those of randomized trials. Freedom of exceptions is granted if single institution results compare favourably with those of randomized trials. Even in this relatively common diagnosis, a concentration of care should be achieved. However it should be mentioned that patients with carotid steno-occlusive disease should not be concentrated in centers that only offer one treatment modality, even with excellent results. Centers offering both treatment modalities on a daily basis are strongly recommended.

A part of the results of this study was published previously in Acta Neurochirurgica [26].

Conclusions

In all subgroup analyses, CEA fared better or at least as well as CAS.

Carotid endarterectomy should still be considered as the preferred procedure over carotid artery stenting. Only in carefully selected cases such as re-stenosis after a previous carotid procedure, carotid dissection, ICA stenosis after radiotherapy, previous major neck surgery, and contralateral cranial nerve palsy or tandem stenosis should stenting be the preferred treatment modailty.

Acknowledgments Supported by grants AZV 16-29148A and MO1012.

Conflict of interest The authors declare that they have no conflict of interest.

References

1. Halm EA, Tuhrim S, Wang JJ, Rockman C, Riles TS, Chassin MR. Risk factors for perioperative death and stroke after carotid endarterectomy: results of the new york carotid artery surgery study. Stroke. 2009;40:221–9.
2. Barnett HJ, Taylor DW, Eliasziw M, Fox AJ, Ferguson GG, Haynes RB, Rankin RN, Clagett GP, Hachinski VC, Sackett DL, Thorpe KE, Meldrum HE, Spence JD. Benefit of carotid endarterectomy in patients with symptomatic moderate or severe stenosis. North American Symptomatic Carotid Endarterectomy Trial Collaborators. N Engl J Med. 1998;339:1415–25.
3. NASCET. Beneficial effect of carotid endarterectomy in symptomatic patients with high-grade carotid stenosis. North American Symptomatic Carotid Endarterectomy Trial Collaborators. N Engl J Med. 1991;325:445–53.
4. NASCET. Clinical alert: benefit of carotid endarterectomy for patients with high-grade stenosis of the internal carotid artery. National Institute of Neurological Disorders and Stroke Stroke and Trauma Division. North American Symptomatic Carotid Endarterectomy Trial (NASCET) investigators. Stroke. 1991;22:816–7.
5. NASCET. North American Symptomatic Carotid Endarterectomy Trial. Methods, patient characteristics, and progress. Stroke. 1991;22:711–20.
6. ECST. MRC European Carotid Surgery Trial: interim results for symptomatic patients with severe (70–99%) or with mild (0–29%) carotid stenosis. European Carotid Surgery Trialists' Collaborative Group. Lancet. 1991;337:1235–43.
7. ECST. Endarterectomy for moderate symptomatic carotid stenosis: interim results from the MRC European Carotid Surgery Trial. Lancet. 1996;347:1591–3.
8. ECST. Randomised trial of endarterectomy for recently symptomatic carotid stenosis: final results of the MRC European Carotid Surgery Trial (ECST). Lancet. 1998;351:1379–87.
9. Warlow CP. Symptomatic patients: the European Carotid Surgery Trial (ECST). J Mal Vasc. 1993;18:198–201.
10. ACAS. Endarterectomy for asymptomatic carotid artery stenosis. Executive Committee for the Asymptomatic Carotid Atherosclerosis Study. JAMA. 1995;273:1421–8.
11. ACAS. Carotid endarterectomy for patients with asymptomatic internal carotid artery stenosis. National Institute of Neurological Disorders and Stroke. J Neurol Sci. 1995;129:76–7.
12. Halliday A, Mansfield A, Marro J, Peto C, Peto R, Potter J, Thomas D. Prevention of disabling and fatal strokes by successful carotid endarterectomy in patients without recent neurological symptoms: randomised controlled trial. Lancet. 2004;363:1491–502.
13. Halliday A, Harrison M, Hayter E, Kong X, Mansfield A, Marro J, Pan H, Peto R, Potter J, Rahimi K, Rau A, Robertson S, Streifler J, Thomas D. 10-year stroke prevention after successful carotid endarterectomy for asymptomatic stenosis (ACST-1): a multicentre randomised trial. Lancet. 2010;376:1074–84.
14. Bonati LH, Ederle J, McCabe DJ, Dobson J, Featherstone RL, Gaines PA, Beard JD, Venables GS, Markus HS, Clifton A, Sandercock P, Brown MM. Long-term risk of carotid restenosis in patients randomly assigned to endovascular treatment or endarterectomy in the Carotid and Vertebral Artery Transluminal Angioplasty Study (CAVATAS): long-term follow-up of a randomised trial. Lancet Neurol. 2009;8:908–17.
15. Brooks WH, McClure RR, Jones MR, Coleman TC, Breathitt L. Carotid angioplasty and stenting versus carotid endarterectomy: randomized trial in a community hospital. J Am Coll Cardiol. 2001;38:1589–95.

16. Brooks WH, McClure RR, Jones MR, Coleman TL, Breathitt L. Carotid angioplasty and stenting versus carotid endarterectomy for treatment of asymptomatic carotid stenosis: a randomized trial in a community hospital. Neurosurgery. 2004;54:318–24; discussion 324–325.
17. CAVATAS. Endovascular versus surgical treatment in patients with carotid stenosis in the Carotid and Vertebral Artery Transluminal Angioplasty Study (CAVATAS): a randomised trial. Lancet. 2001;357:1729–37.
18. Coward LJ, McCabe DJ, Ederle J, Featherstone RL, Clifton A, Brown MM. Long-term outcome after angioplasty and stenting for symptomatic vertebral artery stenosis compared with medical treatment in the Carotid and Vertebral Artery Transluminal Angioplasty Study (CAVATAS): a randomized trial. Stroke. 2007;38:1526–30.
19. Ederle J, Bonati LH, Dobson J, Featherstone RL, Gaines PA, Beard JD, Venables GS, Markus HS, Clifton A, Sandercock P, Brown MM. Endovascular treatment with angioplasty or stenting versus endarterectomy in patients with carotid artery stenosis in the Carotid and Vertebral Artery Transluminal Angioplasty Study (CAVATAS): long-term follow-up of a randomised trial. Lancet Neurol. 2009;8:898–907.
20. Ringleb PA, Allenberg J, Bruckmann H, Eckstein HH, Fraedrich G, Hartmann M, Hennerici M, Jansen O, Klein G, Kunze A, Marx P, Niederkorn K, Schmiedt W, Solymosi L, Stingele R, Zeumer H, Hacke W. 30 day results from the SPACE trial of stent-protected angioplasty versus carotid endarterectomy in symptomatic patients: a randomised non-inferiority trial. Lancet. 2006;368:1239–47.
21. Yadav JS, Wholey MH, Kuntz RE, Fayad P, Katzen BT, Mishkel GJ, Bajwa TK, Whitlow P, Strickman NE, Jaff MR, Popma JJ, Snead DB, Cutlip DE, Firth BG, Ouriel K. Protected carotid-artery stenting versus endarterectomy in high-risk patients. N Engl J Med. 2004;351:1493–501.
22. Bonati LH, Dobson J, Featherstone RL, Ederle J, van der Worp HB, de Borst GJ, Mali WP, Beard JD, Cleveland T, Engelter ST, Lyrer PA, Ford GA, Dorman PJ, Brown MM, International Carotid Stenting Study investigators. Long-term outcomes after stenting versus endarterectomy for treatment of symptomatic carotid stenosis: the International Carotid Stenting Study (ICSS) randomised trial. Lancet. 2015;385:529–38.
23. Brott TG, Howard G, Roubin GS, Meschia JF, Mackey A, Brooks W, Moore WS, Hill MD, Mantese VA, Clark WM, Timaran CH, Heck D, Leimgruber PP, Sheffet AJ, Howard VJ, Chaturvedi S, Lal BK, Voeks JH, Hobson RW II, Investigators C. Long-term results of stenting versus endarterectomy for carotid-artery stenosis. N Engl J Med. 2016;374:1021–31.
24. Ederle J, Davagnanam I, van der Worp HB, Venables GS, Lyrer PA, Featherstone RL, Brown MM, Jager HR, ICSS investigators. Effect of white-matter lesions on the risk of periprocedural stroke after carotid artery stenting versus endarterectomy in the International Carotid Stenting Study (ICSS): a prespecified analysis of data from a randomised trial. Lancet Neurol. 2013;12:866–72.
25. Kuliha M, Roubec M, Prochazka V, Jonszta T, Hrbac T, Havelka J, Goldirova A, Langova K, Herzig R, Skoloudik D. Randomized clinical trial comparing neurological outcomes after carotid endarterectomy or stenting. Br J Surg. 2015;102:194–201.
26. Bradac O, Mohapl M, Kramar F, Netuka D, Ostry S, Charvat F, Lacman J, Benes V. Carotid endarterectomy and carotid artery stenting: changing paradigm during 10 years in a high-volume centre. Acta Neurochir. 2014;156:1705–12.

Tailored Strategies in Carotid Artery Stenting to Avoid Periprocedural Complications

Yusuke Egashira, Yukiko Enomoto, Keita Yamauchi, Masanori Tsujimoto, Shinichi Yoshimura, and Toru Iwama

Abstract Carotid artery stenting (CAS) has been widely accepted as a valuable therapeutic alternative to carotid endarterectomy (CEA) for high-grade carotid stenosis. Because carotid revascularization including CAS is usually performed in patients with minimal or no neurological deficits, utmost care should be taken to avoid periprocedural complications. The major concerns associated with CAS are embolic stroke, hyperperfusion syndrome (HPS), and perioperative myocardial infarction.

Plaque characteristics, cerebral blood flow (CBF) in the affected cerebral hemisphere, and concomitant coronary artery disease prior to CAS are all important to assess the risks of these complications and are routinely evaluated.

Tailored CAS is planned based on findings of preoperative evaluation, as follows. (1) If the plaque component is thought vulnerable, proximal embolic protection methods, use of a closed-cell-type stent, or referral to CEA should be considered to avoid embolic complications. (2) If patients have severe CBF impairment, staged angioplasty is an effective strategy to prevent postoperative HPS. (3) If concomitant cardiac diseases are present, the optimal treatment sequence should be discussed between cardiologists and neurointerventionalists.

These tailored strategies based on preoperative risk evaluations may lead to safer procedures and better clinical outcome in CAS patients.

Y. Egashira, M.D., Ph.D. (✉) · Y. Enomoto, M.D., Ph.D.
K. Yamauchi, M.D. · M. Tsujimoto, M.D., Ph.D.
T. Iwama, M.D., Ph.D.
Department of Neurosurgery, Gifu University Graduate School of Medicine, Gifu, Japan
e-mail: egashi@gifu-u.ac.jp

S. Yoshimura
Department of Neurosurgery, Hyogo College of Medicine, Nishinomiya, Hyogo, Japan

Keywords Carotid artery stenting · Complication · Preoperative evaluation · Tailored strategy

Abbreviations

CAS	Carotid artery stenting
CBF	Cerebral blood flow
CEA	Carotid endarterectomy
CVR	Cerebrovascular reserve
HPS	Hyperperfusion syndrome
MRA	Magnetic resonance angiography
MRI	Magnetic resonance imaging
PTA	Percutaneous transluminal angioplasty
SAP	Staged angioplasty
SPECT	Single-photon emission computed tomography
TOF	Time-of-flight

Introduction

Recent evidence demonstrates that carotid artery stenting (CAS) is a valuable therapeutic alternative to carotid endarterectomy (CEA) for high-grade carotid stenosis [1, 2]. Hence, the application of CAS instead of CEA is steadily increasing in Japan [3]. Carotid revascularization including CAS is usually performed to prevent stroke, and patients present minimal or no neurological deficits. Thus, utmost care should be taken to avoid periprocedural complications when attempting CAS. The major concerns are embolic stroke, postoperative hyperperfusion syndrome (HPS), and perioperative myocardial infarction. Herein, we present a "tailored strategy" for CAS to avoid these complications, and emphasize the importance of preoperative risk evaluation.

G. Esposito et al. (eds.), *Trends in the Management of Cerebrovascular Diseases*, Acta Neurochirurgica Supplement, Vol. 129,
https://doi.org/10.1007/978-3-319-73739-3_15,

Preoperative Risk Evaluation

Plaque Characterization

Time-of-flight magnetic resonance angiography (TOF-MRA) is a simple and reliable method to determine whether the plaque represents a high risk for embolic complications during CAS [4]. A high-intensity signal visualized in the carotid plaque on TOF-MRA indicates vulnerable plaque characteristics such as intraplaque hemorrhage or severe inflammation. Furthermore, plaques with a high-intensity signal on TOF-MRA are significantly associated with new ischemic lesions detectable by diffusion-weighted magnetic resonance imaging or with postoperative ischemic symptoms [4]. According to these findings, we select CEA rather than CAS when plaque is visualized as a high-intensity lesion on TOF-MRA [5].

Measurement of Cerebral Blood Flow

^{123}I *N*-isopropyl-*p*-iodoamphetamine single-photon emission tomography (^{123}I-IMP SPECT) with an acetazolamide challenge is performed on all patients who are scheduled for CAS to measure cerebral blood flow (CBF) and cerebrovascular reserve (CVR) in the affected cerebral hemisphere. Patients with decreased resting CBF (below 80%) relative to the contralateral hemisphere and those with impaired CVR below 20% measured by quantitative ^{123}I-IMP-SPECT are considered high risk for postoperative HPS, according to the SPECT performed after CAS [6].

Screening of Concomitant Cardiac Disease

All patients possibly receiving CAS undergo simultaneous coronary angiography and cerebral angiography before CAS, with collaboration between the cardiologist and the neurointerventionalist [7]. Cardiac ultrasonography is also performed in all patients who are scheduled for CAS.

Tailored CAS Procedures

Algorithm of Treatment Selection

The algorithm used to select the treatment in carotid stenosis is shown in Fig. 1. As previously mentioned, all patients scheduled for CAS undergo quantitative CBF evaluation. In our institution, if the CVR value is less than 10%, then staged

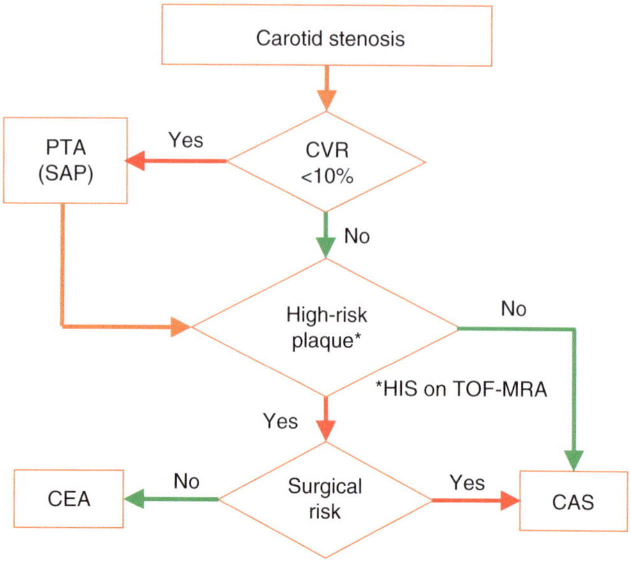

Fig. 1 Algorithm used for the selection of treatment in carotid stenosis. *CVR* cerebrovascular reserve on quantitative single-photon emission computed tomography, *PTA* percutaneous transluminal angioplasty, *SAP* staged angioplasty, *HIS* high-intensity signal, *TOF-MRA* time-of-flight magnetic resonance angiography, *CEA* carotid endarterectomy, *CAS* carotid artery stenting

angioplasty (SAP) is considered. High-risk plaque, visualized by TOF-MRA, is the most important surrogate marker for predicting perioperative embolism. These cases are subjected to CEA, and CAS should be avoided if the patients have minimal or no surgical risks.

Selection of Embolic Protection Devices and Stents to Avoid Embolic Complication

Several kinds of embolic protection devices such as the filter, distal balloon, proximal protection device, and stents are currently available. Several randomized-controlled trials have compared the efficacy of each embolic protection method, revealing significantly fewer embolic complications when proximal protection devices were used compared to distal filter protection devices [8–10]. In contrast to embolic protection devices, a few reports have investigated the relationship between stent design and embolic complications [11]. Although little empirical evidence is available, embolic complications tend to be less frequent when a closed-cell stent is used. We present the following suggestions for performing CAS more safely, especially in cases involving high-risk plaques. (1) Proximal protection is considered better than distal filter protection to avoid embolism during CAS procedures. (2) The closed-cell stent design enables better plaque coverage than open-cell design, which may lead to a reduced risk of embolism. (3) Modest pre- and postdilatation may be atraumatic procedures for fragile plaque.

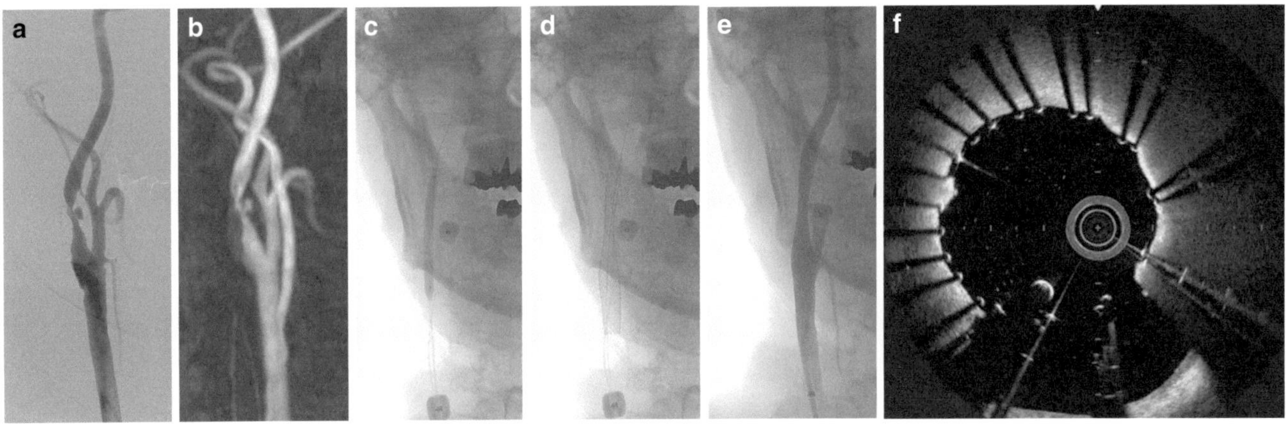

Fig. 2 A 71-year-old male presented with recurrent stroke caused by right carotid stenosis. (**a**) Antero-posterior view of preoperative right carotid angiogram (CAG) showed NASCET 75% stenosis at the origin of right internal carotid artery. (**b**) The plaque was visualized as high intensity by time-of-flight magnetic resonance angiography. Under proximal protection using Mo.Ma system with flow reversal, (**c**) percutaneous transluminal angioplasty, followed by (**d**) Carotid Wallstent® placement. (**e**) Postoperative CAG showed no abnormalities within the stent, although small residual ulceration was noted outside the stent. (**f**) Intravascular imaging using optical coherent tomography revealed no abnormalities within the stent

Staged Angioplasty to Prevent Postoperative Hyperperfusion Syndrome

Despite the low incidence of this complication, HPS including potential risk of subsequent intracranial bleeding is recognized as the most serious complication following carotid revascularization. Even in patients without subsequent intracranial bleeding, the prognosis worsens significantly after HPS. We previously reported the efficacy of SAP using undersized percutaneous transluminal angioplasty (PTA) followed by CAS to prevent postoperative HPS [12]. Technical tips for staged angioplasty are as follows: (1) In the first session, it would be ideal to use a PTA balloon with a diameter ≤3.0 mm. (2) The appropriate interval between PTA and CAS seems to be 1–3 weeks. (3) CAS should be performed in the usual manner. (4) CBF measurements must be performed immediately after each procedure to detect cerebral hyperperfusion phenomenon.

Representative Cases

Case 1

A 71-year-old male presented with recurrent stroke resulting from right carotid stenosis defined as NASCET 75% (Fig. 2a). He had concomitant unstable angina requiring intervention and was referred to our institution for CAS. TOF-MRA clearly demonstrated a high-intensity plaque at the stenotic site (Fig. 2b). We used Mo.Ma Ultra proximal protection device (Medtronic Inc., Santa Rosa, CA, USA) with a flow reversal method. Predilatation was performed using a 3.5 mm diameter PTA balloon, after which a 10 × 31 mm Carotid Wallstent® (Boston Scientific Corp., Natick, MA, USA), a closed-cell stent, was placed. The stenotic site was adequately dilated, and a postoperative angiography showed no abnormalities within the stent (Fig. 2c–e). Intravascular imaging using optical coherent tomography also detected no abnormalities within the stent (Fig. 2f). This intravascular imaging can be very helpful to detect in-stent plaque protrusions or a thrombus [13]. These procedures yielded a successful course of treatment and no perioperative complications occurred.

Case 2

An 84-year-old female suffered recurrent transient ischemic attacks of right hemiparesis and aphasia despite maximal medical treatment, including dual antiplatelet agent and statin. She was referred to our institution for CAS. Her left carotid angiogram showed severe stenosis defined as NASCET 90% (Fig. 3a). TOF-MRA revealed no evidence of high-risk plaque at the stenotic site. CVR value estimated by quantitative SPECT with acetazolamide was −2.6% in the left frontal region after administration of acetazolamide (Fig. 3b). As she was considered to be at risk for HPS after CAS, we selected SAP. She underwent PTA first. We created proximal protection using a 9-French guiding catheter with an occlusion balloon (Optimo; Tokai medical products, Aichi, Japan) and another occlusion balloon (Guardwire Plus; Medtronic Inc.) with a flow reversal system. Then, a 2.5-mm semicompliant PTA balloon was inserted into the stenotic lesion and inflated (Fig. 3c). Following angioplasty,

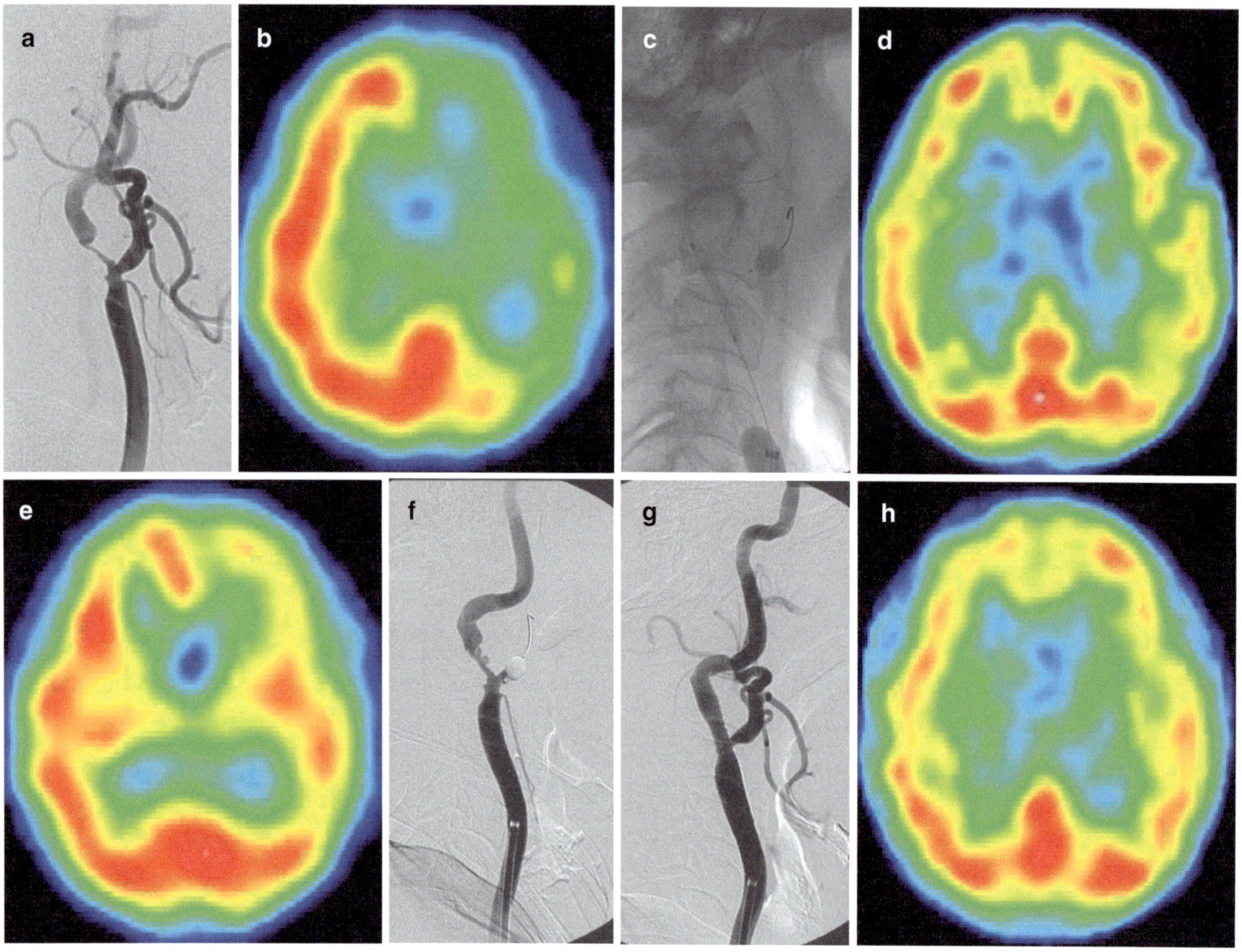

Fig. 3 An 84-year-old female presented with recurrent transient ischemic attacks caused by left carotid stenosis. (**a**) Lateral view of preoperative left carotid angiogram (CAG) showed NASCET 90% stenosis at the origin of the internal carotid artery. (**b**) The cerebrovascular reserve (CVR) value estimated by quantitative single-photon emission computed tomography (SPECT) with acetazolamide challenge was −2.6% in the left hemisphere. (**c**) Under proximal protection with flow reversal, percutaneous transluminal angioplasty (PTA) was performed using a 2.5 mm diameter semicompliant balloon. (**d**) The SPECT taken immediately after the PTA revealed improvement of the CBF in the left hemisphere and no hyperperfusion. (**e**) The SPECT obtained 13 days after PTA showed normalization of the CVR in the affected hemisphere. Carotid artery stenting (CAS) was performed 2 weeks after PTA. Pre-CAS (**f**) and post-CAS (**g**) left CAG showed that the complete dilatation of stenotic site was obtained after CAS. (**h**) The SPECT obtained immediately after CAS showed no hyperperfusion phenomenon

the stenosis improved from 90% to 75%. The SPECT acquired immediately after the procedure revealed improvement of the CBF in the left hemisphere and no hyperperfusion (Fig. 3d). Thirteen days later, ^{123}I-IMP SPECT with acetazolamide showed improvement of the CVR in the affected hemisphere (Fig. 3e). CAS was performed under the same protection system 2 weeks after the first session (Fig. 3f, g). The ^{123}I-IMP SPECT obtained immediately after CAS showed no hyperperfusion phenomenon (Fig. 3h). She did not develop HPS or any symptoms from ischemia in each periprocedural period, and was discharged with no neurological deficits.

Discussion

The major concerns associated with carotid revascularization are neurological complications such as embolic infarction or cerebral HPS. Thus, the evaluation of the CBF in the affected hemisphere and the analysis of the characteristics of the plaque are key elements to assess the risks for these complications. We believe that a tailored strategy (for CAS) based on risks evaluation may contribute to improve CAS safety.

The reported incidence of development of new ischemic lesions (detectable through diffusion weighted-MRI) is more than five times higher after CAS than after CEA [14]. Vulnerable plaque characteristics including intraplaque hemorrhage or lipid-rich core are associated with an increased number of emboli after CAS [15]. Tailored CAS strategies, such as use of proximal protection devices or closed-cell stents, may help reduce the incidence of periprocedural embolism, especially in patients with high-risk plaques. Indeed, the concept of tailored CAS is widely accepted in Japan, and is considered to contribute to excellent treatment results [3, 16].

Cerebral HPS is the most serious potential complication after carotid revascularization. The prognosis of this condition is poor although the incidence of intracranial hemorrhage caused by HPS is relatively low [17]. Development of HPS is also associated with the risk of persistent cognitive impairment. In our experience, SAP by undersized PTA followed by regular CAS is an effective method to prevent HPS, although it does require multiple sessions.

Screening for concomitant cardiac disease prior to CAS is essential, as patients with severe aortic valve stenosis must be excluded from CAS. Approximately half of the patients who schedule a CAS have concomitant coronary artery disease [7]. Thus, screening of concomitant cardiac disease by cardiac US and coronary angiography and consultation with a cardiologist prior to CAS is of importance.

Conclusion

The proposed tailored strategy for CAS is based on preoperative risk evaluation. Plaque characterization, CBF evaluation, and screening for concomitant cardiac diseases prior to CAS are critical, whose pretreatment analysis is important to avoid periprocedural complications.

Conflict of Interest We declare that we have no conflict of interest.

References

1. Rosenfield K, Matsumura JS, Chaturvedi S, Riles T, Ansel GM, Metzger DC, Wechsler L, Jaff MR, Gray W, Investigators AI. Randomized trial of stent versus surgery for asymptomatic carotid stenosis. N Engl J Med. 2016;374:1011–20. https://doi.org/10.1056/NEJMoa1515706.
2. Silver FL, Mackey A, Clark WM, Brooks W, Timaran CH, Chiu D, Goldstein LB, Meschia JF, Ferguson RD, Moore WS, Howard G, Brott TG, Investigators C. Safety of stenting and endarterectomy by symptomatic status in the Carotid Revascularization Endarterectomy Versus Stenting Trial (CREST). Stroke. 2011;42:675–80. https://doi.org/10.1161/STROKEAHA.110.610212.
3. Miyachi S, Taki W, Sakai N, Nakahara I, Japanese CASSI. Historical perspective of carotid artery stenting in Japan: analysis of 8,092 cases in the Japanese CAS survey. Acta Neurochir. 2012;154:2127–37. https://doi.org/10.1007/s00701-012-1508-9.
4. Yoshimura S, Yamada K, Kawasaki M, Asano T, Kanematsu M, Takamatsu M, Hara A, Iwama T. High-intensity signal on time-of-flight magnetic resonance angiography indicates carotid plaques at high risk for cerebral embolism during stenting. Stroke. 2011;42:3132–7. https://doi.org/10.1161/STROKEAHA.111.615708.
5. Yoshimura S, Yamada K, Kawasaki M, Asano T, Kanematsu M, Miyai M, Enomoto Y, Egashira Y, Iwama T. Selection of carotid artery stenting or endarterectomy based on magnetic resonance plaque imaging reduced periprocedural adverse events. J Stroke Cerebrovasc Dis. 2013;22:1082–7. https://doi.org/10.1016/j.jstrokecerebrovasdis.2012.07.018.
6. Kaku Y, Yoshimura S, Kokuzawa J. Factors predictive of cerebral hyperperfusion after carotid angioplasty and stent placement. AJNR Am J Neuroradiol. 2004;25:1403–8.
7. Enomoto Y, Yoshimura S, Yamada K, Kawasaki M, Nishigaki K, Minatoguchi S, Iwama T. Silent coronary artery disease in Japanese patients undergoing carotid artery stenting. J Stroke Cerebrovasc Dis. 2013;22:1163–8. https://doi.org/10.1016/j.jstrokecerebrovasdis.2012.12.013.
8. Cano MN, Kambara AM, de Cano SJ, Pezzi Portela LA, Paes AT, Costa JR Jr, Abizaid AA, Moreira SM, Sousa AG, Sousa JE. Randomized comparison of distal and proximal cerebral protection during carotid artery stenting. JACC Cardiovasc Interv. 2013;6:1203–9. https://doi.org/10.1016/j.jcin.2013.07.006.
9. Bijuklic K, Wandler A, Hazizi F, Schofer J. The PROFI study (Prevention of Cerebral Embolization by Proximal Balloon Occlusion Compared to Filter Protection During Carotid Artery Stenting): a prospective randomized trial. J Am Coll Cardiol. 2012;59:1383–9. https://doi.org/10.1016/j.jacc.2011.11.035.
10. Montorsi P, Caputi L, Galli S, Ciceri E, Ballerini G, Agrifoglio M, Ravagnani P, Trabattoni D, Pontone G, Fabbiocchi F, Loaldi A, Parati E, Andreini D, Veglia F, Bartorelli AL. Microembolization during carotid artery stenting in patients with high-risk, lipid-rich plaque. A randomized trial of proximal versus distal cerebral protection. J Am Coll Cardiol. 2011;58:1656–63. https://doi.org/10.1016/j.jacc.2011.07.015.
11. Timaran CH, Rosero EB, Higuera A, Ilarraza A, Modrall JG, Clagett GP. Randomized clinical trial of open-cell vs closed-cell stents for carotid stenting and effects of stent design on cerebral embolization. J Vasc Surg. 2011;54:1310–1316.e1311.; ; discussion 1316. https://doi.org/10.1016/j.jvs.2011.05.013.
12. Yoshimura S, Kitajima H, Enomoto Y, Yamada K, Iwama T. Staged angioplasty for carotid artery stenosis to prevent postoperative hyperperfusion. Neurosurgery. 2009;64:ons122–8.; ; discussion ons128–129. https://doi.org/10.1227/01.NEU.0000334046.41985.BB.
13. Shindo S, Fujii K, Shirakawa M, Uchida K, Sugiura Y, Saito S, Ando Y, Yoshimura S. Three-dimensional optical frequency domain imaging evaluation of novel dual-layered carotid stent implantation for vulnerable carotid plaque. J Stroke Cerebrovasc Dis. 2016;25:e31–2. https://doi.org/10.1016/j.jstrokecerebrovasdis.2015.11.019.
14. Gargiulo G, Sannino A, Stabile E, Perrino C, Trimarco B, Esposito G. New cerebral lesions at magnetic resonance imaging after carotid artery stenting versus endarterectomy: an updated meta-analysis. PLoS One. 2015;10:e0129209. https://doi.org/10.1371/journal.pone.0129209.

15. Biasi GM, Froio A, Diethrich EB, Deleo G, Galimberti S, Mingazzini P, Nicolaides AN, Griffin M, Raithel D, Reid DB, Valsecchi MG. Carotid plaque echolucency increases the risk of stroke in carotid stenting: the Imaging in Carotid Angioplasty and Risk of Stroke (ICAROS) study. Circulation. 2004;110:756–62. https://doi.org/10.1161/01.CIR.0000138103.91187.E3.
16. Egashira Y, Yoshimura S, Sakai N, Enomoto Y, Japanese Registry of Neuroendovascular Therapy I. Real-world experience of carotid artery stenting in Japan: analysis of 7,134 cases from JR-NET1 and 2 nationwide retrospective multi-center registries. Neurol Med Chir (Tokyo). 2014;54:32–9.
17. Ogasawara K, Sakai N, Kuroiwa T, Hosoda K, Iihara K, Toyoda K, Sakai C, Nagata I, Ogawa A, Japanese Society for Treatment at Neck in Cerebrovascular Disease Study G. Intracranial hemorrhage associated with cerebral hyperperfusion syndrome following carotid endarterectomy and carotid artery stenting: retrospective review of 4494 patients. J Neurosurg. 2007;107:1130–6. https://doi.org/10.3171/JNS-07/12/1130.

Part III

Arteriovenous Malformations and Dural Arteriovenous Fistulas

Surgical Treatment of Arteriovenous Malformations: Role of Preoperative Staged Embolization

Mattia Del Maestro, Sabino Luzzi, Massimo Gallieni, Donatella Trovarelli, Aldo Victor Giordano, Massimo Gallucci†, Alessandro Ricci, and Renato Galzio

Abstract Preoperative embolization is complementary to surgery for large brain arteriovenous malformations (AVMs). From January 2005 to December 2015, 69 patients harboring an AVM were managed in our department by the same surgeon (RG). Forty one were ruptured and 65 were supratentorial. Thirty nine smaller AVMs were treated with surgery stand-alone, whereas, for 30 larger malformations, surgery was combined with adjuvant treatment involving preoperative staged embolization and/or, less frequently, radiosurgery. In all patients treated with surgery alone, complete resection of AVM was achieved. A successful preoperative partial endovascular obliteration of AVM was obtained in 24 out of 27 more complex cases, with a zero mortality rate and a very low morbidity. Here, embolization was of a certain utility in the handling of deeper feeders and nidus excision, also facilitating intraoperative hemostasis. In three cases of residuals, radiosurgery was performed. In those patient treated with a combined approach, a good overall outcome, 0–2 modified Rankin Scale (mRS), was achieved in 25 cases. Preoperative embolization proved to be a reasonable option complementary to high-grade AVMs surgery, reducing the frequency of breakthrough hemorrhages, aiding the elimination of deep feeders, and making the nidus dissection easier.

Keywords AVMs embolization · AVMs surgery · Brain AVMs · Intracranial arteriovenous malformations · Onyx embolization

Introduction

Brain arteriovenous malformations (AVMs) are complex, dynamic structures composed of a network of abnormal arteries and veins lacking a capillary bed and eventually resulting in high-flow arteriovenous shunts. Each AVM is different in location, size, involvement of eloquent areas, angio-architecture, and flow characteristics and so always represent challenging lesions. AVMs are congenital and most often nonfamiliar. Clinical onset is usually related to seizures and/or spontaneous cerebral hemorrhage; headache and focal neurological deficit may also be seen. It has been estimated that the yearly risk of hemorrhage related to an untreated AVM ranges between 2 and 4%, with a mortality of 18% [1, 2]. Nowadays, treatment options for AVMs include microsurgical resection, endovascular embolization, and radiosurgery. These modalities may be used alone in smaller lesions or in various types of combinations for high-grade ones. The literature indicates that an incomplete treatment of an AVM is not only unhelpful but also increases the risk of bleeding up to four times [3, 4], and therapy must aim for a complete exclusion of the lesion. This study report experience gained over 10 years in the surgical management of this complex pathology, focusing on the combined endovascular-surgical treatment of high-grade AVMs in the brain in terms of usefulness and limits.

† Deceased

M. Del Maestro, M.D. (✉) · M. Gallieni
Department of Life, Health and Environmental Sciences (Me.S.V.A.), University of L'Aquila, L'Aquila, Italy
e-mail: mattiadelmaestro@gmail.com

S. Luzzi · A. Ricci
Department of Neurosurgery, "San Salvatore" L'Aquila City Hospital, L'Aquila, Italy

D. Trovarelli
Department of Anesthesiology, "San Salvatore" L'Aquila City Hospital, L'Aquila, Italy

A. V. Giordano · M. Gallucci
Department of Neuroradiology, "San Salvatore" L'Aquila City Hospital, L'Aquila, Italy

R. Galzio
Department of Life, Health and Environmental Sciences (Me.S.V.A.), University of L'Aquila, L'Aquila, Italy

Department of Neurosurgery, "San Salvatore" L'Aquila City Hospital, L'Aquila, Italy

G. Esposito et al. (eds.), *Trends in the Management of Cerebrovascular Diseases*, Acta Neurochirurgica Supplement, Vol. 129,
https://doi.org/10.1007/978-3-319-73739-3_16, © Springer International Publishing AG, part of Springer Nature 2018

Materials and Methods

Between 2005 and 2015, a cohort of 83 patients harboring an AVM were managed in our department and retrospectively reviewed. All AVMs were classified according to the Martin–Spetzler classification system [5] and AVM volume was calculated with the method described by Pasqualin et al. (V = width × height × length × 0.52) [6]. All the patients underwent four vessels brain digital subtraction angiography (DSA) and, in selected cases of cortical AVM, a further detailed study of both external carotid arteries was carried out. T1- and T2-weighted conventional MRI with angio-MRI sequences was obtained in all patients. Functional MRI was performed on all patients harboring lesions in eloquent areas. A preoperative neurophysiological baseline assessment was also performed on all patient candidates for neurophysiological intraoperative monitoring with evaluation of motor evoked potentials (MEP) and somatosensory evoked potential (SSEP). All endovascular procedures were performed using ethylene-vinyl alcohol copolymer (Onyx) with a viscosity index of 18 cP [centipoise]. In multistaged embolizations, the time interval between each was 10–15 days and the surgical step was carried out after 7–10 days from the last embolization. Surgical approaches were tailored for each lesion according to site, size, and AVM architecture. Outcome evaluation was expressed as modified Ranking Score (mRS).

Results

Out of 83 AVMs, 69 patients were surgically managed. In 27 selected cases, a single or multistaged preoperative embolization was performed. Eighteen patients were males and 9 females, age between 16 and 55 years (mean 34 years). All 27 AVMs were supratentorial. Three patients harbored a Spetzler–Martin (SM) grade V AVM, 8 patients grade IV, 13 patients grade III, and 3 patients grade II. The volume of the malformations ranged between 5.3 and 29.6 mL (mean 14 mL). Hemorrhagic onset was seen in 14 cases (52%). In the remaining 13 cases of unruptured AVMs, epilepsy was the only symptom in 6 cases and headache in 4 cases. In three cases the AVM was an incidental finding. One patient was pretreated 2 years before with partial embolization of a left frontotemporal SM IV AVM and was admitted to our department because of a left frontotemporal intraparenchymal hemorrhage. The mean number of embolizations was 1.6 (range 1–3), thus achieving an obliteration rate ranging between 35 and 90%. Angiographic results showed an average obliteration rate of 61% of the entire volume of the AVMs (range 20–90%). After the last endovascular stage but before surgery, three minor neurological deficits, consisting of a slight nondisabling hemiparesis, were observed. In the remaining 24 patients, neurological status was unchanged. The overall mortality related to the embolization was zero. As planned, all 27 patients underwent surgery, achieving a complete excision in 24 AVMs. Postoperative angiography was performed in all patients at 6-month follow-up. Ten patients with SM IV–V grade underwent an early postoperative angiography during the same recovery, before discharge. No relapsed AVMs were evident. During surgery, preoperative embolization proved very useful to manage the deeper feeders of the AVM, made nidus excision easier, and, finally, facilitated the hemostasis leading to a reduced blood loss (explicative cases are reported in Figs. 1 and 2). In three cases of residuals, documented by angiography, patients were referred to radiosurgery. A good overall outcome, 0–2 modified Rankin Scale (mRS), was achieved in 25 patients, 14 of whom suffered from intraparenchymal hemorrhage. A moderate disability (3 mRS) was seen in two hemorrhagic patients. Improved outcomes were especially evident for ruptured AVMs. Two patients with grade IV SM AVM suffered from a worsening, and one patient with a grade V AVM improved (Table 1).

Discussion

Treatment for a patient diagnosed with an AVM must be tailored according to the natural history of this complex pathology, considering several factors such as patient's age, comorbidities, neurological status, site and size of lesion, involvement of eloquent areas, and presence of symptoms attributable to the AVM. Another factor to consider is the intrinsic complexity of the proposed treatment option that, especially for high-grade AVMs, frequently consists of combined approaches. Suppression of seizures and the elimination of the bleeding risk are the main goals of the treatment, achievable only with the complete excision of the AVM. Despite the evolution of endovascular techniques, nowadays microsurgery still plays the most important role in the management of these lesions, because embolization has not gained for AVMs the same role achieved for aneurysms. Surgery is considered the best treatment for small and medium-sized AVMs, especially when superficial and located in noneloquent areas (SM grades I and II). Surgery is also the best treatment option for low-grade ruptured or symptomatic lesions in eloquent areas. For high-grade AVMs (SM grade III-IV-V), a multidisciplinary approach based on microsurgery, embolization, and radiosurgery is often chosen. In 1990, Taki and Terada first proposed embolization of an intracranial AVM with ethylene vinyl alcohol containing embolic agents (Onyx), thus starting the modern era of neuroradiological intervention for brain AVMs [7, 8]. Although some series claim Onyx embolization alone to be a curative option for low-grade brain AVMs (SM I–II) [9–11], it has been shown that the sole endovascular approach is frequently ineffective and even associated with increased morbidity [12–14].

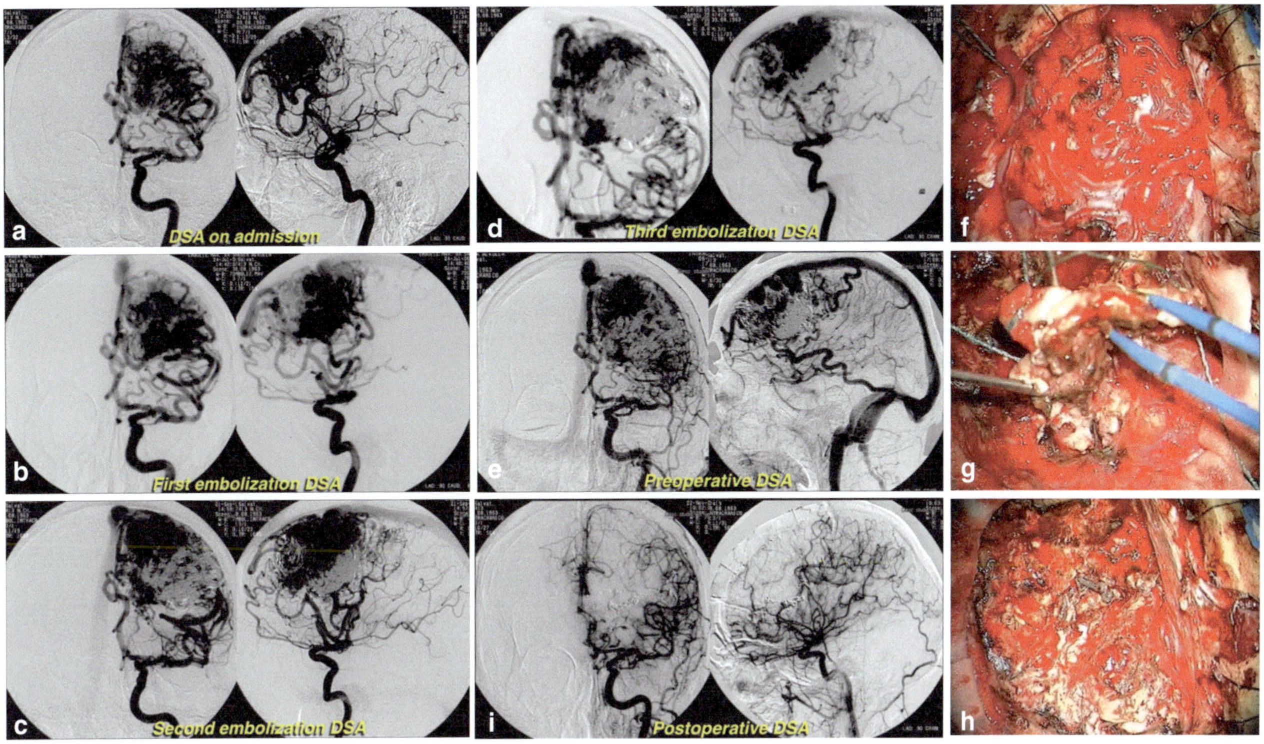

Fig. 1 Male, 43 years old, with history of seizures. Anterior and lateral projections of a four-vessel DSA showing a left fronto-parietal SM grade V, unruptured AVM (**a**). Patient underwent three consecutive procedures of embolization with Onyx (**b–d**). Preoperative DSA showed an obliteration percentage of 70% (**e**). Intraoperative pictures showing the superficial aspect of the lesion (**f**), its removal (**g**), and the surgical field at the end of the procedure, with the complete excision of the AVM (**h**). Sixth-month post-operative DSA documented the complete removal of the lesion (**i**)

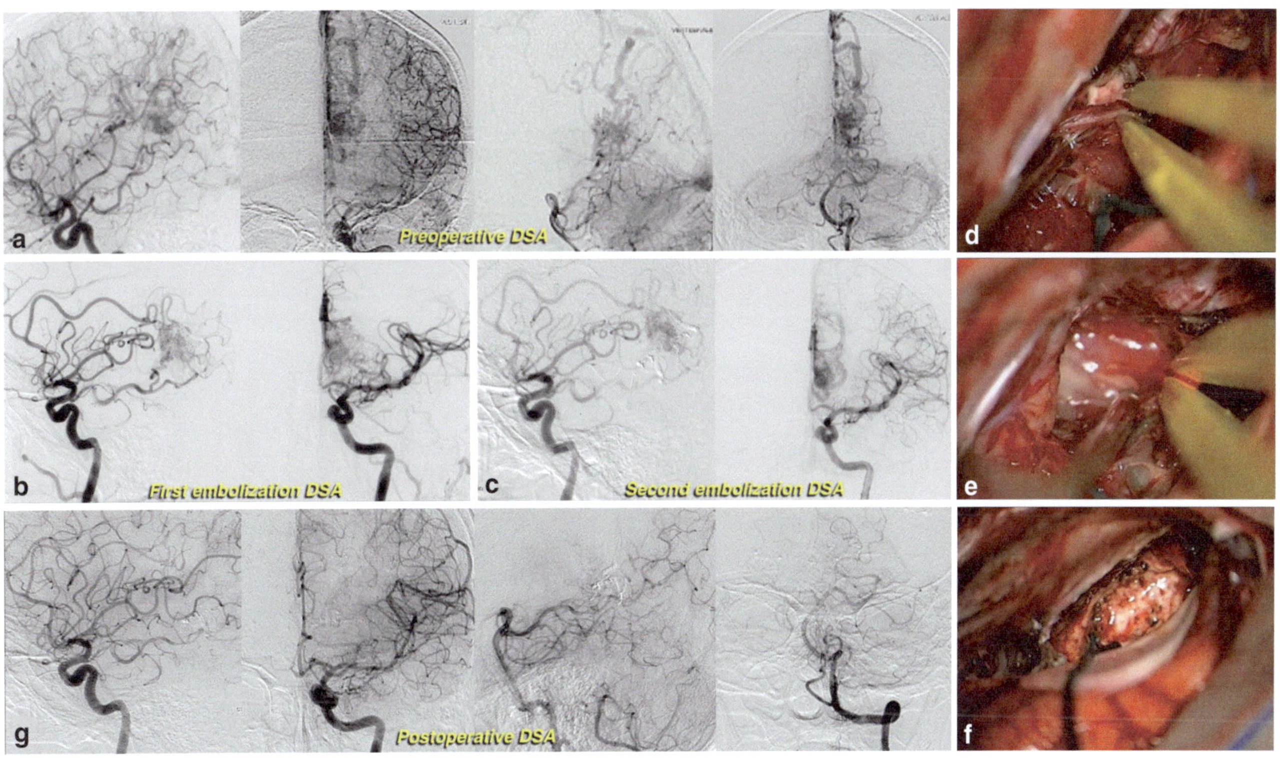

Fig. 2 Male, 52 years old, with history of headache. Anterior and lateral projections of a four-vessel DSA on admission showing a left mesial parietal lobe SM grade IV, unruptured AVM (**a**). Patient underwent two consecutive procedures of embolization with Onyx, achieving an obliteration rate of 50% (**b**, **c**). The lesion was exposed through a right posterior interhemispheric trans-falcine approach (**d**) and the nidus was isolated and completely removed (**e**, **f**). Postoperative anterior and lateral projection of a four-vessel DSA documented the removal of the lesions (**g**)

Table 1 Characteristics, treatment, and outcome of arteriovenous malformations

Patient No.	Age/sex	Symptoms	Ruptured/ unruptured	AVM location	AVMs volume (mL)	Spetzler-Martin grade	Embolizations with Onyx	Obliteration (%)	Radiosurgery	Postop mRS (6 months)
1	40/F	Epilepsy	Unruptured	Left frontal	15.4	IV	2	50	–	1
2	28/F	None	Unruptured	Left occipital	7.2	II	1	80	–	0
3	38/F	Epilepsy	Ruptured	Left Sylvian	25.6	V	2	40	–	1
4	35/M	Headache	Ruptured	Right occipital	19.3	IV	2	50	yes	1
5	44/F	Headache	Unruptured	Left frontal	20.3	V	3	70	–	2
6	22/M	ICH	Ruptured	Left parietal	13.5	IV	2	60	–	3
7	44/M	Epilepsy	Ruptured	Left Insula	16.7	IV	3	60	yes	1
8	20/M	Headache	Unruptured	Right Sylvian	12.1	III	1	35	–	0
9	19/M	Headache	Ruptured	Left temporo-parietal	6.4	III	2	60	–	1
10	34/M	Epilepsy	Ruptured	Left frontal	12.5	III	1	40	–	1
11	31/F	Headache	Ruptured	Right Sylvian	19.3	IV	2	20	–	0
12	22/M	IVH-ICH	Ruptured	Right lateral ventricle	24.7	IV	3	70	–	1
13	26/F	Headache	Ruptured	Right temporal	9.5	III	1	75	–	0
14	37/M	None	Unruptured	Left frontal	7.4	III	1	80	–	0
15	51/M	ICH	Ruptured	Left thalamus	29.6	V	2	40	–	3
16	55/F	Headache	Ruptured	Left fronto-insular	9.3	III	1	20	–	2
17	31/M	Epilepsy	Unruptured	Left fronto-parietal	8.4	III	2	65	yes	1
18	38/M	Epilepsy	Unruptured	Left temporal	11,8	III	2	90	–	1
19	16/M	Headache	Ruptured	Left paracallosal	8.9	III	1	80	–	0
20	46/M	Epilepsy	Unruptured	Left occipital	18.0	IV	2	50	–	1
21	40/M	None	Unruptured	Left occipital	10.0	III	1	75	–	0
22	52/M	Epilepsy	Unruptured	Left parietal	21.4	IV	2	50	–	1
23	25/F	Headache	Unruptured	Left temporal	5.3	II	1	90	–	0
24	19/M	ICH	Ruptured	Right occipital	11.6	III	1	70	–	2
25	37/F	ICH	Ruptured	Right parietal	4.8	II	1	75	–	0
26	26/M	Epilepsy	Unruptured	Left temporal	6.8	III	1	60	–	0
27	42/M	Headache	Unruptured	Right frontal	10.5	III	2	70	–	0

Moreover, a partial palliative treatment of an AVM with embolization alone should always be avoided because it seems to increase the early and long-term risk of bleeding [3, 4].

In the authors' experience, embolization can be considered as complementary to surgery for high-grade AVMs. It should be noted that the unique on-label indication of approval by the Food and Drug Administration for Onyx, in the United States is, indeed, for the preoperative embolization of these lesions [15]. The rationale for its use is the ability to avoid, or at least reduce, the frequency of breakthrough phenomena and the hyperemic complications that may follow the single-stage excision of large high-flow malformations [16, 17]. The major benefit of embolization is the elimination of deep feeding arteries thought to be the limiting factor in the morbidity and surgical resectability of large AVMs [17, 18]. It also facilitates hemostasis, reducing intraoperative blood loss and making nidus dissection easier [19]. Some drawbacks must also be considered. First, preoperative embolization may increase the risk of hemorrhage and further hemodynamic complications. These complications can be avoided if the obliteration of the AVM is pursued with a progressive decrease of the flow inside the AVM by means of two or more different procedures (staged embolization). Besides, the effects of preoperative embolization do not last both because the feeders may reopen and because new feeders can be recruited. This aspect reveals a scheduled, not long-lasting window between the embolization procedures (no more than 2–3 weeks) and between the last embolization and surgery (no more than 7–10 days). Finally, the embolization of large superficial feeders may cause the recruitment or enhancement of the deeper feeders, eventually making surgery more difficult.

The authors reserved radiosurgery to two cases of grade IV and one case of grade III AVM characterized by a small postoperative residual of nidus.

The herein presented data suggest that staged preoperative embolization is a safe and useful adjunct tool in the surgical management of both ruptured and unruptured high-grade AVMs.

Conflict of Interest Statement The authors have no conflict of interest.

References

1. Ellis JA, Lavine SD. Role of embolization for cerebral arteriovenous malformations. MDCVJ. 2014;10(4):234–9.
2. Natarajan SK, Ghodke B, Britz GW, Born DE, Sekhar LN. Multimodality treatment of brain arteriovenous malformations with microsurgery after embolization with Onyx: single-center experience and technical nuances. Neurosurgery. 2008;62:1213–25.
3. Hashimoto N, Nozaki K, Takagi Y. Surgery of cerebral arteriovenousmalformation. Neurosurgery. 2007;61:375–89.
4. Miyamoto S, Hashimoto N, Nagata I. Posttreatment sequelae of palliatively treated cerebral arteriovenousmalformations. Neurosurgery. 2000;46:589–94.
5. Spezler RF, Martin NA. A proposed grading system for arteriovenous malformations. J Neurosurg. 1986;65:476–83.
6. Pasqualin A, Barone G, Cioffi F, Rosta L, Scienza R, Da Pian R. The relevance of anatomic and hemodynamic factors to a classification of cerebral arteriovenous malformations. Neurosurgery. 1991;28:370–9.
7. Taki W, Yonekawa Y, Iwata H, Uno A, Yamashita K, Amemiya H. A new liquid material for embolization of arteriovenous malformations. AJNR Am J Neuroradiol. 1990;11:163–8.
8. Terada T, Nakamura Y, Nakai K, Tsuura M, Nishiguchi T, Hayashi S, Kido T, Taki W, Iwata H, Komai N. Embolization of arteriovenous malformations with peripheral aneurysms using ethylene vinyl alcohol copolymer. Report of three cases. J Neurosurg. 1991;75:655–60.
9. Mounayer C, Hammami N, Piotin M, Spelle L, Benndorf G, Kessler I, Moret J. Nidal embolization of brain arteriovenous malformations using Onyx in 94 patients. AJNR Am J Neuroradiol. 2007;28:518–23.
10. van Rooij WJ, Sluzewski M, Beute GN. Brain AVM embolization with Onyx. AJNR Am J Neuroradiol. 2007;28:172–8.
11. Weber W, Kis B, Siekmann R, Kuehne D. Endovascular treatment of intracranial arteriovenous malformations with Onyx: technical aspects. AJNR Am J Neuroradiol. 2007;28:371–7.
12. Frizzel RT, Fisher WS. Cure, morbidity, and mortality associated with embolization of brain arteriovenous malformations: a review of 1246 patients in 32 series over a 35-year period. Neurosurgery. 1995;37:1031–9.
13. Lundqvist C, Wikholm G, Svendsen P. Embolization of cerebral arteriovenous malformations: part II—aspects of complications and late outcome. Neurosurgery. 1996;39:460–7.
14. Nataraj A, Mohamed MB, Gholkar A, Vivar R, Watkins L, Aspoas R, Gregson B, Mitchell P, Mendelow AD. Multimodality treatment of cerebral arteriovenous malformations. World Neurosurg. 2014;82(1/2):149–59.
15. Crowley RW, Ducruet AF, McDougall CG, Albuquerque FC. Endovascular advances for brain arteriovenous malformations. Neurosurgery. 2014;74:S74–82.
16. Pasqualin A, Zampieri P, Nicolato A, Meneghelli P, Cozzi F, Beltramello A. Surgery after embolization of cerebral arteriovenous malformation: experience of 123 cases. Acta Neurochir Suppl. 2014;119:105–11.
17. Vinuela F, Duckwiler G, Guglielmi G. Contribution of interventional neuroradiology in the therapeutic management of brain arteriovenous malformations. J Stroke Cerebrovasc Dis. 1997;6:268–71.
18. Hurst RW, Berenstein A, Kupersmith MJ, Madrid M, Flamm ES. Deep central arteriovenous malformations of the brain: the role of endovascular treatment. J Neurosurg. 1995;82:190–5.
19. Jafar JJ, Davis AJ, Berenstein A, Choi IS, Kupersmith MJ. The effect of embolization with N-butyl cyanoacrylate prior to surgical resection of cerebral arteriovenous malformations. J Neurosurg. 1993;78:60–9.

Multimodal Interventional Treatment and Outcomes for Unruptured Arteriovenous Malformations

Daisuke Maruyama, Tetsu Satow, Hiroharu Kataoka, Hisae Mori, Eika Hamano, Yoji Orita, Seiichiro Eguchi, and Jun C. Takahashi

Abstract *Background.* This study aimed to evaluate the selection and outcomes of multimodal interventional treatment for unruptured brain arteriovenous malformations (uAVMs) in ARUBA-eligible patients in a single institution.

Methods. We retrospectively reviewed the data of 94 patients with uAVMs treated between 2002 and 2014. They were divided into an intervention group and a conservative group. The primary outcome was defined as the composite of death or symptomatic stroke. Functional outcome was assessed using the modified Rankin Scale (mRS).

Results. The intervention and conservative groups included 75 and 19 patients, respectively, with mean follow-up periods of 59.2 ± 41.6 and 72.8 ± 39.2 months ($P = 0.20$), among whom the primary outcome occurred in 9 (12.3%) and 3 (17.6%) patients, respectively ($P = 0.91$). The proportion of patients with an mRS score ≥ 2 at last follow-up was not significantly different between the two groups (6.9% vs. 11.7%). In the intervention group, the incidence of death or stroke was lower and functional outcomes were better among patients with grade I/II AVMs than among patients with grade III AVMs.

Conclusion. For patients with uAVMs, interventional treatment is not inferior to medical treatment alone, and careful selection should be made for patients with grade III AVMs.

Keywords ARUBA · Interventional therapy · Medical management · Stroke · Unruptured brain arteriovenous malformation

D. Maruyama, M.D. (✉) · T. Satow, M.D., Ph.D. · H. Kataoka, M.D., Ph.D. · H. Mori, M.D. · E. Hamano, M.D. · Y. Orita, M.D. S. Eguchi, M.D., Ph.D. · J. C. Takahashi, M.D., Ph.D.
Department of Neurosurgery, National Cerebral and Cardiovascular Center, Suita, Japan

Introduction

The optimal management of unruptured arteriovenous malformations (uAVMs) is controversial. Currently, A Randomized trial of Unruptured Brain Arteriovenous Malformations (ARUBA) is the only prospective randomized controlled study concerning this issue, which concluded that medical management alone is superior to medical management with interventional therapy for the prevention of death or stroke [1]. Several reports have documented the problems of this study, such as inappropriate study design, recruitment bias because of the low enrollment rate, short follow-up period, and inadequate surgical strategy [2, 3].

In our institution, interventional treatment of AVMs, including surgical resection, embolization, and radiosurgery, is carried out in a single neurosurgical department. Our therapeutic principles for uAVMs are as follows: (1) Younger patients or symptomatic cases with uAVMs are thought to be candidates for intervention. (2) Radiosurgery is primarily considered for eloquent lesions. (3) Surgical resection is considered in cases of superficial lesions distal to, or sometimes near or within, eloquent areas. (4) Transarterial embolization is either a presurgical or a preradiosurgical option to obliterate deep feeders difficult to reach surgically, to utilize embolization materials as intraoperative landmarks, or to reduce volume.

This study aimed to evaluate the selection and outcomes of multimodal interventional treatment for uAVMs in ARUBA-eligible patients in a single institution.

Materials and Methods

Study Population

This was a single-center, retrospective cohort study. Among consecutive patients who were admitted to our institute with a diagnosis of AVMs between April 2002 and March 2014,

G. Esposito et al. (eds.), *Trends in the Management of Cerebrovascular Diseases*, Acta Neurochirurgica Supplement, Vol. 129,
https://doi.org/10.1007/978-3-319-73739-3_17,

ARUBA-eligible patients were enrolled. ARUBA inclusion and exclusion criteria were used to define ARUBA eligibility. Inclusion criteria were patients aged 18 years or older and uAVMs diagnosed by standard neurovascular imaging protocols with a modified Rankin Scale (mRS) score of 0 or 1 at examination [1]. Exclusion criteria were the same as those used in the ARUBA study. Patients' baseline characteristics, therapeutic strategies, and clinical outcome were obtained by reviewing medical records. Patients were divided into two groups—intervention group or conservative group. Interventional therapy was defined as microsurgical resection, transarterial embolization, or radiosurgery. Conservative treatment included medical treatment for seizure or other comorbidities.

Outcomes and Follow-Up

The primary outcome was time to the composite event of death from any cause or symptomatic stroke. Stroke was defined as a clinically symptomatic event associated with imaging findings, hemorrhage, or infarction and poor functional outcome as clinical impairment at last follow-up with an mRS score of 2 or higher. The follow-up period was counted from the day of last elective surgery in the intervention group and at discharge from the hospital for observation in the conservative group.

Therapeutic Procedures

Microsurgical resection was performed with neurophysiological monitoring, indocyanine green videoangiography [4], or intraoperative cerebral angiography. Endovascular embolization was conducted using two liquid embolic agents, Onyx (ev3 Neurovascular, Irvine, California), and *N*-butyl-2 cyanoacrylate. Single or multiple sessions of embolization were conducted before surgical resection or radiosurgery. The final session was performed within 48 h before surgery. Radiosurgical treatment was performed with the Gamma Knife (Elekta, Stockholm, Sweden).

Statistical Analysis

Continuous variables are presented as mean ± standard deviation. Categorical data are reported as frequencies (percentages). Categorical variables were compared by Fisher's exact test. The two-sided unpaired t-test and Mann–Whitney U test were used to analyze normally and nonnormally distributed continuous variables, respectively. The rates of stroke or death in the intervention and conservative groups were compared using Kaplan–Meier survival analysis and the log-rank test. Cox proportional-hazards regression models were used to estimate hazard ratios (HR), adjusting for size of nidus, eloquence, venous drainage, patient age, and sex. We compared the proportion of patients with mRS score of 2 or higher at last follow-up in the intervention and conservative groups with Fisher's exact test. In the intervention group, a subgroup analysis was carried out to compare the outcome between Spetzler–Martin grades I/II and III cases. Statistical significance was defined as a P values <0.05. Analyses were performed with the JMP software package (version 11.0.0; SAS Institute, Cary, NC).

Results

Between April 2002 and March 2014, 270 patients aged 18 years or older with suspected AVMs were admitted to our institute. Among them, 94 patients with uAVMs were included in this study (Fig. 1). Seventy-five patients (79.8%) were assigned to the intervention group, and 19 patients (20.2%) to the conservative group. Table 1 summarizes the baseline characteristics of the study cohort. The mean age was significantly younger (40.8 ± 13.9 vs. 48.4 ± 18.4, $P = 0.049$), the frequency of females was significantly higher (41.3% vs. 15.7%, $P = 0.02$), and the proportion of eloquent lesions was significantly lower (42.7% vs. 68.4%, $P = 0.044$) in the intervention group than in the conservative group.

Clinical Outcomes

The mean follow-up period was 65.9 ± 40.1 months in the entire study cohort, 64.2 ± 40.4 months in the intervention group, and 72.8 ± 39.2 months in the conservative group ($P = 0.20$). A total of 12 patients had a stroke or died during the follow-up period (12.8%). This primary outcome was observed in nine patients (12.3%) in the intervention group, all with intracranial hemorrhage, three of whom died, and in three patients (17.6%) in the conservative group, all with intracranial hemorrhage. Using Kaplan–Meier survival analysis and the log-rank test, there was no significant difference in the rate of death or stroke, either in the first 5 years ($P = 0.18$) or over the entire follow-up period ($P = 0.91$) between the two groups (Fig. 2). Cox regression analysis revealed that the HR of the intervention group

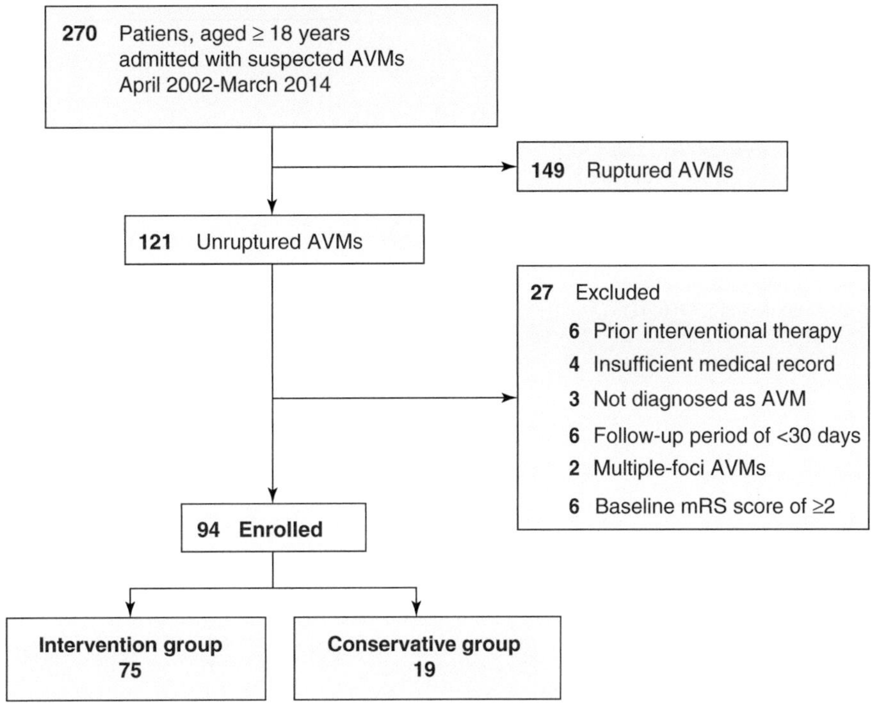

Fig. 1 Participant flow. *AVM* arteriovenous malformation

Table 1 Baseline clinical characteristics of the study cohort

	Total *N* = 94 (%)	Intervention group *N* = 75 (%)	Conservative group *N* = 19 (%)	*P* value
Age	42.3 ± 15.1	40.8 ± 13.9	48.4 ± 18.4	0.049
Female sex	34 (36.1)	31 (41.3)	3 (15.7)	0.029
Clinical presentations				0.91
Seizure	24 (25.5)	19 (25.3)	5 (26.3)	
Focal deficits	1 (1.1)	1 (1.3)	0	
Asymptomatic	69 (73.3)	55 (73.3)	14 (73.6)	
Modified Rankin score				0.16
0	53 (56.3)	45 (60.0)	8 (42.1)	
1	41 (43.6)	30 (40.0)	11 (57.9)	
Spetzler–Martin grade				0.47
I	23 (24.4)	19 (25.3)	4 (21.1)	
II	37 (39.4)	32 (42.7)	5 (26.3)	
III	27 (28.7)	19 (25.3)	8 (42.1)	
IV	6 (6.4)	4 (5.3)	2 (10.5)	
V	1 (1.1)	1 (1.3)	0	
AVM morphology				
Maximum size ≥3 cm	32 (34.1)	24 (32.0)	8 (42.1)	0.40
Eloquent location	44 (46.8)	32 (42.7)	13 (68.4)	0.044
Deep venous drainage	32 (34.4)	26 (35.1)	6 (31.6)	0.77
Lobar	83 (88.3)	67 (89.3)	16 (84.2)	0.31
Infratentorial	8 (8.5)	5 (6.7)	3 (15.7)	0.26

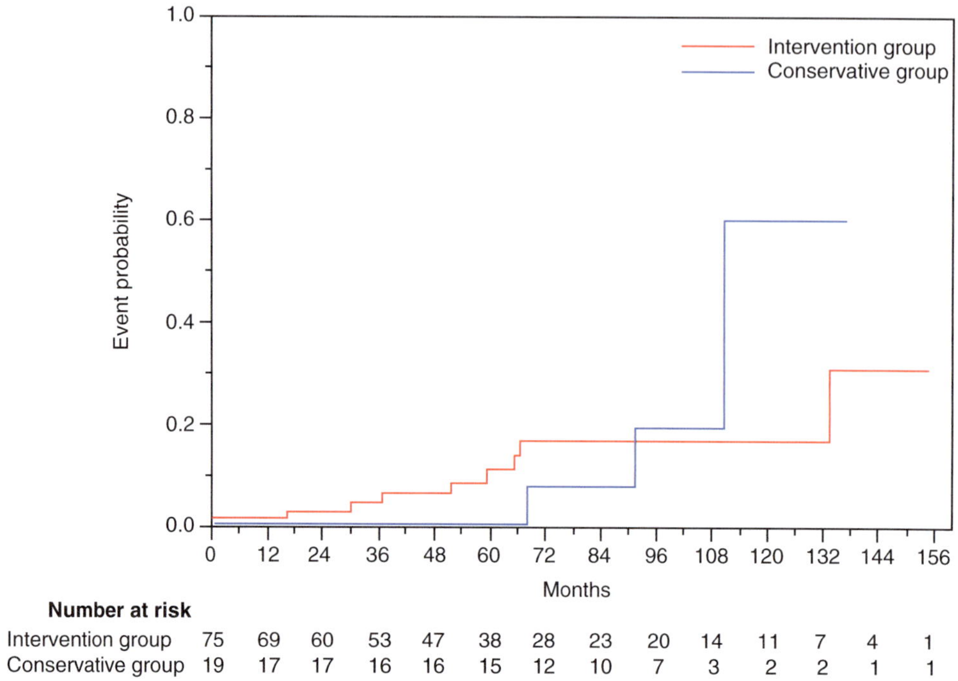

Fig. 2 Kaplan–Meier survival estimates of any death or symptomatic stroke in the entire cohort. Events were observed after a period of 5 years in the conservative group. There was no significant difference in the rate of death or stroke between the interventional and conservative groups, either in the first 5 years ($P = 0.18$) or over the entire follow-up period ($P = 0.91$)

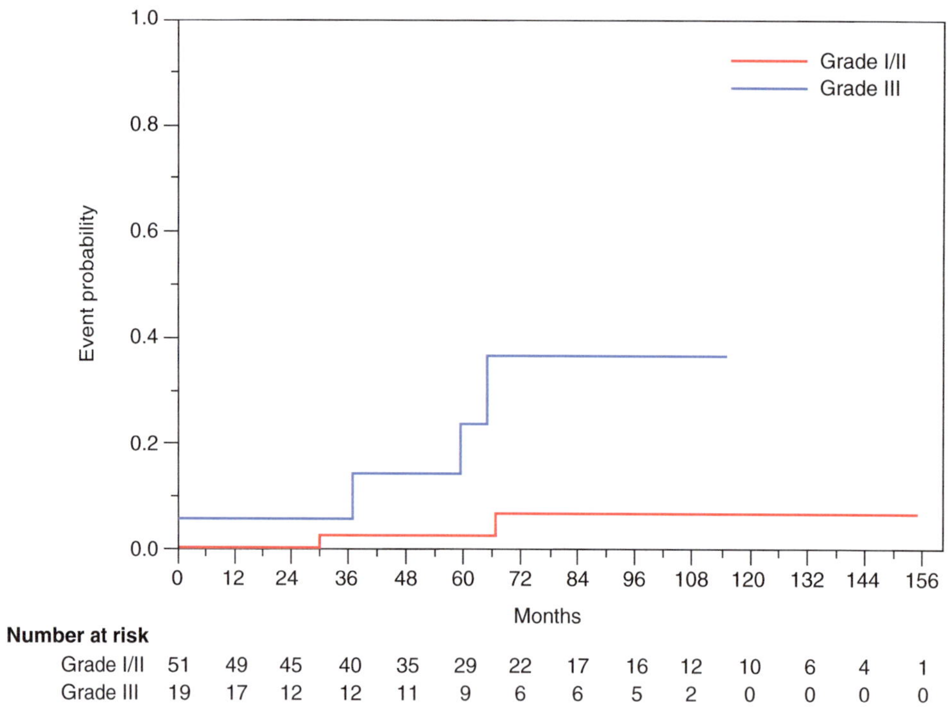

Fig. 3 Kaplan–Meier survival estimates of any death or symptomatic stroke in subgroups of the intervention group. In the intervention group, the incidence of death or stroke was lower among patients with Spetzler–Martin grade I/II uAVMs than among patients with grade III uAVMs ($P = 0.007$)

compared with the conservative group was 2.34 (95% confidence interval [CI], 0.59–11.9) in the entire follow-up period ($P = 0.23$). Poor functional outcome at last follow-up was observed in five patients (6.9%) in the intervention group and two patients (11.7%) in the conservative group ($P = 0.50$) (Table 2).

Subgroup Analysis in the Intervention Group

In the intervention group, 14 patients (18.7%) underwent resection and 61 (81.3%) radiosurgery. Pretreatment embolization was conducted in ten of the patients who underwent resection (71.4%) and two who underwent radiosurgery

Table 2 Proportion of patients who had a stroke, died, or had poor functional outcome

	Total $N = 94$ (%)	Intervention group $N = 75$ (%)	Conservative group $N = 19$ (%)	P value
Mean follow-up period (months)	65.9 ± 40.1	64.2 ± 40.4	72.8 ± 39.2	0.20
Symptomatic stroke or death	12 (12.8)	9 (12.3)	3 (17.6)	0.91
Hemorrhagic stroke	12 (12.8)	9 (12.3)	3 (17.6)	
Death	3 (3.2)	1 (4.0)	0	
mRS ≥ 2 at last follow-up	7 (7.4)	5 (6.9)	2 (11.7)	0.50

(3.3%). There were no cases of embolization alone. Surgical resection was performed on 21.6% of patients with Spetzler–Martin grade I/II AVMs and 15.8% with grade III AVMs. By contrast, all the patients with grade IV/V AVMs were treated with radiosurgery. The incidence of death or stroke was lower and functional outcomes were better among patients with grade I/II AVMs than among patients with grade III AVMs (4.1% vs. 20%, log-rank $P = 0.007$; HR 0.12, 95% CI 0.01–0.65, $P = 0.014$, and 2.0% vs. 15.7%, $P = 0.04$, respectively) (Fig. 3).

Complete AVM obliteration was documented by catheter angiography in 92.9% of cases after resection. One patient had incompletely resected AVM. Regarding radiosurgery, complete obliteration at 3 years was documented by either catheter angiography or MR angiography in 72.3%.

Discussion

This study demonstrated the following in 94 ARUBA-eligible patients with uAVM. (1) Interventional treatment was selected in almost 80% of cases, with 20% involving surgical resection and 80% gamma-knife radiosurgery. (2) Interventional treatment was not inferior to medical treatment alone, either in the incidence of any death or symptomatic stroke followed up for 66 months or in the proportion of patients with a mRS score ≥ 2 at last follow-up. (3) In the intervention group, the incidence of death or stroke was lower and functional outcomes were better among patients with grade I/II AVMs than among those with grade III AVMs.

In this study, the incidence of any death or stroke in the intervention group was 12.3%, which dropped to 4.1% in patients with Spetzler–Martin grade I/II AVMs. These rates appear to be superior to those of the ARUBA interventional therapy group, and relatively comparable to those of the ARUBA medical management group (36.7 and 30.8%, 8.0 and 4.2%, as treated, respectively) [1], in spite of the longer follow-up. Our surgical results for ARUBA-eligible patients are comparable with those of other institutions [5, 6], and not in conflict with the recent reports of good surgical outcomes for AVMs of Spetzler–Martin grades I/II [7, 8]. As reflected in our therapeutic principles, correct choice of resection or radiosurgery with curative intent and adjunctive use of transarterial embolization are considered key factors for a good surgical outcome. Based on this study, careful selection should be made for patients with grade III AVMs to optimize the surgical outcomes.

This study has several limitations. First, selection bias may exist because of the nonrandom choice of treatment and the retrospective nature of the study. The length of the study may also have influenced selection bias. However, a unified treatment strategy was adopted throughout the study, and long-term follow-up was achieved in a single institution. Second, the study population was small, especially for the conservative group, and there were significant differences in age and sex between the intervention and conservative groups. These factors may have reduced the statistical power to analyze the differences between therapies, but it reflects the results of our therapeutic selection over a 10-year period in Japan.

The ARUBA study was important for demonstrating the medical outcomes of uAVMs, with a spontaneous rupture rate of 2.2% per year not predicted by Spetzler–Martin grade. With appropriate selection of patients and low surgical morbidity, multimodal interventional treatment for uAVMs could overcome those outcomes of long-term management.

Conclusion

This study found that for patients with uAVMs, interventional treatment is not inferior to medical treatment alone over a long-term follow-up. Multimodal interventional treatment exhibited good outcomes, especially in patients with Spetzler–Martin grade I/II AVMs. However, careful selection is required for patients with grade III AVMs. With appropriate selection of patients and low surgical morbidity, multimodal interventional treatment for uAVMs might be an optimal therapy for long-term management.

Compliance with Ethical Standards

Conflicts of interest: The authors declare that they have no conflict of interest.

Ethical approval: All procedures performed in studies involving human participants were in accordance with the ethical standards of the institutional and/or national research committee and with the 1964 Helsinki declaration and its later amendments or comparable ethical standards. For this type of study, formal consent is not required.

References

1. Mohr JP, Parides MK, Stapf C, Moquete E, Moy CS, Overbey JR, Al-Shahi Salman R, Vicaut E, Young WL, Houdart E, Cordonnier C, Stefani MA, Hartmann A, von Kummer R, Biondi A, Berkefeld J, Klijn CJ, Harkness K, Libman R, Barreau X, Moskowitz AJ. Medical management with or without interventional therapy for unruptured brain arteriovenous malformations (ARUBA): a multicentre, non-blinded, randomised trial. Lancet. 2014;383:614–21.
2. Amin-Hanjani S. ARUBA results are not applicable to all patients with arteriovenous malformation. Stroke. 2014;45:1539–40.
3. Magro E, Gentric JC, Darsaut TE, Ziegler D, Bojanowski MW, Raymond J. Responses to ARUBA: a systematic review and critical analysis for the design of future arteriovenous malformation trials. J Neurosurg. 2016;29:1–9.
4. Fukuda K, Kataoka H, Nakajima N, Masuoka J, Satow T, Iihara K. Efficacy of FLOW 800 with indocyanine green videoangiography for the quantitative assessment of flow dynamics in cerebral arteriovenous malformation surgery. World Neurosurg. 2015;83:203–10.
5. Nerva JD, Mantovani A, Barber J, Kim LJ, Rockhill JK, Hallam DK, Ghodke BV, Sekhar LN. Treatment outcomes of unruptured arteriovenous malformations with a subgroup analysis of ARUBA (A Randomized Trial of Unruptured Brain Arteriovenous Malformations)-eligible patients. Neurosurgery. 2015;76:563–70.
6. Rutledge WC, Abla AA, Nelson J, Halbach VV, Kim H, Lawton MT. Treatment and outcomes of ARUBA-eligible patients with unruptured brain arteriovenous malformations at a single institution. Neurosurg Focus. 2014;37:E8.
7. Potts MB, Lau D, Abla AA, Kim H, Young WL, Lawton MT. Current surgical results with low-grade brain arteriovenous malformations. J Neurosurg. 2015;122:912–20.
8. Steiger HJ, Fischer I, Rohn B, Turowski B, Etminan N, Hanggi D. Microsurgical resection of Spetzler-Martin grades 1 and 2 unruptured brain arteriovenous malformations results in lower long-term morbidity and loss of quality-adjusted life-years (QALY) than conservative management—results of a single group series. Acta Neurochir. 2015;157:1279–87.

Falcotentorial Location of Dural Arteriovenous Fistulas Derived from the Neural Crest as a Risk Factor for Aggressive Clinical Course

Michihiro Tanaka

Abstract The topographical distribution of dural arteriovenous fistulas (DAVFs) was analyzed based on the embryological anatomy of the dural membrane. Sixty-six consecutive cases of intracranial and spinal DAVFs were analyzed based on the angiography, and each shunt point was identified according to the embryological bony structures. The area of dural membranes was categorized into three different groups: a ventral group located on the endochondral bone (VE group), a dorsal group on the membranous bone (DM group), and a falcotentorial group (FT group) in the falx cerebri, tentorium cerebelli, falx cerebelli, and diaphragma sellae. The FT group was derived from the neural crest and designated when the dural membrane was formed only with the dura propria (meningeal layer of the dura mater) and not from the endosteal dura. Olfactory groove, falx, tent of the cerebellum, and nerve sleeve of spinal cord were categorized in the FT group, which presented later in life and which had a male predominance, more aggressive clinical presentations, and significant cortical and spinal venous reflux. The FT group was formed only with the dura propria that was considered as an independent risk factor for aggressive clinical course and hemorrhage of DAVFs.

Keywords Dorsal mesoderm · Dura propria · Dural arteriovenous fistulas · Endochondral bone · Membranous bone · Neural crest · Paraxial mesoderm

Abbreviations

CT	Computed tomography
DAVFs	Dural arteriovenous fistulas
DM group	Dorsal membranous bone group
DSA	Digital subtraction angiography
FT group	Falcotentorial group
MRI	Magnetic resonance imaging
VE group	Ventral endochondral group

M. Tanaka, M.D., Ph.D. (✉)
Department of Neurosurgery, Kameda Medical Center, Kamogawa, Chiba, Japan

Introduction

The most popular classifications of dural arteriovenous fistulas (DAVFs) in the literature are hemodynamic classifications based on angiographic findings [1–3]. Geibprasert et al. [4] reported a new classification for DAVFs based on craniospinal epidural venous anatomy and that significant differences existed between groups with regard to biological and/or developmental characteristics according to the epidural region [4]. They suggested that DAVFs had heterogeneous pathology and that susceptibility to shunt formation on the surface of dura mater varied according to this classification. The shunt point of DAVFs is usually located on a certain area of dural membrane, such as the transverse sigmoid sinus, carotid cavernous sinus, cribriform plate of the olfactory groove, falcotentorial surface, and anterior condylar confluence; these areas are vulnerable to DAVF formation [4–14].

Embryologically, the intracranial dural membrane is derived from two types of bony structures—endochondral bone with cartilaginous ossification and membranous bone based on the intramembranous ossification [6, 7, 13–19].

By contrast, the falcotentorial dural membrane is independent from bony structures [13]. This means several different anatomical domains of dural membrane exist. This study retrospectively analyzed the topographical features of shunt points on DAVFs in terms of embryological domains of bony structures corresponding to these two different dural compartments derived from neural crest and paraxial mesoderm.

G. Esposito et al. (eds.), *Trends in the Management of Cerebrovascular Diseases*, Acta Neurochirurgica Supplement, Vol. 129, https://doi.org/10.1007/978-3-319-73739-3_18,

Materials and Methods

Sixty-six consecutive DAVFs (32 men and 34 women; age range 38–80 years; mean age, 68.4 years) were analyzed with selective and superselective digital subtraction angiography, three-dimensional (3D) rotational angiography, and high-resolution cone beam computed tomography (CT). Based on these imaging modalities, each shunt point was identified and categorized into one of three different dural compartments related to the embryologic bony structures:

1. Ventral group of endochondral bone from the dura propria and osteal dura (VE group)
2. Dorsal group of membranous bone from the dura propria and osteal dura (DM group)
3. Falx and tent of the cerebellum group only from the dura propria (FT group)

Patients were diagnosed in our hospital between January 2006 and December 2014. All patients underwent digital subtraction angiography with selective catheterization to identify the shunt points. 3D rotational angiography and/or high-resolution cone beam CT were performed when it was difficult to identify the precise location of the shunt point. Each shunt point was plotted on the map of the dural membrane to define the anatomical distribution on its surface. In the cases of multiple shunts of DAVFs, superselective angiography from the dominant feeder was performed, and the highest flow compartment was defined as the primary shunt point.

The topographical distribution was then categorized into three different domains on the surface of the dural membrane derived from three different embryological structures, as follows:

1. VE group: ventral group on the surface of endochondral bone

   The carotid cavernous sinus, sigmoid sinus, and anterior condylar confluence belong to the VE group. This dural membrane consists of the osteal dura and the dura propria. (Fig. 1, red area)
2. DM group: dorsal group on the surface of membranous bone

   The transverse sinus, confluence (torcular Herophili), marginal sinus (dorsal portion), medial occipital sinus, and accessory epidural sinuses on the dorsal surface of posterior fossa belong to the DM group. This dural membrane consists of the osteal dura and dura propria (Fig. 1, yellow area)
3. FT group: falx and tent of the cerebellum group were defined as the dural membrane that was apart from the bony structures (Fig. 1, green area)

   The olfactory groove (paramedian surface of crista galli), superior sagittal sinus, tent of the cerebellum, cerebral falx, falcine sinus, and inferior sagittal sinus belong to the FT group. They are derived from part of the neural crest cells and form the dural membrane that is apart from the skull base and cranial vault [13–16, 18, 20].

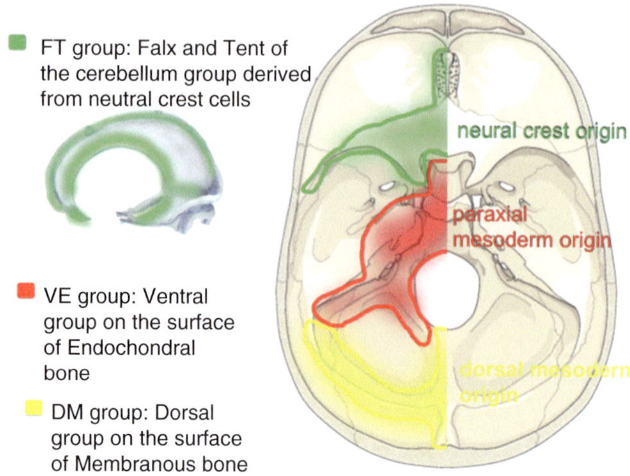

Fig. 1 Embryological classification of DAVFs. FT group is derived from neural crest. VE group is derived from paraxial mesoderm associaed with endochondral bone. DM group is derived from dorsal mesoderm associated with membranous bone

Based on anatomical considerations, the falx and tent of the cerebellum arise from two folding layers of the dura propria, distinguishing this group from the other two groups [6, 13, 15]. Spinal cord DAVFs are also categorized in this group. The shunt point of spinal DAVF is located on the nerve sleeve that corresponds to the border zone between the vertebral body (endochondral bone) and the paired laminae of the vertebra arch (membranous bone). As the FT group is formed relatively apart from the major bony structures during the embryological stage and consists of dura propria alone, the FT group is independent from both the VE and DM groups in terms of embryological domain on the dural membrane. In fact, the spinal dura mater consists only of dura propria and lacks the periosteal layer of the cranial dura (Fig. 2).

Clinical manifestations, existence of cortical venous reflux, angioarchitecture of the terminal feeding arteries, initial venous outlet, and types of Borden's classification were investigated retrospectively. Sixty-two of 66 patients underwent management via the endovascular approach. The other four patients underwent only diagnostic angiography, which showed no indication for intervention (Fig. 3).

Statistical data were processed with Stat Plus **R**software (a free statistical analysis application for the Macintosh operating system). A p-value of less than 0.05 was used to indicate statistical significance.

Fig. 2 The topographical character of FT group that consists only from the dura propria. Olfactory groove, falx, tent of the cerebellum, and lateral spinal dura are derived from neural crest. Spinal cord is covered with only dura propria and there is no periosteal dura in the spinal canal

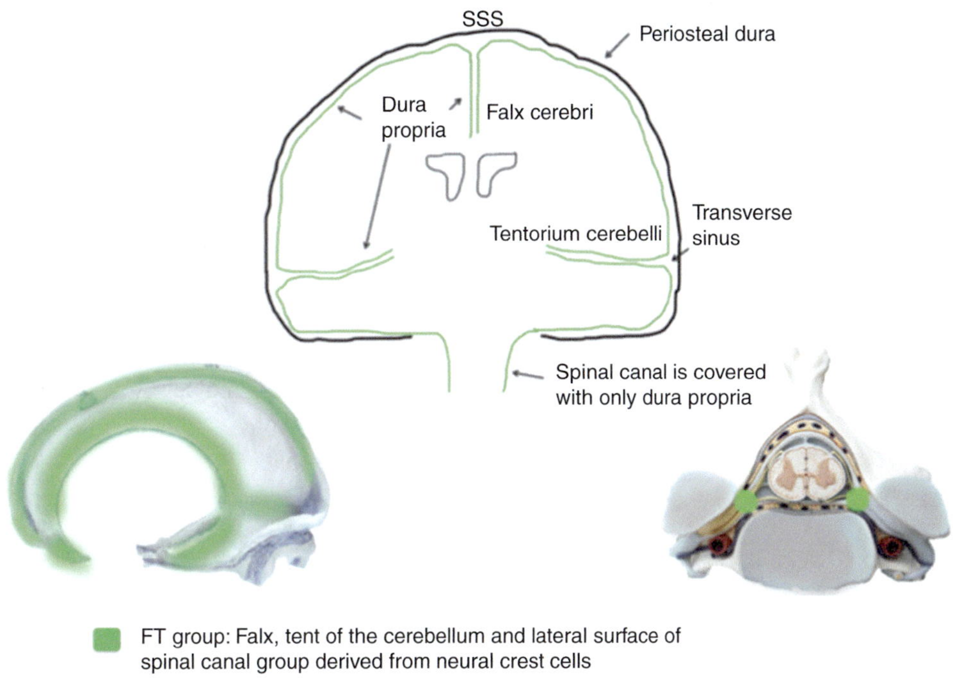

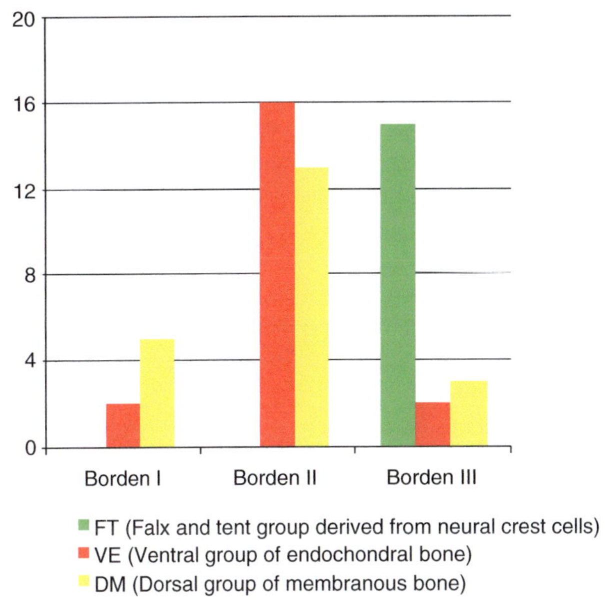

Fig. 3 Correlation between the anatomical location of DAVFs and Borden classification. All of FT group presented with aggressive clinical course

Results

Thirty patients (45.5%) had lesions classified in the VE group. This group consisted of 8 men and 22 women, indicating a female predominance (22 of 30 [73%]; $P < 0.001$). Mean age was 72.1 years. Shunt points were at the carotid cavernous sinus in 19 patients, the sigmoid sinus in 8, and the anterior condylar confluence in 3.

For carotid cavernous lesions, the majority of shunt points were located at the level of the posterior clinoid processes that belonged to the endochondral bony structure of clivus. All these shunt points were localized at the paramedian unilateral posterior compartment of the cavernous sinus rather than at the midline.

Twenty-one patients (31.8%) had lesions classified to the DM group. These included 16 patients with transverse sinus DAVFs and 5 with confluence DAVFs. There was no marked sex predominance (male: female ratio = 13:8; $P = 0.383$), and mean age was 54.5 years.

There were 15 patients (22, 7%) who had lesions classified to the FT group. These included three patients with olfactory groove DAVFs, three with cerebellar tentorium DAVFs, five with superior sagittal sinus DAVFs, and four with spinal cord DAVFs. There was a strong male predominance (13 of 15 [87%]; $P < 0.001$), and mean age was 75.2 years, which was significantly older than the other two groups (Table 1).

Clinical Manifestations and Cortical Venous Reflux in Terms of Angiosemiology

In the FT group, 12 of 15 (80%) patients presented with aggressive clinical symptoms ($P < 0.001$). There were five patients with neurological deficit associated with perifocal edema caused by the cortical venous reflux, three with intracerebral hemorrhage, and four with spinal cord DAVFs who

Table 1 Correlation of each group and population, cortical venous reflux, clinical manifestation as the semiology

	FT: Falx and tent of the cerebellum derived from neural crest cells associated with dura propria (olfactory groove, falx, tentorium cerebelli, lateral spinal)	VE: Ventral group derived from paraaxial mesoderm associated with endochondoral bone. (cavernous sinus, anterior condylar confluence, sigmoid sinus)	DM: Dorsal group derived from dorsal mesoderm associated with membranous bone (transverse sinus, occipital sinus, confluence)
N (male/female)	15 (87%/13%)	30 (27%/73%)	21 (62%/38%)
Mean age (years)	65.1	78.4	59.8
Cortical venous reflux	93%	37%	52%
Major symptoms	Headache, neurological deficit associated with venous infraction, hemorrhage, paraplegia (central myelopathy)	Diplopia, chemosis, bruit	Headache, tinnitus

FT group represented aggressive clinical course

presented with progressive myelopathy. Regarding the angioarchitecture of this group, the venous outlet of the arteriovenous (AV) shunts was independent from the main sinus and, therefore, 100% of shunt flow created reflux directly into the pial vein of the brain or spinal cord.

This was the main reason the FT group showed an aggressive clinical course (i.e., Cognar types III, IV, and V, and Borden's classification type 3) (Fig. 3).

Discussion

Dural membrane is formed by the following two layers:

1. Dura propria: inner meningeal layer, forming falx cerebri, tentorium cerebelli continuous inferiorly with the dural sac of the spinal cord
2. Endosteal dura: outer endosteal layer, continuous via sutures and foramina with the periosteum

The dural membrane is the outermost tough connective tissue covering the arachnoid membrane, and it attaches to the inner surface of the cranial vault and skull base. The dura mater, arachnoid mater, and pia mater develop from the meninx primitive, which is one of the meningeal mesenchymes containing the mesodermal and neural crest [13, 16, 18, 20]. At the level of the skull, the outer dural layer forms the inner periosteum of the skull, and the inner dural layer forms the dural folds (falx and tentorium) containing the dural sinuses [9, 10, 13, 15]. The cranial dura mater is a tough, fibrous membrane consisting of two connective tissue layers: an external periosteal layer and an inner meningeal layer. These are fused together, except for where the dural venous sinuses are located (e.g., superior sagittal sinus). The periosteal layer of the dura mater adheres to the inner surface of the skull bone and is highly vascular and innervated. The dura propria (meningeal layer of the dura) is smooth and avascular and is lined by mesothelium (a single layer of squamous-like, flattened cells) on its inner surface. At the foramen magnum (a large opening at the base of the occipital bone through which the medulla is continuous with the spinal cord), the dura propria joins the spinal dura. The spinal dura mater consists of only the dura propria and lacks the osteal dura (periosteal layer of the cranial dura). At the level of the spinal cord, the dura mater is separated from the periosteum of the vertebral canal by an epidural space. This means there is no interdural space at the spinal cord level. In fact, there are no dural sinuses in the spinal canal. The definition of the craniospinal epidural venous system by Geibprasert is the venous structures locating in the epimeningeal layer of dural membrane that corresponds to dura propria [4, 13, 15].

The histology of the dural membrane is affected by the differences of bony structures. Both mesenchymal and neural-crest-derived cells appear to be involved in the formation of the primary meninx that differentiates during embryonic development [4, 13, 15, 17, 20]. The tent of cerebellar and falcine sinus (FT group) is formed in this early stage, but these develop relatively independently from the bony structure because the topographical location of the FT group is apart from the bony structures. The vulnerability of the dural membrane can be presumed and predicted from the process of development in the early stage of embryo in terms of shunt formation [13, 18].

Geibprasert et al. reported a new classification of DAVFs according to the craniospinal epidural venous anatomical bases and clinical correlations [4]. These investigators introduced three different types of epidural spaces at which the shunt points are located, the groups of ventral epidural shunts, of dorsal epidural shunts, and of lateral epidural shunts. They showed that ventral epidural shunts were linked to the vertebral body, basioccipital, sigmoid sinus, petrous pyramid, basisphenoid (cavernous sinus) and adjacent sphenoid wings, and related dural structures. Dorsal epidural shunts were associated with the transverse sinus, occipital sinus, and superior sagittal sinus. Lateral epidural shunts were related to spinal dural AV shunts, marginal sinus (lateral portion of the foramen magnum) with the emissary-bridging vein to the condyloid vein, falcotentorial (vein of Galen), petrosal and basitentorial, sphenoparietal sinus, paracavernous region (embryonic tentorial sinus remnants), intraorbital shunts, and lamina cribriformis. Their ventral epidural shunts corresponded to our VE group, and their dorsal epidural shunts partly corresponded to our DM group. Their ventral epidural group included the sigmoid sinus, but the sigmoid sinus was surrounded with membranous bone and was therefore categorized in the DM group in our classification.

The main difference between their classification and ours was with regard to lateral epidural shunts. There was some controversy in that anterior condylar confluence DAVFs were defined as lateral epidural shunts despite the fact that the hypoglossal canal belongs to the basioccipital bone that was categorized as a ventral epidural shunt. We categorized the anterior condylar confluence DAVFs within the VE group simply because the shunt points were located at the level of the hypoglossal canal from endochondral bony structures. Additionally, there were some common characteristics between anterior condylar confluence DAVFs and carotid cavernous DAVFs. Both DAVFs had meningeal dural supply and intraosseous terminal feeding arteries not usually observed in the FT group [5, 10–14].

The FT group was defined as an embryological domain of the dural membrane that consisted of only dura propria and that was considered as the structures derived from neural crest cells. This topographical area contained the entire falx, the tent of the cerebellum, and the dural membrane covering the nerve sheaths of the spinal cord. The olfactory groove (lamina cribriformis) also belongs to this system as the most anterior part of the falx. This concept is consistent with there being a strong male predominance and symptoms presenting later in life in patients with spinal cord, olfactory groove, falx and tent of cerebellum DAVFs among this FT group (Table 1).

Because of the aggressive clinical presentations, it was evident that transarterial embolization is indicated for the management of patients in the FT group [2, 5, 8, 12–14].

There are three major weak points of this study. First is that the vulnerability of dural membrane at the level of interdural space has not yet been proven histologically. Second is that the initial trigger of shunt formation and its mechanism are still unknown. Third is that the reason for male predominance with elder generations in the FT group cannot be explained. Regardless, characteristics of angioarchitecture and the natural history of DAVFs could be predicted according to classification based on the embryological domains of intracranial and spinal cord dural membrane. Further investigation of this concept may provide additional information to clarify the pathoetiology of DAVFs.

Conclusions

The classification presented based on the concept of embryological domain is useful to clarify the pathoetiology and epidemiology of DAVFs. Segmental vulnerability of the dural membrane might be related to the biological and/or hormonal differences influenced by the embryological bony structures associated with neural crest and paraxial mesoderm. The falcotentorial location of DAVFs was considered as an independent risk factor for an aggressive clinical course and hemorrhage of DAVFs.

Acknowledgments The author thanks Dr. Giuseppe Esposito and Prof. Tetsuya Tsukahara for their proposal and organization to publish this chapter.

Conflicts of interest disclosure: The author reports no conflict of interest concerning the materials or methods used or the findings specified in this study.

References

1. Borden JA, Wu JK, Shucart WA. A proposed classification for spinal and cranial dural arteriovenous fistulous malformations and implications for treatment. J Neurosurg. 1995;82:166–79.
2. Cognard C, Casasco A, Toevi M, Houdart E, Chiras J, Merland JJ. Dural arteriovenous fistulas as a cause of intracranial hypertension due to impairment of cranial venous outflow. J Neurol Neurosurg Psychiatry. 1998;65:308–16.
3. Cognard C, Gobin YP, Pierot L, Bailly AL, Houdart E, Casasco A, et al. Cerebral dural arteriovenous fistulas: clinical and angiographic correlation with a revised classification of venous drainage. Radiology. 1995;194:671–80.
4. Geibprasert S, Pereira V, Krings T, Jiarakongmun P, Toulgoat F, Pongpech S, et al. Dural arteriovenous shunts: a new classification of craniospinal epidural venous anatomical bases and clinical correlations. Stroke. 2008;39:2783–94.
5. Agid R, Terbrugge K, Rodesch G, Andersson T, Söderman M. Management strategies for anterior cranial fossa (ethmoidal) dural arteriovenous fistulas with an emphasis on endovascular treatment. J Neurosurg. 2009;110:79–84.
6. Aurboonyawat T, Suthipongchai S, Pereira V, Ozanne A, Lasjaunias P. Patterns of cranial venous system from the comparative anatomy in vertebrates. Part I, introduction and the dorsal venous system. Interv Neuroradiol. 2007;13:335–44.
7. Aurboonyawat T, Pereira V, Krings T, Toulgoat F, Chiewvit P, Lasjaunias P. Patterns of the cranial venous system from the comparative anatomy invertebrates. Part III. The ventricular system and comparative anatomy of the venous outlet of spinal cord and its homology with the five brain vesicles. Interv Neuroradiol. 2008;14:125–36.
8. Awad IA, Little JR, Akarawi WP, Ahl J. Intracranial dural arteriovenous malformations: factors predisposing to an aggressive neurological course. J Neurosurg. 1990;72:839–50.
9. Baltsavias G, Parthasarathi V, Aydin E, Al Schameri RA, Roth P, Valavanis A. Cranial dural arteriovenous shunts. Part 1. Anatomy and embryology of the bridging and emissary veins. Neurosurg Rev. 2014;38(2):253–64. https://doi.org/10.1007/s10143-014-0590-2.

10. Baltsavias G, Kumar R, Avinash KM, Valavanis A. Cranial dural arteriovenous shunts. Part 2. The shunts of the bridging veins and leptomeningeal venous drainage. Neurosurg Rev. 2014;38(2):265–72. https://doi.org/10.1007/s10143-014-0594-y.
11. Baltsavias G, Valavanis A. Endovascular treatment of 170 consecutive cranial dural arteriovenous fistulae: results and complications. Neurosurg Rev. 2014;37(1):63–71.
12. Lasjaunias P, Chiu M, ter Brugge K, Tolia A, Hurth M, Bernstein M. Neurological manifestations of intracranial dural arteriovenous malformations. J Neurosurg. 1986;64:724–30.
13. Tanaka M. Embryological consideration of dural arteriovenous fistulas. Neurol Med Chir (Tokyo). 2016;56(9):544–51. https://www.jstage.jst.go.jp/article/nmc/advpub/0/advpub_oa.2015-0313/_article.
14. Tanaka M. Embryological consideration of dural AVF. In: Tsukahara T, Pasqualin A, Esposito G, Regli L, Pinna G, editors. Trends in cerebrovascular surgery, vol. 123. Cham: Springer; 2016. p. 169–76. https://doi.org/10.1007/978-3-319-29887-0_24.
15. Adeeb N, Mortazavi MM, Tubbs RS, Cohen-Gadol AA (2012) The cranial dura mater: a review of its history, embryology, and anatomy. Childs Nerv Syst 28(6):827–837. http://www.ncbi.nlm.nih.gov/pubmed/18635840.
16. Friede H. Normal development and growth of the human neurocranium and cranial base. Scand J Plast Reconstr Surg. 1981;15(3):163–9.
17. Griessenauer CJ, Raborn J, Foreman P, Shoja MM, Loukas M, Tubbs RS. Venous drainage of the spine and spinal cord: a comprehensive review of its history, embryology, anatomy, physiology, and pathology. Clin Anat. 2015;28:75–87. http://www.ncbi.nlm.nih.gov/pubmed/24677178.
18. Mitsuhashi Y, Aurboonyawat T, Pereira VM, Geibprasert S, Toulgoat F, Ozanne A, et al. Dural arteriovenous fistulas draining into the petrosal vein or bridging vein of the medulla: possible homologs of spinal dural arteriovenous fistulas. Clinical article. J Neurosurg. 2009;111:889–99.
19. Opperman LA. Cranial sutures as intramembranous bone growth sites. Dev Dyn. 2000;219:472–85.
20. Noden DM, Trainor PA. Relations and interactions between cranial mesoderm and neural crest populations. J Anat. 2005;207:575–601. http://www.pubmedcentral.nih.gov/articlerender.fcgi?artid=1571569&tool=pmcentrez&rendertype=abstract.

Part IV

Miscellaneous

Training of Cerebrovascular Specialists: The Surgeon's View

Hans-Jakob Steiger

Abstract The key to becoming an expert in a surgical field is mainly practice and perseverance. The old-fashioned system of teaching from one older person to a younger one, by simple demonstration, imitation, and practice, cannot be replaced in the surgical field by more modern didactic tools. Structured and explicit concepts, however, can accelerate the learning process. Structured concepts consist of a system of specifics—for example, types of aneurysms in the field of vascular pathology—and standard operating procedures. It is important to realize that the teaching requirements of the surgical disciplines differ substantially from those of the conservative disciplines. The number of procedures performed is probably the most critical factor for competence. At our center we have used the target number of 100 microsurgical aneurysm cases treated under supervision before sufficient competence is considered to have been achieved for independent surgery. Following initial training a certain amount of practice is required to remain current or competent. The proficiency requirements accepted in aviation could be seen as a guide for proficiency requirements in neurosurgery. In aviation, a minimum of 12 per year is specified for most critical procedures.

Keywords Cerebrovascular surgery · Training · Teaching · Training curriculum

Introduction

The key to becoming an expert is—according to Malcom Gladwell (in *Outliers*) and Daniel Levitin (in *This Is Your Brain on Music*)—perseverance [1, 2]. They propagated the "10,000-Hour Rule," claiming that the key to achieving world-class expertise in any skill is, to a large extent, a matter of practicing the correct way, for a total of around 10,000 h. This perspective puts weight much more on perseverance than on talent as critical factor for success. As provocative as the rule may look at first sight, the study of multiple biographies of successful personalities in all fields—be it arts, science, or politics—obviously supports this view. It is, however, simplistic. There are multiple examples of people doing the same things for years and remaining at a low level—for example, a school rock band performing popular songs at the level of three chords. Ten thousand hours of practice may be the most important factor, but it is not enough. Just doing it—unguided practice—leads to flat improvement and an early plateau. Good technical and conceptual guidance accelerates progress and improves the final level.

The Master-and-Apprentice Concept

Old-fashioned teaching has always conveyed knowledge and competence from one generation to the next, frequently from an older person to a younger one, by simple demonstration, imitation, and practice (Fig. 1). The advancing complexity of our world calls for an improved didactic concept to make learning more efficient. The didactic concepts developed for teaching knowledge are not sufficient for teaching practical skills. Here, modern concepts have, rather, emerged from findings in neuroscience and rehabilitation medicine. A surgeon can, by demonstration of a procedure, convey more technical details than he or she may actually realize. Correspondingly, the resident may adopt skills by observation more than he or she cognitively realizes. The concept of mirror neurons in our brains is an attractive explanation for these phenomena. These cells were first described in macaques by the Italian Giacomo Rizzolatti and his coworkers in 1992 [3]. In these investigations it was noticed that neurons in field F5c of the cerebrum reacted both when certain target–motor–hand–object interactions were carried out by the monkey and when the monkey observed the same

H.-J. Steiger, M.D. (✉)
Department of Neurosurgery, Heinrich Heine University, Düsseldorf, Germany
e-mail: steiger@uni-duesseldorf.de

G. Esposito et al. (eds.), *Trends in the Management of Cerebrovascular Diseases*, Acta Neurochirurgica Supplement, Vol. 129,
https://doi.org/10.1007/978-3-319-73739-3_19,

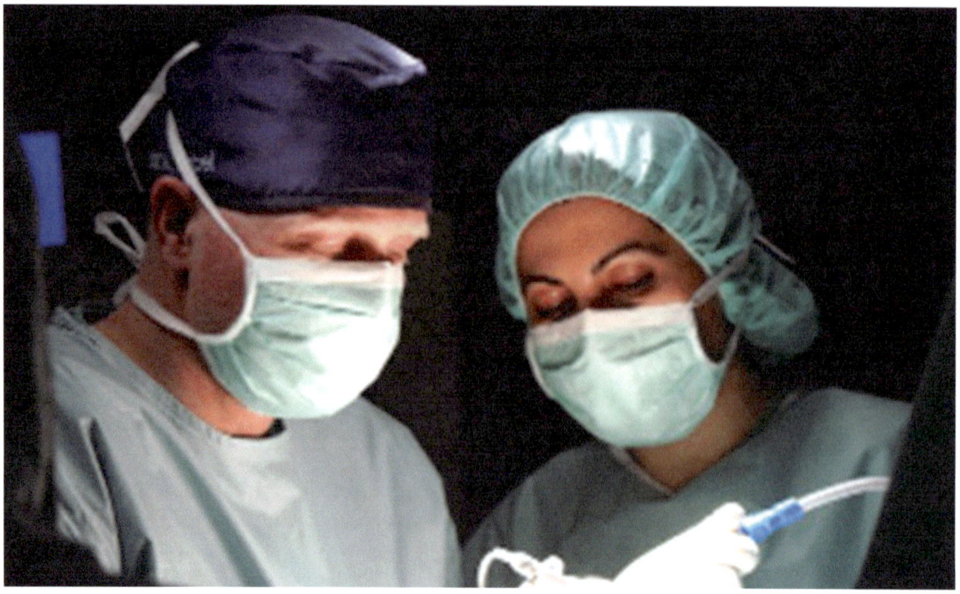

Fig. 1 The traditional tandem approach to teaching is still the mainstay of conveying surgical technique to the next generation. Not everything conveyed can be framed in words and sentences, but a logical framework with explicit concepts helps to teach more efficiently

interaction in another animal—or even in a human being. In 2002 the possibility of a mirror neuron system in Brodmann's area 44 was discussed in humans, which was supposed to be associated with recognition of actions and imitation. More recently the function of these mirror neurons has been judged a bit more critically. It is important, at this point, to note that the teaching requirements of the surgical disciplines differ substantially from those of the nonsurgical/noninvasive disciplines—a fact that does not always receive the necessary consideration.

The Need for Structured Teaching

Just watching an "expert" can teach us to recognize common events and learn common procedures and manipulations. There is, however, little doubt that clearly defined learning objectives and content can accelerate the learning process. For common procedures, structured concepts probably accelerate learning, but without such concepts the learning process also advances, though more slowly and arguably plateauing at a lower level than within a structured teaching environment.

While they are helpful to teach reactions to common events, structured concepts are absolutely necessary to convey recognition of, and responses to, rare events, i.e., emergency processes. As an illustration, let us consider the following scenario. An apprentice in customs control at the airport learns to identify smugglers. Illegal importation of cigarettes, alcohol, and other banned or restricted goods appears to be common and is done by around 20% of travelers, according to a recent UK report [4]. Just accompanying an experienced customs officer may teach the apprentice to identify the look, the gait, etc., of the most likely smugglers. The smugglers identified by the experienced officer are the training data set for the novice. If the problem of terrorism at the airport is considered, the situation looks entirely different. Terrorists are still extremely rare. Therefore, the knowledge to identify them cannot be learned in the same way as that used to identify smugglers. This situation calls for definition of a risk score based on certain characteristics. In neurosurgery the same is true for rare events, including emergencies and disasters.

Teaching Issues

The following three factors are the cornerstones of a framework for effective teaching:

- The training environment
- Teacher dedication
- A structured syllabus (standard operating procedures [SOPs])

The training environment—also meaning the training culture or training tradition—is a central aspect. For neurosurgery this means essentially that it is acceptable that a procedure done by a resident under supervision may take longer, provided that the result is the same as, or better than, the result achieved by a more experienced surgeon. Furthermore, teaching must be accepted as important by staff members. Although teaching dedication varies widely between hospitals and individuals, once established, a teaching environment survives when faculty members realize the mutual benefit of the teaching environment, such as accompanying scientific studies and publications.

The question of the need for SOPs has undergone significant variations in perspective during the last two decades. SOPs have appeared progressively since the beginning of the millennium. They have usually been written after discussion with the involved parties and review of the evidence. After publication they have usually been—and still are—put in some sort of archive, with the implicit expectation that everybody knows and follows the rules. With the increasing number of SOPs it has become very clear that this is an illusion. SOPs cannot replace continuing oral teaching—the teaching culture. SOPs have some value and should be maintained. In my experience, SOPs are more important for the people who have written them than they are for novices. It turns out that routine procedures tend to drift over the years. This is particularly common regarding aspects of care where no clear evidence exists and where no national or international guidelines have been formulated. Let us consider the following example. Our standard initial procedure to treat a cranial cerebrospinal fluid (CSF) leak is use of spinal drainage for 5 days, except in the presence of accepted contraindications such as occlusive hydrocephalus. I recently realized that drainage was prescribed for only 3 days, and I was uncertain for a second whether we had written "3 days" or "5 days" in the SOP. The SOP reads "Following CT to exclude occlusive hydrocephalus and subdural hygroma, a lumbar CSF drainage is inserted for 5 days and 6 to 20 mL are drained six times per day." Therefore, the SOPs may be, in the end, more important for the teacher than for the trainee. Oral teaching during rounds cannot be replaced by SOPs.

Despite the limitations, SOPs are important to establish a general concept of care beyond the available evidence. Many things can be written in SOPs that we do not have evidence for and where multiple ways of doing things may be acceptable. Here, SOPs help to standardize processes and prevent chaos.

In order to illustrate the value of written standards, Richard Sennet presented, in his book *The Craftsman*, the example of Antonio Stradivari (1648–1737) [5]. Stradivari had elaborated ingenious techniques to create his violins, involving special methods of tarnishing, etc. The culture was lived daily in the atelier, but SOPs were never written up. After Stradivari's death the special techniques resulting in exceptional acoustic quality were forgotten, which is the reason why these violins are still highly valued today.

Regarding Conceptual Structure

In conservative medicine, everything is about decision making. In a surgical field, half of it is about decision making and half is about how to do things. Both scenarios require analysis and consequences. Analysis requires a series of criteria—an ontology or classification of situations and constellations. Therefore, it is important to classify surgical pathology and intraoperative situations. As an example, our classification of aneurysm projections will be considered briefly [6]. On the basis of hemodynamic concepts, we have defined four main projections of the aneurysm dome with regard to the afferent artery. The projection of the dome determines, to a large degree, specific problems with the approach and also the manner of clip application. For an anterior communicating artery aneurysm, the classification is as follows (see Fig. 2): type 1 aneurysms project downward to the optic chiasm and often adhere to this structure. This is important, since elevation of the orbital cortex with a brain retractor during the approach may lead to traction on the aneurysm dome and premature intraoperative rerupture. Type 2 aneurysms project essentially forward as an elongation of the dominant A1 segment. Although they do not adhere to the chiasm, they lie within the interhemispheric fissure, and formal splitting of the fissure between the gyri recti is therefore hazardous with these aneurysms. The dome of type 3 aneurysms lies approximately within the plane of the A2 segments. Although the initial approach is less problematic than with type 1 and 2 projections, type 3 aneurysms require more upward dissection and retraction because of the higher position of the aneurysm neck. Furthermore, type 3 aneurysms are in close vicinity to the perforators originating from the distal A1 and proximal A2 segments. Type 4 aneurysms lie above the plane of the A1 segments and behind the plane of the A2s. These aneurysms require access to the neck above the A1s, which is between the perforators. Type 4 aneurysms are also in close vicinity to the hypothalamus, and this structure is hurt by aneurysmal hemorrhage and surgical manipulations more easily than with the other projections. Therefore, type 4 projections are associated with a less favorable functional outcome than the other projections.

Because the pre- and intraoperative decisions become intelligible for the trainee, teaching on the basis of structured concepts, such as the example mentioned above, is more efficient.

Cerebrovascular Subspecialty Training Curricula

In contrast to residencies, for which exact numbers of performed procedures are defined in many countries, the curricula of fellowships most often represent only a list of

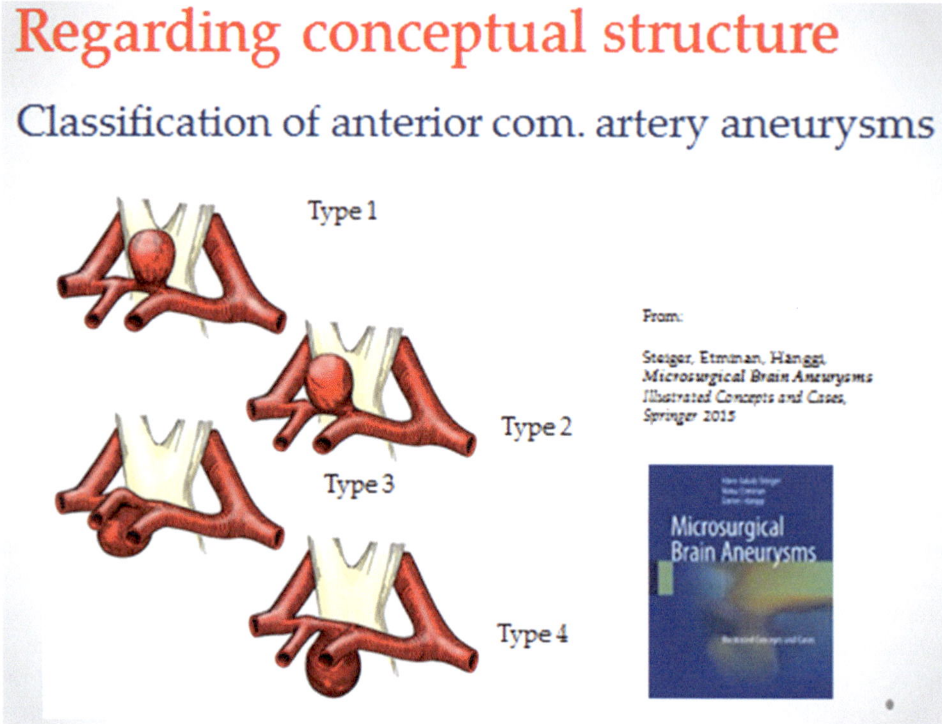

Fig. 2 Development of explicit criteria for pre- and intraoperative decisions is necessary for efficient neurosurgical teaching. The example here is our classification of anterior communicating artery aneurysms. The classification is based on hemodynamic concepts of aneurysm development, suggesting that there are principally dominant projection angles with regard to the afferent artery. Each of these angles is associated with specific caveats and details of the approach and clipping method

learning objectives. The typical example of a cerebrovascular fellowship curriculum illustrates this issue. Its learning objectives are as follows:

- Achievement of competence with treatment decisions for neurovascular disease
- Familiarization with current guidelines and pertinent key literature on neurovascular pathology and treatment
- Exposure to a large number of microsurgical vascular procedures
- Proficiency in interdisciplinary treatment decision making with neuroradiological and neurological vascular specialists
- Participation in laboratory and clinical research
- Participation in undergraduate training together with staff and fellows from neurosurgery, neurology, neuroradiology, and intensive care

It must be assumed that the resulting competence varies widely from fellowship to fellowship. Although some fellows certainly learn more quickly than others, a framework with regard to the number of procedures necessary to gain sufficient competence should be mandatory.

The Learning Curve of Aneurysm Surgery

Several studies have shown that procedural outcomes are better at high-volume institutions, possibly because of greater physician experience (learning) or practice (repetition). However, there are no reliable numbers with regard to the personal learning experience necessary to achieve an acceptable level of competence. Singh and coworkers tried to analyse the learning curve for endovascular treatment of unruptured aneurysms [7]. They found that complications occurred in 53% of the first five cases that each physician treated, and in 10% of later cases. After adjustment for all other predictors, the odds of a complication decreased with increasing physician experience, with an odds ratio of 0.69 for every five cases treated. This would imply that after 20–30 cases an acceptable level of competence is achieved; that is, the risk associated with personal competence becomes small compared with aneurysm- and patient-related factors.

Most of us would agree that microsurgical treatment requires a larger number of procedures than endovascular therapy to achieve an acceptable level of competence. At our

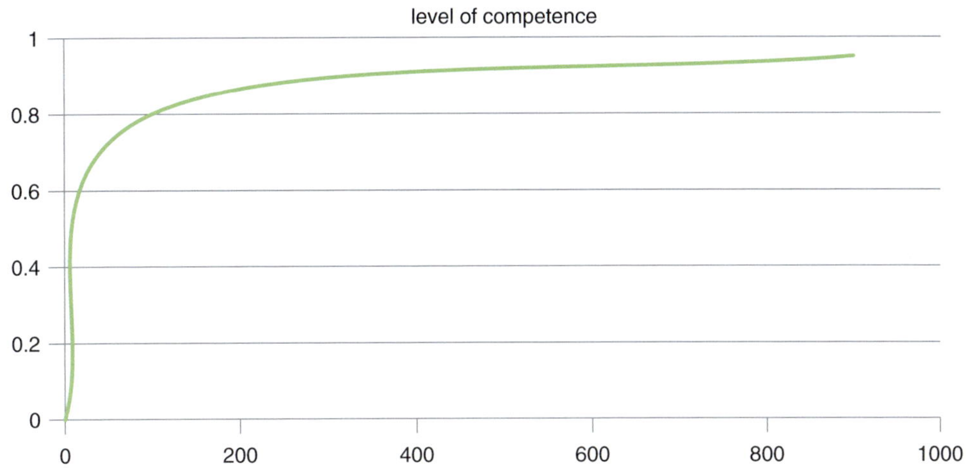

Fig. 3 Empirical correlation between the level of competence and the performed number of microsurgical procedures for brain aneurysms. The learning curve has the typical characteristics, with a steep initial phase, followed by a longer period of increasing perfection. The number needed to achieve sufficient competence depends on the specific procedure. The higher the number of anatomic and technical variables, the higher the number needed for for competence. Experience with some 100 cases, on average, appears to result in a sufficient level of competence for trainees to be allowed unsupervised performance of procedures

center we have been using the target number of 100 cases done under supervision before microsurgical aneurysm procedures are performed independently. At first glance this number appears high, but since the specific anatomic conditions differ substantially between individual locations, sufficient experience must be gained at all common aneurysm sites. We estimate that 100 cases are necessary to reach some 80% of the possible competence (Fig. 3).

What to Do with Orphan Procedures

The learning curve to achieve initial competence is one aspect of practical proficiency. Continuing practice is the other side. Here, "scientific" analysis is even scarcer than with regard to the learning curve. Therefore, I have personally used the proficiency requirement accepted in aviation. Here, for most critical procedures—such as total annual flight hours as a pilot in command, takeoff and landing carrying passengers during the night, instrument approaches, etc.—a number of 3 per 3 months or 12 annually has been specified [8]. These numbers for currency are generally considered low in the community, and it is well known that higher numbers are necessary for proficiency. Translated to neurosurgery this would mean that a dozen aneurysm procedures per neurosurgeon and year are necessary, or a dozen operations for cavernomas or arteriovenous malformations or dural fistulas or extracranial–intracranial (EC–IC) bypasses. Here, things get more complicated, since fewer than a dozen arteriovenous malformations and dural fistulas per year are encountered at many neurosurgical centers—not to mention bypass surgery. In these situations the only solution is to allocate all procedures to one person. Nonetheless, if the number of procedures is single-digit per year, these rare procedures finally tend to become obsolete procedures. For example, at our center we do not perform surgical treatment of basilar artery aneurysms anymore; therefore, we no longer teach the relevant techniques to the younger generation.

Postmortem: Can We Learn from Mistakes?

Regular morbidity and mortality (M&M) conferences are firmly established in training programs in the USA and Europe. The initial aims were obviously to learn from mistakes and specifically to prevent similar occurrences in the future. The efficacy in this respect, however, is difficult to prove. Following the introduction of regular M&M conferences at our center in 2003, we have tracked the frequencies of the typical neurosurgical complications up to the present. At the time of an interim analysis the spectrum of complications was as follows [9]: postoperative hemorrhage requiring surgical revision and additional neurological deficits were the most common adverse events (23% and 25%, respectively). Other complications accounted for some 10% each. They were incomplete result of surgery, CSF fistula, implant misplacement, infection of implants, and other infections.

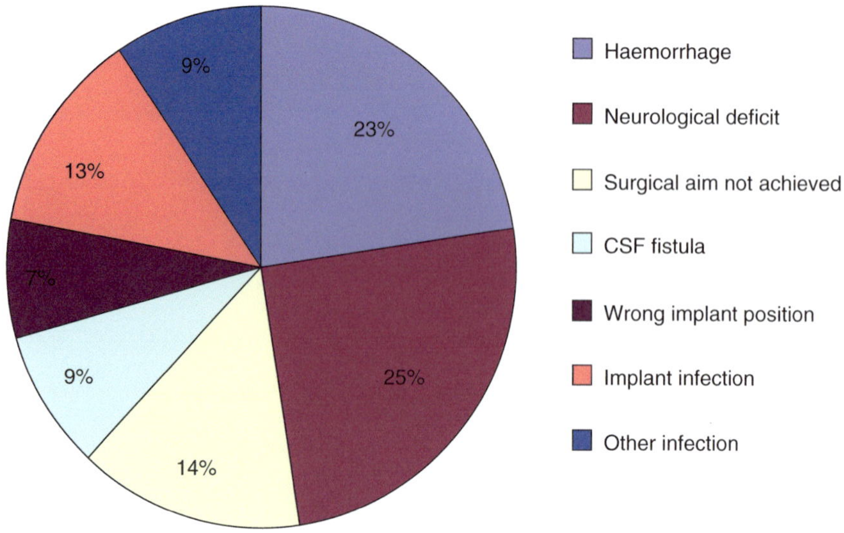

Fig. 4 Spectrum of complications for all neurosurgery at Heinrich Heine University (HHU) from 2003 to the present. In an HHU retrospective subanalysis (2003–2009), the human factor played the dominant role in complications. Fifty-eight percent of mistakes were classified as unconscious mistakes and 40% as proficiency failures. Just 2% of all mishaps were classified as "ill fate." No mishaps had to be considered a consequence of willful deviation or a consequence of physical incapacitation

There was no definitive trend toward lower complication rates over the years (Fig. 4).

A secondary analysis regarding the human factor involved showed that 60% of complications were due to unconscious mistakes and 40% to lack of proficiency. Conscious mistakes and physical incapacitation did not play a role. Just 2% of complications were attributed to "ill fate."

The stable rate of complications over the years should not lead to the conclusion that M&M conferences are devoid of any effect. Regular discussion of typical complications is probably necessary to control complications at a given level. The M&M conference must therefore be seen mainly as a teaching forum for residents and fellows.

Conclusions

- For neurosurgeons, teaching should be an art rather than a science.
- The master-and-apprentice concept remains the mainstay of the teaching of surgical procedures.
- Formalization of concepts accelerates learning.
- Microsurgical experience in treating some 100 aneurysms is a good rule of thumb for "sufficient" competence.
- Rare procedures done only a few times per year tend to disappear completely.

Disclosure The author declares that there are no conflicts of interest pertinent to the work reflected in this manuscript.

References

1. Gladwell M. Outliers—the story of success. London: Penguin Books; 2008. p. 35–68.
2. Levitin D. This is your brain on music. London: Atlantic Books; 2006. p. 193–225. ISBN 978 0 85789 514 1.
3. Rizzolatti G, Fabbri-Destro M. Mirror neurons: from discovery to autism. Exp Brain Res. 2010;200:223–37. ISSN 1432-1106, PMID 19760408, doi: https://doi.org/10.1007/s00221-009-2002-3
4. TravelMail. A nation of smugglers. 2014. http://www.dailymail.co.uk/travel/article-2621329/One-five-travellers-ignores-customs-sneaks-cigarettes-alcohol-UK.html
5. Sennet R. The craftsman. London: Penguin Books; 2008. p. 53–80.
6. Steiger HJ, Etminan N, Hänggi D. Microsurgical brain aneurysms—illustrated concepts and cases. New York: Springer; 2015.
7. Singh V, Gress DR, Higashida RT, Dowd CF, Halbach VV, Johnston SC. The learning curve for coil embolization of unruptured intracranial aneurysms. Am J Neuroradiol. 2002;23:768–71.
8. FAA. Code of Federal Regulations, Part 61 certification: pilots, flight instructors, and ground instructors, subpart A—general. 2016. http://rgl.faa.gov/Regulatory_and_Guidance_Library/rgFar.nsf/FARSBySectLookup/61.57
9. Steiger HJ, Stummer W, Hänggi D. Can systematic analysis of morbidity and mortality reduce complication rates in neurosurgery? Acta Neurochir. 2010;152(12):2013–9.

Potential of Hybrid Assistive Limb Treatment for Ataxic Gait Due to Cerebellar Disorders Including Hemorrhage, Infarction, and Tumor

Hiroshi Abe, Takashi Morishita, Kazuhiro Samura, Kenji Yagi, Masani Nonaka, and Tooru Inoue

Abstract Cerebellar hemorrhage (CH) is a severe life-threatening disorder, and surgical treatment is often required in an emergency situation. Even in cases in which the surgical procedure is successful, functional recovery is likely to be delayed because of cerebellar symptoms such as ataxia and gait disturbance. Here, we briefly review the efficacy of hybrid assistive limb (HAL) treatment in neurosurgical practice and propose a new comprehensive treatment strategy for CH to facilitate early neurological recovery. We have experienced cases of ataxic gait due to various etiologies, treated with rehabilitation using the HAL, and our data showed that HAL treatment potentially improves ataxic gait and balance problems. HAL treatment seems to be an effective and promising treatment modality for selected cases. Future studies should evaluate gait appearance and balance, in addition to walking speed, to assess improvement in cerebellar symptoms.

Keywords Hybrid assistive limb · Cerebellar hemorrhage · Neurorehabilitation · Ataxic gait

Introduction

Cerebellar hemorrhage (CH) is a severe life-threatening disorder, and surgical treatment is often required in an emergency situation. CH is frequently associated with hypertension in elderly patients. In surgical cases of CH, the conventional approach is suboccipital craniotomy (or craniectomy) for evacuation of the hematoma. However, suboccipital craniotomy may be too time consuming in an emergency situation and too invasive for elderly patients. On the other hand, a recent development in neuroendoscopy has enabled a burr-hole approach to CH [1], and we use this approach in our practice.

Even following a successful surgical procedure, functional recovery is likely to be delayed because of cerebellar symptoms such as ataxia and gait disturbance. Early initiation of high-quality rehabilitation is essential for preservation and recovery of brain functions [2, 3]. Among various treatment modalities, robotic rehabilitation has attracted increasing attention in the field of neurorehabilitation [4, 5]. In recently published stroke rehabilitation guidelines, the American Heart Association/American Stroke Association stated that "robot-assisted movement training to improve motor function and mobility after stroke in combination with conventional therapy may be considered" [6]. Therefore, we considered that the combination of minimally invasive endoscopic surgery and robotic rehabilitation may be a desirable approach to CH treatment. We compared activities of daily living scores (the Barthel Index and the Functional Independence Measure) and walking speed (10 m walking test) pre- and post-HAL treatment. The outcomes are summarized in Table 1.

Among various robots, the hybrid assistive limb (HAL; Cyberdyne Inc., Tsukuba, Japan) has the potential to change the rehabilitation approach to stroke. The HAL is an exoskeleton-type robot developed by Sankai and colleagues for neurorehabilitation based on the "interactive biofeedback (iBF)" theory [6, 7]. The HAL is designed to detect bioelectrical signals (BESs) to predict and assist in the movement produced by the muscles of affected limbs. This system makes the HAL robot unique among various rehabilitation robots, as most robotic ambulation trainers allow passive movements for patients. According to the iBF theory, the motor signals are generated in the central nervous system (CNS) and conducted via peripheral nerves to initiate muscle activity; these BESs then trigger the motion through interaction with the HAL supporting the paretic

H. Abe, M.D., Ph.D. · T. Morishita (✉), M.D. · K. Yagi, M.D., Ph.D.
M. Nonaka, M.D., Ph.D. · T. Inoue, M.D., Ph.D.
Department of Neurosurgery, Fukuoka University Faculty of Medicine, Fukuoka, Japan
e-mail: tmorishita@fukuoka-u.ac.jp

K. Samura, M.D., Ph.D.
Department of Neurosurgery, International University of Health and Welfare, School of Medicine, Narita, Japan

G. Esposito et al. (eds.), *Trends in the Management of Cerebrovascular Diseases*, Acta Neurochirurgica Supplement, Vol. 129,
https://doi.org/10.1007/978-3-319-73739-3_20,

Table 1 Clinical outcomes comparing pre- and post-hybrid assistive limb (HAL) rehabilitation in 14 cases

Case	Age (years)	Sex	Diagnosis	Lesion location	Number of HAL sessions	Barthel index		Functional independence measure		10 m walking test(s)	
						Pre	Post	Pre	Post	Pre	Post
1	42	F	Tumor	Cerebellum	2	60	60	92	92	20	17
2	69	M	Tumor	Cerebellum	2	100	100	126	126	12	11
3	65	M	Tumor	Cerebellum	8	95	100	122	125	8	7
4	28	M	Tumor	Medulla	5	60	95	83	121	12	10
5	37	F	Tumor	Pons	7	40	55	44	79	23	21
6	13	F	Tumor	Fourth ventricle	2	80	NA	99	NA	11	11
7	53	F	Infarction	Medulla	7	65	90	93	118	14	8
8	59	M	Infarction	Medulla	7	20	65	60	92	9	8
9	44	M	Infarction	Medulla	6	40	85	69	110	21	10
10	37	F	Infarction	Cerebellum	4	55	75	78	111	21	13
11	57	F	Hemorrhage	Cerebellum	3	75	90	98	107	16	10
12	95	M	Hemorrhage	Cerebellum	4	25	65	44	81	32	26
13	68	M	Hemorrhage	Cerebellum	8	65	100	80	109	19	7
14	46	M	Hemorrhage	Pons	12	50	90	86	117	14	8
Mean ± SD	49.5 ± 20.3	M 8, F 6			5.5 ± 2.9	59.3 ± 23.6	82.3 ± 16.3	83.9 ± 24.5	106.8 ± 15.9	16.6 ± 6.5	11.9 ± 5.6
P value						0.034		0.034		0.001	

A Wilcoxon signed-rank test was performed for statistical analysis. *F* female, *M* male, *NA*, *SD* standard deviation

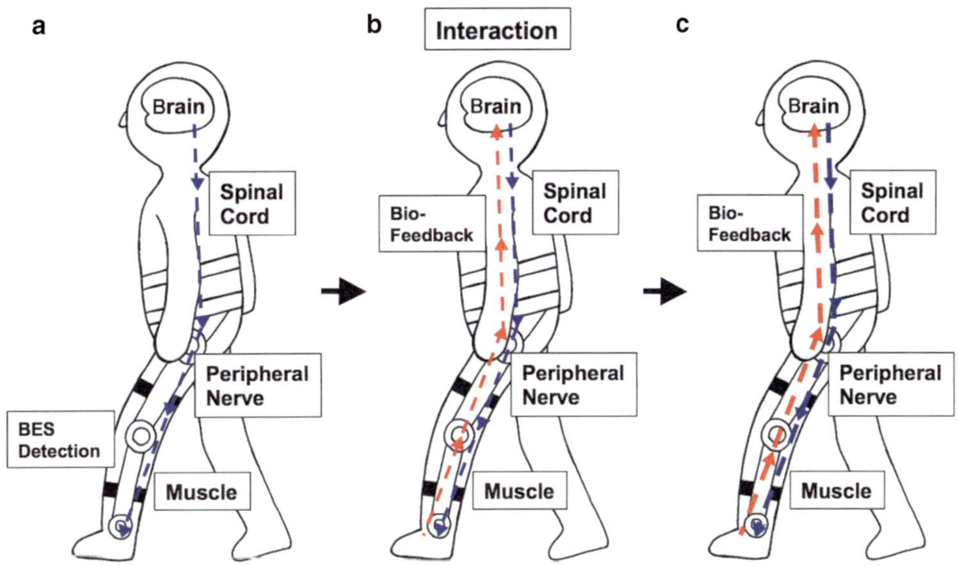

Fig. 1 Conceptualization of the closed-loop system formed by interactive biofeedback. (**a**) The bioelectrical signal from the impaired corticospinal tract is detected and the voluntary muscle movement is assisted by the hybrid assistive limb (HAL). (**b**) Then, the sensory signal is sent back to the brain. (**c**) The brain–machine interaction strengthens the signal from the corticospinal tract. (Adapted from Morishita and Inoue [19], with permission)

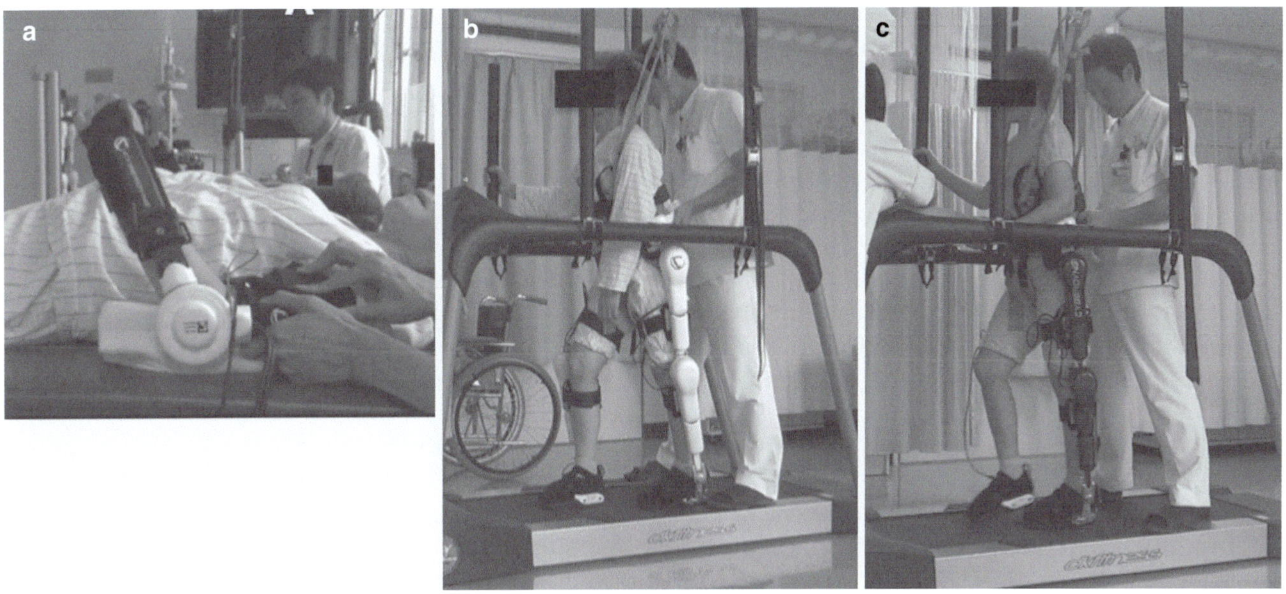

Fig. 2 Overview of rehabilitation of the representative case. (**a**) Single-joint (SJ) version of hybrid assistive limb (HAL) for upper extremity training. (**b**) Bilateral-leg (BL) version of HAL. (**c**) Single-leg (SL) version of HAL. (Adapted from Morishita and Inoue [19], with permission)

limb. Sensory input is then sent back to the CNS to activate the impaired neuronal networks (via biofeedback), and the CNS in turn enhances motor output. The formation of this closed loop is believed to activate the brain and facilitate recovery (Fig. 1). Currently, the following three types of HAL robot are available for rehabilitation: a bilateral-leg type (BL), a single-leg type (SL), and a single-joint type (SJ) (Fig. 2) [7, 8].

The HAL has been widely applied to various neurological disorders and shown to be effective. HAL therapy has been approved for medical use in patients with gait disability due to spinal cord injury in Germany since 2013. It should be noted that the use of the HAL was approved for national insurance coverage to treat rare neurological disorders on the basis of the favorable outcomes of a clinical trial (study NCY-3001; Japan Medical Association Center for Clinical Trials [JMACCT] ID: JMA-ILA00156); these disorders include spinal muscular atrophy, spinal and bulbar muscular atrophy, amyotrophic lateral sclerosis, Charcot–Marie–Tooth disease, distal myopathy, inclusion body myositis, congenital myopathy, and muscular dystrophy. Additionally, a randomized controlled trial to test the efficacy of gait training using the HAL for stroke patients is now under way in Japan (HIT-2016 trial).

In these proceedings, we briefly review the efficacy of HAL treatment in neurosurgical practice and present an idea for a new comprehensive treatment strategy for CH to facilitate early neurological recovery.

Stroke Rehabilitation Using Hybrid Assistive Limb Therapy

The size and location of the stroke lesion determines the severity of neurological deficits, and medical and surgical interventions in the acute phase seek to minimize damage to the brain. Motor paresis following a stroke is thought to result from damage to the corticospinal tract (CST), and the preservation of motor performance depends on CST integrity [9]. Another factor preventing motor recovery is related to an interhemispheric imbalance of excitability due to maladaptive compensatory changes in the contralesional hemisphere [10, 11]. Increased excitability in the contralesional somatosensory cortex has been demonstrated following induction of small ischemic lesions in several animal studies of acute and chronic stroke [12, 13]. In addition, hyperactivity of the contralesional hemisphere after a stroke has recently been shown by functional magnetic resonance imaging (fMRI) studies, and these studies suggested that the hyperactive contralesional hemisphere might inhibit the activities of the lesional hemisphere [10]. Another fMRI study also showed increased functional connectivity between the bilateral primary motor cortices following a stroke [14]. Interhemispheric imbalances may be aggravated by nonuse of the paretic limb as well [11].

After the limb is paralyzed because of the stroke lesion, neuroplasticity is induced use-dependently in the process of motor recovery [11]. The potential for rehabilitation using the HAL has been shown by several studies since the first feasibility study evaluating the risks associated with HAL-supported rehabilitation in acute stroke cases using the HAL was undertaken [15]. We also retrospectively reviewed the clinical data of acute stroke patients who underwent neurorehabilitation using either the HAL-BL or HAL-SL to determine the cases where HAL treatment was effective for ambulatory training [16]. For patients with mild to moderate hemiparesis, improvements were seen in activities of daily living scores. Additionally, we recently published a paper reporting favorable outcomes of rehabilitation for acute stroke, using multiple types of HAL robot [8].

Cerebellar symptoms following hemorrhage can manifest as ataxia, dysmetria, and balance problems, rather than paresis. The cerebellum contributes to various functions associated with tactile sensations and processing of sensory events. In this context, sensory feedback from HAL therapy may promote neuroplasticity in the cerebellum and neural network reorganization. The HAL may be a promising treatment tool for cerebellar symptoms. We have recently published three cases where HAL treatment was effective for ataxic gait due to brain stem infarction [17]. In addition, we have successfully performed HAL therapy in cerebellar ataxia cases due to brain tumor and stroke, including three CH cases (Table 1).

To maximize the clinical outcomes of HAL rehabilitation, patient selection is important [16, 18]. Intact cognitive function is important for treatment efficacy, as the patient is required to follow commands given by the therapist. A recent report emphasized the importance of evaluating cognitive function prior to the initiation of HAL rehabilitation from the perspective of HAL suitability as defined by clinical efficacy [18]. Secondly, it should be noted that patients with complete paralysis are unable to use the HAL system, as the HAL requires BESs generated by voluntary muscle movement [16]. The same study demonstrated that intracerebral hemorrhage cases with severe hemiplegia were at higher risk of orthostatic hypotension, despite the fact that HAL therapy was performed safely [15].

Rehabilitation Protocol

The full details of our rehabilitation protocol have been described elsewhere [8, 19]. Briefly, for upper extremity training, elbow extension and flexion exercises are repeated 100–150 times during each session. Concerning gait disability, we perform rehabilitation step by step according to the severity. For lower extremity training, we start with the HAL-SJ at the bedside to facilitate knee joint movement prior to ambulation training. Once the patient achieves a sitting position, we begin using the HAL-BL for gait training. When the HAL-BL supports both legs, the patient learns how the robot supports the paretic limb, by moving the non-paretic limb. In addition to ambulation training, the patient practices the extension and flexion of the paretic leg in a seated position and repeats the exercise in standing and seated positions.

Case Presentation

This patient was a 68-year-old man brought to the emergency department with complaints of nausea, vomiting, and vertigo. He was alert and oriented to time, place, and name but had slurred speech and right cerebellar ataxia (Fig. 3a). He was diagnosed with CH and subsequently underwent a small craniotomy for endoscopic evacuation of a hematoma (Fig. 3b). A conventional rehabilitation program was started

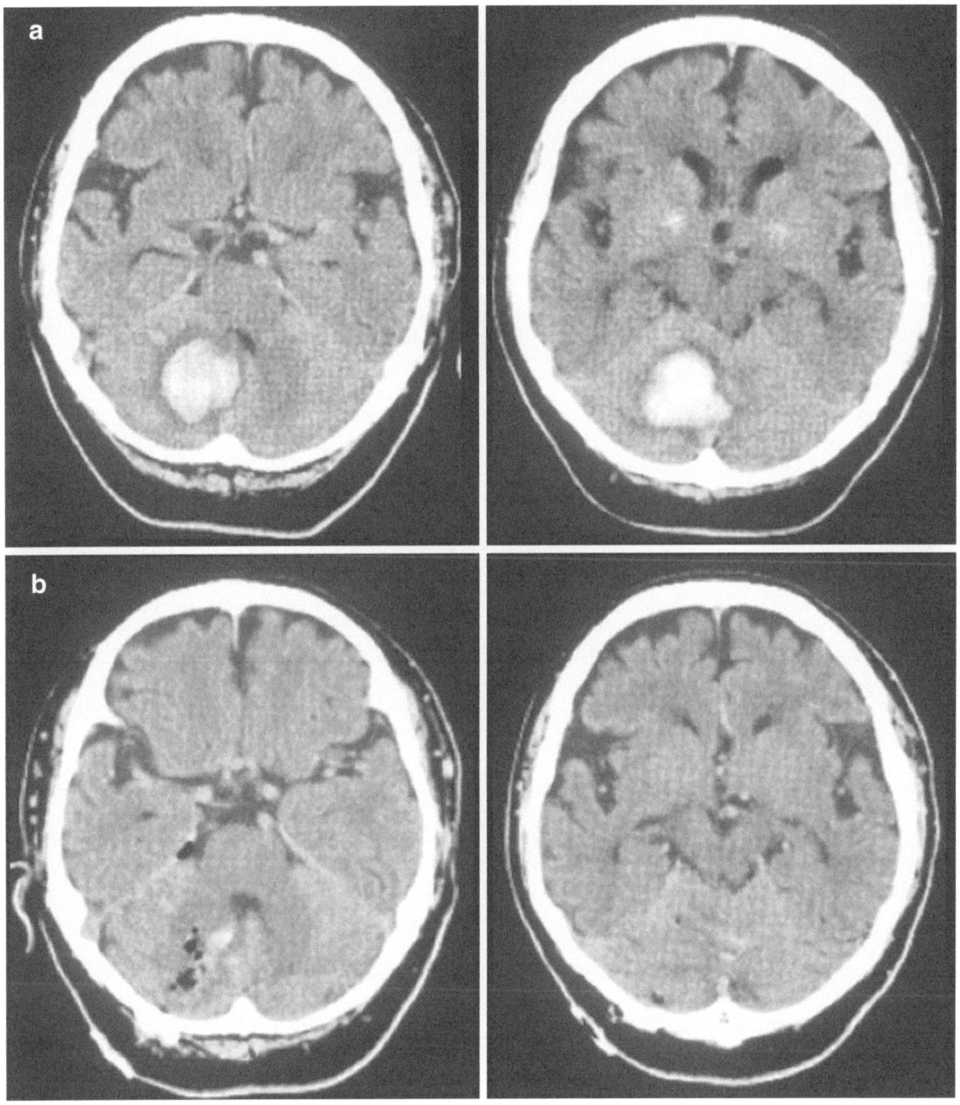

Fig. 3 Computed tomography (CT) image showing pre- (**a**) and postevacuation (**b**) of a hematoma in the representative case

on postoperative day (POD) 1, and HAL training was started on POD 4. The patient completed five and seven sessions of upper and lower extremity training, respectively, using the HAL. The patient returned to work on POD 42 without permanent neurological deficits.

Conclusions

In this chapter, we have presented the concept and our preliminary experience of HAL therapy for CH. iBF therapy using the HAL system seems to be an effective and promising treatment modality for selected cases, as our data have shown improvements in ataxic gait and balance problems due to cerebellar disorders. However, since clinical evidence for the use of the HAL after stroke currently consists only of case series [19], randomized controlled trials with larger samples are warranted. Formation of a multicenter registry for stroke cases managed with HAL rehabilitation may also help improve our understanding of its mechanisms of action and clinical outcomes, as suggested in our previous paper [19]. In future studies, we advocate assessment of walking appearance and balance ability, rather than mere measurement of walking speed, in cases with cerebellar symptoms.

Acknowledgements This study was in part supported by a Japan Society for the Promotion of Science Grant-in-Aid for young scientists [(B) 15 K19984], the Takeda Science Foundation, the Uehara Memorial Foundation, the Central Research Institute of Fukuoka University [No. 161042], and the Clinical Research Promotion Foundation in Japan.

Conflict of Interest The authors have no conflicts of interest to report.

References

1. Yamamoto T, Nakao Y, Mori K, Maeda M. Endoscopic hematoma evacuation for hypertensive cerebellar hemorrhage. Minim Invasive Neurosurg. 2006;49:173–8.
2. Jauch EC, Saver JL, Adams HP Jr, Bruno A, Connors JJ, Demaerschalk BM, Khatri P, McMullan PW Jr, Qureshi AI, Rosenfield K, Scott PA, Summers DR, Wang DZ, Wintermark M, Yonas H, American Heart Association Stroke Council, Council on Cardiovascular Nursing, Council on Peripheral Vascular Disease, Council on Clinical Cardiology. Guidelines for the early management of patients with acute ischemic stroke: a guideline for healthcare professionals from the American Heart Association/American Stroke Association. Stroke. 2013;44:870–947.
3. Morgenstern LB, Hemphill JC 3rd, Anderson C, Becker K, Broderick JP, Connolly ES Jr, Greenberg SM, Huang JN, MacDonald RL, Messe SR, Mitchell PH, Selim M, Tamargo RJ, American Heart Association Stroke Council, Council on Cardiovascular Nursing. Guidelines for the management of spontaneous intracerebral hemorrhage: a guideline for healthcare professionals from the American Heart Association/American Stroke Association. Stroke. 2010;41:2108–29.
4. Basteris A, Nijenhuis SM, Stienen AH, Buurke JH, Prange GB, Amirabdollahian F. Training modalities in robot-mediated upper limb rehabilitation in stroke: a framework for classification based on a systematic review. J Neuroeng Rehabil. 2014;11:111.
5. Norouzi-Gheidari N, Archambault PS, Fung J. Effects of robot-assisted therapy on stroke rehabilitation in upper limbs: systematic review and meta-analysis of the literature. J Rehabil Res Dev. 2012;49:479–96.
6. Winstein CJ, Stein J, Arena R, Bates B, Cherney LR, Cramer SC, Deruyter F, Eng JJ, Fisher B, Harvey RL, Lang CE, MacKay-Lyons M, Ottenbacher KJ, Pugh S, Reeves MJ, Richards LG, Stiers W, Zorowitz RD, American Heart Association Stroke Council, Council on Cardiovascular and Stroke Nursing, Council on Clinical Cardiology, Council on Quality of Care and Outcomes Research. Guidelines for adult stroke rehabilitation and recovery: a guideline for healthcare professionals from the American Heart Association/American Stroke Association. Stroke. 2016;47:e98–e169.
7. Suzuki K, Mito G, Kawamoto H, Hasegawa Y, Sankai Y. Intention-based walking support for paraplegia patients with robot suit HAL. Adv Robot. 2007;21:1441–69.
8. Fukuda H, Morishita T, Ogata T, Saita K, Hyakutake K, Watanabe J, Shiota E, Inoue T. Tailor-made rehabilitation approach using multiple types of hybrid assistive limb robots for acute stroke patients: a pilot study. Assist Technol. 2016;28:53–6.
9. Stinear CM, Barber PA, Smale PR, Coxon JP, Fleming MK, Byblow WD. Functional potential in chronic stroke patients depends on corticospinal tract integrity. Brain. 2007;130:170–80.
10. Grefkes C, Fink GR. Connectivity-based approaches in stroke and recovery of function. Lancet Neurol. 2014;13:206–16.
11. Xerri C, Zennou-Azogui Y, Sadlaoud K, Sauvajon D. Interplay between intra- and interhemispheric remodeling of neural networks as a substrate of functional recovery after stroke: adaptive versus maladaptive reorganization. Neuroscience. 2014;283:178–201.
12. Mohajerani MH, Aminoltejari K, Murphy TH. Targeted mini-strokes produce changes in interhemispheric sensory signal processing that are indicative of disinhibition within minutes. Proc Natl Acad Sci U S A. 2011;108:E183–91.
13. Takatsuru Y, Fukumoto D, Yoshitomo M, Nemoto T, Tsukada H, Nabekura J. Neuronal circuit remodeling in the contralateral cortical hemisphere during functional recovery from cerebral infarction. J Neurosci. 2009;29:10081–6.
14. Liu J, Qin W, Zhang J, Zhang X, Yu C. Enhanced interhemispheric functional connectivity compensates for anatomical connection damages in subcortical stroke. Stroke. 2015;46:1045–51.
15. Ueba T, Hamada O, Ogata T, Inoue T, Shiota E, Sankai Y. Feasibility and safety of acute phase rehabilitation after stroke using the hybrid assistive limb robot suit. Neurol Med Chir (Tokyo). 2013;53:287–90.
16. Fukuda H, Samura K, Hamada O, Saita K, Ogata T, Shiota E, Sankai Y, Inoue T. Effectiveness of acute phase hybrid assistive limb rehabilitation in stroke patients classified by paralysis severity. Neurol Med Chir (Tokyo). 2015;56:487–92.
17. Hamada O, Samura K, Abe H, Fukuda H, Ogata T, Nonaka M, Higashi T, Shiota E, Inoue T. Three cases with ataxic gait disorder improved by using a hybrid assistive limb robot suit. Jpn J Neurosurg. 2015;24:413–9.
18. Chihara H, Takagi Y, Nishino K, Yoshida K, Arakawa Y, Kikuchi T, Takenobu Y, Miyamoto S. Factors predicting the effects of hybrid assistive limb robot suit during the acute phase of central nervous system injury. Neurol Med Chir (Tokyo). 2016;56:33–7.
19. Morishita T, Inoue T. Interactive bio-feedback therapy using hybrid assistive limbs for motor recovery after stroke: current practice and future perspectives. Neurol Med Chir (Tokyo). 2016;56(10):605–12.

Author Index

https://doi.org/10.1007/978-3-319-73739-3,

Subject Index

G. Esposito et al. (eds.), *Trends in the Management of Cerebrovascular Diseases*, Acta Neurochirurgica Supplement, Vol. 129, https://doi.org/10.1007/978-3-319-73739-3, © Springer International Publishing AG, part of Springer Nature 2018

MIX
Papier aus verantwortungsvollen Quellen
Paper from responsible sources
FSC® C105338

If you have any concerns about our products,
you can contact us on
ProductSafety@springernature.com

In case Publisher is established outside the EU,
the EU authorized representative is:
Springer Nature Customer Service Center GmbH
Europaplatz 3, 69115 Heidelberg, Germany

Printed by Libri Plureos GmbH
in Hamburg, Germany